Community Oral Health Practice
for the Dental Hygienist

Third Edition

Community Oral Health Practice

for the Dental Hygienist

Kathy Voigt Geurink, RDH, MA
Clinical Associate Professor
Department of Dental Hygiene
School of Health Professions
University of Texas Health Science Center at San Antonio
San Antonio, Texas

ELSEVIER
SAUNDERS

3251 Riverport Lane
St. Louis, Missouri 63043

COMMUNITY ORAL HEALTH PRACTICE
FOR THE DENTAL HYGIENIST

ISBN: 978-1-4377-1351-0

Library of Congress Cataloging-in-Publication Data

Community oral health practice for the dental hygienist / [edited by] Kathy Voigt Geurink.—3rd ed.
    p. ; cm.
  Rev. ed. of: Community oral health practice for the dental hygienist / Kathy Voigt Geurink. 2nd ed. c2005.
  Includes bibliographical references and index.
  ISBN 978-1-4377-1351-0 (pbk. : alk. paper)
  1. Dental public health.   2. Community dental services.   3. Dental hygienists.   I. Geurink, Kathy Voigt.   II. Geurink, Kathy Voigt. Community oral health practice for the dental hygienist.
  [DNLM: 1. Community Dentistry—United States.   2. Dental Hygienists—United States.   WU 113]
  RK52.G48 2012
  362.19'76—dc22

2011001986

Acquisitions Editor: Kristin R Hebberd
Developmental Editor: Joslyn Dumas and Laurie Vordtriede
Publishing Services Manager: Anitha Raj
Project Manager: Sukanthi Sukumar and Gayle May
Design Direction: Margaret Reid

Printed in the United States of America

Last digit is the print number: 9 8 7 6 5 4 3

This text is dedicated to dental health professionals who have participated in community efforts to improve the oral health of all citizens. Oral health, as an integral component of the overall health and well-being of individuals, must be an entity available and attainable by all populations. Throughout my many years of working in the field of community oral health, I have observed the dedication and commitment of dental health professionals working toward this goal. They need to be commended and thanked and told to keep up their efforts. Many worthwhile programs and services have been provided, but there is still much to be done.

Contributors

Linda M. Altenhoff, DDS
Manager, Oral Health Branch/State Dental
  Director
Family and Community Health Service Division
Texas Department of State Health Services
Headquarters: Austin, Texas
Oral Health Programs in the Community

Robin Brocato, MHS
Health Program Specialist
Office of Head Start
Washington, D.C.
*Planning a Student Community Project with Head
  Start*

Diane Brunson, RDH, MPH
Director, Public Health and Community
  Outreach
University of Colorado School of Dental
  Medicine
Aurora, Colorado
Social Responsibility

Magda A. de la Torre, RDH, MPH
Assistant Professor
Department of Dental Hygiene
School of Health Professions
University of Texas Health Science Center at
  San Antonio
San Antonio, Texas
Cultural Competency

Kathy Voigt Geurink, RDH, MA
Clinical Associate Professor
Department of Dental Hygiene
School of Health Professions
University of Texas Health Science Center at
  San Antonio
San Antonio, Texas
*People's Health; Careers in Public Health for the
  Dental Hygienist; Oral Health Programs in the
  Community; Planning a Student Community
  Project with Head Start; Test-Taking Strategies
  and Community Cases*

Sheranita Hemphill, RDH, MPH, MS
Professor
Dental Health Sciences
Sinclair Community College
Dayton, Ohio
Service-Learning

Beverly Isman, RDH, MPH, ELS
Dental Public Health Consultant
Davis, California
Health Promotion and Health Communication

Sherry R. Jenkins, RDH, BS
Clinical Professor
Department of Dental Hygiene
University of Texas Health Science Center at
  San Antonio
Program Dental Hygienist
School-Based Dental Program
Methodist Healthcare Ministries
San Antonio, Texas
Oral Health Programs in the Community

Sharon Logue, RDH, MPH
Sealant Program Coordinator
Division of Dental Health
Virginia Department of Health
Richmond, Virginia
Careers in Public Health for the Dental Hygienist

**Jane E. M. Steffensen, RDH, BS, MPH,
  CHES**
Associate Professor
Department of Community Dentistry, Dental
  School
University of Texas Health Science Center at
  San Antonio
San Antonio, Texas
*Assessment in the Community; Measuring Progress
  in Oral Health; Population Health*

Stacy A. Weil, RDH, MS
Associate Director
Clinical Operations
Pharmaceutical Product Development
Austin, Texas
Research

Chapter 2 Mini-Profiles

Lynn A. Bethel, RDH, MPH
Director of Office of Oral Health
Massachusetts Department of Public Health
Boston, Massachusetts

Diann Bomkamp, RDH, BSDH, CDHC
President, American Dental Hygienists'
   Association (2008–2009)
St. Louis, Missouri

Matt Crespin, RDH, MPH
Oral Health Project Manager
Children's Health Alliance of Wisconsin
Milwaukee, Wisconsin

Kathy Lituri, RDH, MPH
Oral Health Promotion Director, Clinical
   Instructor
Division of Community Health Programs
Department of Health Policy and Health
   Services Research
Boston University Henry M. Goldman School of
   Dental Medicine
Adjunct Faculty
Forsyth School of Dental Hygiene
Massachusetts College of Pharmacy and Health
   Sciences
Boston, Massachusetts

Ginger Melton, RDH, BS
Dental Hygienist, Director of Dental
   Administration
Healthy Smiles Dental Center of the
   Portsmouth Community Health Center
Portsmouth, Virginia

Kathy Phipps, RDH, MPH, DrPH
Oral Health Research Consultant
Morro Bay, California

Leonor Ramos, RDH
Hospital Dentistry Dental Hygienist
Department of Defense
United States Air Force
Wilford Hall Medical Center
Lackland Air Force Base
San Antonio, Texas

JoAnn W. Wells, RDH, BS
Regional Dental Hygienist
Virginia Department of Health
Division of Dental Health
Chesterfield County Health District
Chesterfield, Virginia

Reviewers

Shaunda L. Clark, CDA, RDH, MEd
Program Director
Dental Hygiene Program
Kirkwood Community College
Cedar Rapids, Iowa

Michelle Oristian Fellona, RDH, MSDH
Associate Professor, Baccalaureate Programs
College of Health Science
St. Petersburg College
St. Petersburg, Florida

Katherine J. Hamman, RN, BSN
Professor of Nursing, Dental Assisting, and
    Dental Hygiene
Flint Hills Technical College
Emporia, Kansas

Julie A. Nocera, RDH, MS
Associate Professor of Dental Hygiene
Tunxis Community College
Farmington, Connecticut

Debra Schultz, RDH, PhD
Professor, Dental Auxiliaries Programs
Grand Rapids Community College
Grand Rapids, Michigan

Preface

"Why do I need to know anything about Community Oral Health?"

This is the question that many dental hygiene instructors hear from their students at the beginning of the Community Oral Health course. The purpose of this text is to provide students with information about community oral health that is relevant to dental hygiene. It is my intention that, through reading the chapters and participating in the suggested activities, dental hygiene students can find the answer to this question and develop an understanding of the importance of this integral component of their education and future profession. Although this text is written specifically for dental hygiene students, it also is a valuable resource for all oral health professionals practicing their professional responsibility of improving the oral health of their community.

Community Oral Health is a required course for dental hygiene accreditation. The Commission on Dental Hygiene Accreditation states that the curriculum in dental hygiene schools must include content in the following general areas: general education, biomedical sciences, dental sciences, and dental hygiene science. These areas must be incorporated with sufficient depth, scope, sequence of instruction, quality, and emphasis to ensure achievement of the curriculum's competencies.

According to Accreditation Standard 2-14,

Dental hygiene science content must include oral health education and preventive counseling; health promotion; patient management; clinical dental hygiene; provision of services for and management of patients with special needs; **community dental/oral health;** *medical and dental emergencies, including basic life support; legal and ethical aspects of dental hygiene practice; infection and hazard control management; and the provision of oral health care services to patients with bloodborne infectious diseases.*

The American Dental Education Association (ADEA), Section on Dental Hygiene Education Competency Development Committee, developed dental hygiene competencies to assist dental hygiene schools in meeting accreditation standards. The competency statements are meant to serve as guidelines for individual programs in defining the abilities they want their graduates to possess. The competency statements are presented in the following five domains:

Core Competencies (C)
Health Promotion/Disease Prevention (HP)
Community (CM)
Patient/Client Care (PC)
Professional Growth and Development (PGD)

The ADEA Community Dental/Oral Health Competencies are as follows:

CM.1 Assess the oral health needs of the community and the quality of resources and services

CM.2 Provide screening, referral, and educational services that allow clients to access the resources of the health care system

CM.3 Provide community oral health services in a variety of settings

CM.4 Facilitate client access to oral health services by influencing individuals and organizations for the provision of oral health care

CM.5 Evaluate reimbursement mechanisms and their impact on the patient's or client's access to oral health care

CM.6 Evaluate the outcomes of community-based programs and plan for future activities

At the end of each chapter in this book, competencies from all domains that are relevant to the chapter content and knowledge application activities are listed. The complete document of competencies for entry into the profession of dental hygiene, approved and adopted by the ADEA House of Delegates in 2003, can be found in Appendix B and on the Evolve website that accompanies this text. Therefore the instructor and student can apply the information within *Community Oral Health Practice for the Dental Hygienist* to the goal of developing competencies in the profession of dental hygiene.

Chapter 1 defines community oral health for students through examples of public health problems and solutions. The core public health functions and essential public health services are defined. Chapter 2, on careers in public health, enables students to envision the future use of the information they are learning about in the book and in the community course; it features profiles of dental hygienists who practice within the field of community oral health. Reviewing these featured career choices allows students to comprehend the relevance of the content in the forthcoming chapters.

Chapter 3, on assessment, and Chapters 4 and 5, on measuring oral health, emphasize the importance of these crucial steps in planning community oral health programs. Dental hygienists involved in public health need to be knowledgeable about and proficient in using the tools of assessment and measurement of oral health. *Healthy People 2020* oral health objectives are discussed as an important framework for assessment of community oral health programs. These chapters are appropriately placed within the book as a preparation for Chapter 6, on community oral health programs, which discusses the planning, implementation, and evaluation phases of program development. Successful community oral health programs at the local, state, and national levels are featured. Internet websites and updates on state oral health programs are included.

Chapter 7 covers statistics in a relevant, organized format, with application to community oral health. Criteria for reviewing dental literature are included. Chapter 8 explains theories of health promotion and identifies strategies for delivering health information to the public. The dental hygienist's social responsibility with respect to cultural competency and the dental hygienist's role in improving access to care for underserved populations are addressed in Chapter 9. A case study is provided to initiate discussion on the dental hygienist's roles, values, and beliefs.

Chapter 10, on cultural competency, not only defines the term for students but also provides models of how to incorporate cultural competency into interactions with patients and in our community health promotion endeavors.

Chapter 11, on service-learning, defines the importance of the collaboration between the needs of the community and student learning. The benefits of service-learning for students, communities, dental hygiene programs, academic institutions, and the nation's oral health are discussed.

Chapter 12 (new to this edition) describes the steps needed to set up a student community project and uses the participants in the Head Start program as the target population.

Chapter 13 provides the student with practice in answering community oral health test questions similar to those on the Dental Hygiene National Board Examination. These community cases test the student's understanding of content in the textbook. The practice test assists the student in successfully answering this type of question. Teachers who use this textbook should anticipate improved scores on the national board examination in the area of community oral health. Students are provided with the information they need to begin their profession with a positive attitude toward community dental health and a willingness to contribute to the oral health of all persons in their community.

A vocabulary of terms is unique to community oral health practice, therefore a Glossary is located at the end of this textbook for reference. Appendix A contains websites for oral health resources, Appendix B lists the dental hygiene competencies, and Appendix C and D include valuable information for forming community partnerships and performing community health assessments, respectively.

Sample community cases with test questions can be found at the end of each chapter. These cases assist students in their mastery of the material in each chapter and provide additional practice in answering case-type questions similar to those on the Dental Hygiene National Board Examination. Instructors will find the answers/rationales on the Evolve website, which contains supplemental information and learning activities related to *Community Oral Health Practice for the Dental Hygienist.*

ACKNOWLEDGMENTS

Over the course of preparing this text for publication, many people have provided their support, guidance, and assistance in researching information pertinent to oral health in the community. I want to acknowledge with sincere appreciation the following persons for their contributions and support:

From the Department of Dental Hygiene, School of Allied Health Sciences, University of Texas Health Science Center at San Antonio:

Faculty and staff

Juanita Wallace, RDH, PhD, Department Chair

Taline Dadian-Infante, RDH, MS, Program Director

Health professionals and faculty who reviewed selected chapters:

Ladonia Franke, RDH, BS

Bea Hicks, RDH, MA

Kimberly Burk, BBA, MSHC

Carol Nguyen, RDH, MS

Rebecca Wright, RDH, MS

Appreciation to my family who continually support my professional endeavors with understanding and love:

Parents, Peg and Jim Voigt; husband, Terry; daughters, Kelly and Kimberly

Kathy Voigt Geurink

Contents

People's Health

Kathy Voigt Geurink, RDH, MA

Objectives

Upon completion of this chapter, the student will be able to:
* Define the terms *health*, *public health*, and *dental public health*.
* Define the term *population health*.
* Identify public health problems within a community.
* Identify public health measures or solutions.
* Define dental disease as a public health problem with public health solutions.
* Explain the role of the government in public health solutions.
* Discuss the 10 greatest public health achievements of the twentieth century.
* Identify core functions of public health and the essential public health services.
* Describe the relation of public health to the roles of the dental hygienist.

Key Terms

Community	Population health	Assessment
Health	Fluoridation	Policy development
Public health	Department of Health and	Assurance
Public	Human Services (DHHS)	
Dental public health		

Opening Statements

What Is Public Health?
* Influenza immunizations save lives and money.
* Vaccine research of the human immunodeficiency virus (HIV) is a top priority to end the epidemic.
* Community water fluoridation is listed as one of the 10 greatest public health achievements of the twentieth century.
* Evidence links dental disease to life-threatening systemic diseases such as heart disease, respiratory ailments, and diabetes.
* The website of the world's largest tobacco company acknowledges that smoking tobacco causes serious health risks.
* Improved water sanitation controls infectious diseases.
* The White House and the American Dental Hygienists' Association (ADHA) team together to provide dental insurance to children.
* Bioterrorism has put public health officials on alert for unusual diseases.

HEALTH, PUBLIC HEALTH, AND DENTAL PUBLIC HEALTH

Becoming familiar with the Opening Statements will set you on the right track to begin your journey in developing an understanding of the importance of people's health. The connection between people's health and **community** oral health will become apparent throughout the text. Thinking of specific examples, such as those in the Opening Statements, will enable you to envision what is meant by the topics of health, public health, and dental public health. It is also necessary to review the more formal definitions of these terms that occur in most texts on the topics. Various definitions exist for these terms; however, the following definitions should suffice for use within the scope of community oral health practice for the dental hygienist:

> **Health** has been described by the World Health Organization (WHO) as follows: "Health comprises complete physical and social well-being and is not merely the absence of disease."[1]
>
> **Public health,** as described by Winslow, is "the science and art of preventing disease, prolonging life, and promoting physical health and efficiency through organized community efforts."[2] It is concerned with lifestyle and behavior, the environment, human biology, and organizations of health programs and systems.[3] The **public** pertains to the community, state, or nation. Public health is people's health.[4]
>
> **Dental public health** has been described by the American Board of Dental Health as the science and art of preventing and controlling dental disease and promoting dental health through organized community efforts. It is that form of dental practice which serves the community as the patient rather than the individual. It is concerned with the dental education of the public, applied dental research, and the administration of group dental care programs, as well as prevention and control of dental diseases on a community basis.[2]

In this text, the terms *public health* and *community health* are used synonymously, and both refer to the "effort that is organized by society to protect, promote and restore the health and quality of life of the people."[3]

The term **population health** has been defined as "the health outcomes of a group of individuals, including the distribution of such outcomes within the group."[5] It is an approach to health with a goal to improve the health of the entire population. One major step in achieving this goal is to reduce the health disparities among population groups. The field of population health includes health outcomes, patterns of health determinants, and policies and interventions. These topics and their correlations are discussed further in the book in various chapters.

THE PUBLIC HEALTH PROBLEM AND THE PUBLIC HEALTH SOLUTION

Public Health Problem

Upon reading these definitions carefully, you are ready to view two concepts of importance to your comprehension of public or people's health: (1) the public health problem and (2) the public health solution. The public health problem, as perceived by the public, usually brings to mind an infectious disease such as acquired immunodeficiency syndrome (AIDS) or the swine flu (N1H1). The spectrum of problems, however, is vast and more extensive than one might first realize. Examples of public health problems include the following:

1. Diseases caused by the pollution of the country's air and water systems
2. Chronic diseases of the expanding population of older adults
3. Inadequate funding for dental disease in indigent children
4. An increase in violence among youth of today

Studying examples of public health problems appears to be the easiest means of developing an understanding of what constitutes public health. Public health problems, as described by Burt and Ecklund, must meet the following criteria[6]:

1. A condition or situation that is a widespread actual or potential cause of morbidity or mortality
2. An existing perception that the condition is a public health problem on the part of the public, the government, or public health authorities

The history of public health demonstrates that once the problem is identified and knowledge and expertise have been developed to solve the problem, the community must unify to find social and political support to proceed with the public health solutions.

Public Health Solution

Examples of solutions to public health problems that most persons are familiar with include immunizations, tobacco cessation programs, fluoridation of drinking water, and seat belts and air bags in cars to prevent injuries and mortality. These public health solutions are concerned with health promotion and disease prevention. They address the problems of the community at large and are effective measures that follow seven characteristics (see Guiding Principles).

GUIDING PRINCIPLES

Seven Characteristics of Public Health Solutions
- Not hazardous to life or function.
- Effective in reducing or preventing the targeted disease or condition.
- Easily and efficiently implemented.
- Potency maintained for a substantial time period.
- Attainable regardless of socioeconomic status.
- Effective immediately upon application.
- Inexpensive and within the means of the community.

Community water **fluoridation** has proved to be a safe, cost-effective solution for reducing dental decay in children. It is easily implemented by adding fluoride to the water supply, and it reaches all people regardless of socioeconomic status. It is effective immediately upon initiation and costs far less than the financial burden of restorative treatment. It meets all seven characteristics to be considered an effective solution to the problem of dental decay.

DENTAL DISEASE AS A PUBLIC HEALTH PROBLEM

Dental Caries

Dental disease is a universal problem that does not undergo remission if left untreated. For many Americans, especially children from minority, racial, and ethnic groups, dental caries is common and widespread. About 99% of adults have had tooth decay by the time they reach their early 40s. Sixty percent of adults older than 75 years of age have had root caries.[7] The extent and severity of dental caries warrant the need for treatment and prevention programs throughout the

United States. Dental decay, if left untreated, continues to escalate and results in expensive surgical procedures. Therefore it is important to focus on prevention of the disease.

Community water fluoridation is the perfect example of a dental public health solution to the problem of dental decay. Organized community efforts have brought fluoridated drinking water to more than 144 million people, and the results have shown a significant reduction in the amount of dental decay. Dental disease, however, still exists as a public health problem of the twenty-first century. More community dental health education needs to be performed with the implementation of additional dental health promotion and prevention programs.

Chapters 6 and 8 describe various programs and health promotion efforts that can be implemented and expanded upon within communities nationwide. The 2000 Surgeon General's report on oral health emphasizes the need for these programs and addresses the importance of oral health to the general health of the public.[8] Dental disease is discussed as a dental public health problem of universal prevalence that can be alleviated, and even prevented, with future public health measures. Dental professionals, both those employed in the field of public health and those employed in private practice, must work together to educate the community and to provide the necessary programs to treat and prevent further disease.

Public Health/Private Practice

Programs to treat dental disease can be conducted on a community (public health) or individual (private practice) level. On the community level, the dental professional treats the community as a patient rather than as an individual. **Table 1-1** demonstrates the similarities of community oral health practice to private practice. The community oral health steps parallel steps conducted in the private practice. Community oral health practice extends the role of the dental hygienist in private practice to include the people of the community as a whole. The public health facility (e.g., hospital, community clinic, school, or agency), rather than the private dental office, becomes the environment in which the service of oral health care is provided. The patient's dental examination parallels the community survey as a means of assessment of the situation or problem.

The treatment plan and the plan for the community are similar; both include the many facets of preparation, such as determining various methods, strategies, and costs of choosing a plan that will work best for the patient or community. The treatment and the program operation occur during the actual implementation of the plan. Payment for dental services is equated with program funding. Various methods of payment are often explored in both cases.

Evaluation of the treatment is similar to the program appraisal and should occur during the implementation and at the end of the treatment or operation.[6] This comparison should help the

Table 1-1 **Comparison of Components in Private Practice and Public Health**

Private Practice	Public Health
Patient	Community
Examination	Survey
Diagnosis	Analysis
Treatment planning	Program planning
Treatment	Program implementation
Fee/payment	Budget/financing
Patient evaluation	Program evaluation

private practice hygienist become comfortable with the concepts of community program planning, implementation, and evaluation (see Chapter 6).

GOVERNMENT'S ROLE IN PUBLIC HEALTH

Government Agencies

As a dental hygienist, you may contribute to the health of people in the community through participating in community health promotion activities. You may choose to present an educational program at a school or conduct a cancer screening at a facility for older residents (see Chapter 8). The more formal public health programs, however, generally fall under the aegis of the government. Both prevention and the delivery of services are concerns within the programs developed by government agencies.

The federal government's role in participating in dental health-related activities falls under the jurisdiction of the US **Department of Health and Human Services** (DHHS). *Healthy People 2020,* a publication of the DHHS, lists health objectives for the United States, including oral health, that need to be achieved by the year 2030 (see Chapter 4).

The US Public Health Service (PHS) is one of four major agencies within the DHHS. The PHS promotes health standards, ensures that the highest level of health care is available for all citizens, and cooperates with other nations on health projects. There are eight operating agencies under the PHS (**Figure 1-1**). Agencies that are important because they are involved in oral health programs include the following:

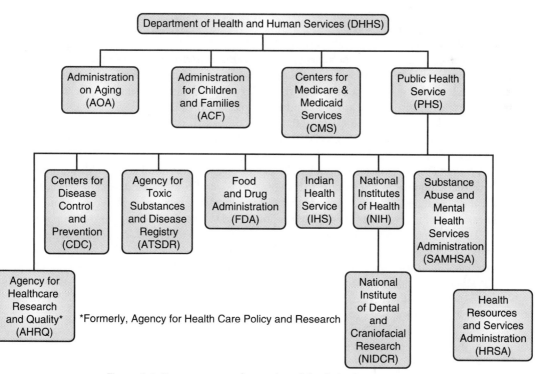

Figure 1-1 Departments and agencies of the federal government.

- Centers for Disease Control and Prevention (CDC)
- Health Resources and Services Administration (HRSA)
- National Institutes of Health (NIH), National Institute of Dental and Craniofacial Research (NIDCR)
- Agency for Healthcare Research and Quality (AHRQ)[9]

In 2009, the HRSA of the DHHS awarded contracts to the National Academy of Sciences to study oral health care in the United States and to provide a plan that would expand access to oral health care and make recommendations for improvement in the quality of oral health care. This plan can be reviewed at www.iom.edu/Reports.aspx.

At the state level, public health agencies have been charged with the task of developing oral health programs within their states. These programs increase the awareness of oral health issues, promote sound oral health policy development, and support initiatives for the prevention and control of dental disease. At the local level, dental programs vary throughout the nation. As an example, local community health centers provide services for low income families and school-based programs provide oral health education on and disease prevention services to children (see Chapter 6). As a result of a decline in funding at all levels, there has been less involvement at this level in recent years, and fewer data have been collected to determine needs.[10]

National Initiatives

Whether an oral health program has national, state, or local impact, its objectives should be tied in with the National Oral Health Initiatives, which have the following common goals:

- Promoting oral health
- Improving the quality of life
- Eliminating oral health disparities

The 2000 Surgeon General's Report, *Oral Health in America,* is a 300-page document with a focus exclusively on oral health issues. The major message of the Report is that oral health is essential to the general health and well-being of all Americans and can be achieved by all Americans; however, there are profound and consequential disparities within the US population.[8] Several federal, state, and local initiatives were developed in response to the Surgeon General's Report, including *Healthy People 2010,* the 2003 *National Call to Action to Promote Oral Health,* and *Healthy People 2020.*

Healthy People 2010 is a comprehensive set of disease prevention and health promotion objectives that contains an oral health focus area and 17 oral health objectives.[11] Every 10 years, the DHHS leverages scientific insights and lessons learned from the past decade, along with new knowledge of current data, trends, and innovations, to create the *Healthy People* reports.

The *National Call to Action to Promote Oral Health,* to create the *Healthy People* reports was a combined effort of a broad coalition of public and private organizations and individuals who generated five principal actions and implementation strategies to be undertaken to ensure that all Americans achieve optimum oral health. As health care providers we are called to participate in the following five actions:

- Change perceptions of oral health
- Overcome barriers by replicating effective programs
- Build the science and accelerate science transfer
- Increase oral health workforce diversity, capacity, and flexibility
- Increase collaborations[12]

The successful execution of these five actions requires partnerships and collaborations focused on the common goals.

Healthy People 2020 reflects assessments of major risks to health and wellness, changing public health priorities, and emerging issues related to our nation's health preparedness and prevention (see Chapter 5). *Healthy People 2020* provides a framework to address risk factors and determinants of health and the diseases and disorders that affect our communities. Oral health is included with objectives and guidance for reaching the new targets for the next 10 years.[13]

The public, health care providers, policymakers, communities, and anyone interested in the improvement of oral health must work together to achieve the vision, goals, and objectives of the National Initiatives.

Core Functions of Public Health

Federal, state, and local programs have been charged with improving the health of the people through **assessment, policy development,** and **assurance.** These core public health functions of assessment, policy development, and assurance were identified in an Institute of Medicine (IOM) report in 1988. This report states that the core public health functions were developed to protect and promote health, wellness, and the quality of life and to prevent disease, injury, disability, and death.[14] **Box 1-1** presents these core functions.

BOX 1-1 Core Functions of Public Health Agencies at All Levels of Government

Assessment
- Every public health agency regularly and systematically collects, assembles, analyzes, and makes available information on the health of the community, including statistics on health status, community health needs, and epidemiologic and other studies of health problems. Not every agency is large enough to conduct these activities directly; intergovernmental and interagency cooperation is essential. Nevertheless, each agency bears the responsibility for seeing that the assessment function is fulfilled. This basic function of public health cannot be delegated.

Policy Development
- Every public health agency exercises its responsibility to serve the public interest in the development of comprehensive public health policies by promoting use of the scientific knowledge base in decision making about public health and by leading in developing public health policy. Agencies must take a strategic approach, developed on a base of positive appreciation for the democratic political process.

Assurance
- Public health agencies assure their constituents that services necessary to achieve agreed upon goals are provided, either by encouraging actions by other entities (private or public sector), by requiring such action through regulation, or by providing services directly.
- Each public health agency involves key policymakers and the general public in determining a set of high-priority personal and community-wide health services that governments will guarantee to every member of the community. This guarantee should include subsidization or direct provision of high-priority personal health services for people unable to afford them.

Reprinted with permission from National Academy of Science. The Future of the Public's Health in the 21st Century. Washington, DC: National Academies Press; 2002.

BOX 1-2 **Essential Public Health Services in the United States**

Public Health
- Prevents epidemics
- Protects against environmental hazards
- Prevents injuries
- Promotes and encourages healthy behaviors
- Responds to disasters and assists communities in recovery
- Ensures the quality and accessibility of health services

Essential Public Health Services
- Monitor health status to identify community health problems
- Diagnose and investigate health problems and health hazards in the community
- Inform, educate, and empower the public about health issues
- Mobilize community partnerships to identify and solve health problems
- Develop policies and plans to support individual and community health efforts
- Enforce laws and regulations that protect the public's health and ensure safety
- Link policies to needed personal health services
- Ensure a competent public health and personal health care workforce
- Evaluate effectiveness, accessibility, and quality of personal and population-based health services
- Conduct research for new insight and innovative solutions to health problems

From Public Health in America. Washington, DC: Public Health Functions Steering Committee; 1994.

The public health functions have been further delineated since the publication of the IOM report. Through a consensus development process, a number of organizations and agencies produced a document entitled *Public Health in America*. This document lists essential public health services necessary to accomplish the core public health functions (**Box 1-2**). **Figure 1-2** demonstrates the relationship of the essential public health services to the core public health functions. Successful provision of these services requires collaboration among private and public partners within the community and across various levels of government. These services are essential to achievement of healthy people in healthy communities.[15]

Building on the framework of the core public health functions and the essential public health services, the Association of State & Territorial Dental Directors (ASTDD) developed essential public health services for oral health. These essential public health services for oral health provide guidelines for state oral health programs within state health departments (see Chapter 6). The core public health functions, the essential public health services, and the essential public health services for oral health provide guidance for all dental public health professionals working at national, state, and local levels.

FUTURE OF DENTAL PUBLIC HEALTH

What Needs to Be Done

Over the years, the number of dental public health programs at federal, state, and local levels has declined as a result of tight budgets and diminishing resources. Dental disease persists as a public health problem that can be alleviated and possibly eliminated. The knowledge exists, but because

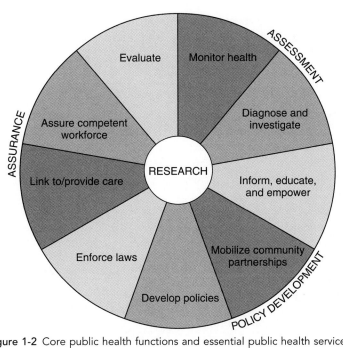

Figure 1-2 Core public health functions and essential public health services.

of restraints and a lack of resources, this knowledge is not being applied toward the goal of communities free from dental disease. The ongoing need to emphasize the importance of oral health has never been stronger. It is the responsibility of dental health professionals to emphasize the connection of oral health to people's general health to the policymakers of our nation (see Chapter 9). Corbin and Marten's report[16] on the future of dental health states that although oral health needs are documented, oral health is given a low priority by health planners. The report emphasizes goals to meet for improved dental public health (see Guiding Principles).

GUIDING PRINCIPLES

Goals to Be Met to Improve Dental Public Health[14]
- Earn support from the public.
- Earn support from the policymakers.
- Earn support from program administrators.
- Earn support from the dental community.
- Ensure recruitment and professional development of dental public health personnel.
- Ensure collaboration with colleagues.

Going in the Right Direction

Although the dental profession must continue to seek legislation and funding for health programs and to educate the public on the relationship of oral health to general health, the profession appears to be moving in the direction of success. A 1999 report by the CDC lists the 10 most important public health accomplishments of the twentieth century.[17] This list is encouraging and supportive to the efforts of all public health professionals (see Guiding Principles).

GUIDING PRINCIPLES

The 10 Greatest Public Health Accomplishments of the Twentieth Century[15]
- A significant decline in deaths from coronary heart disease and stroke as a result of behavior modification, a decrease in smoking, and early intervention programs.
- The 1964 Surgeon General's acknowledgment of tobacco as a health hazard and resultant antismoking campaigns that have changed the public health perceptions about the habit.
- Vaccination, which has helped eradicate smallpox and manage diseases such as measles, rubella, and tetanus.
- Improved motor vehicle safety, with greater emphasis placed on personal responsibility for reducing motor vehicle–related fatalities caused by drinking and reckless driving.
- Control of infectious diseases, which has been aided by improved water sanitation and better understanding of the science of microbiology.
- Safer workplaces, which have contributed to a higher standard of living and a 40% reduction in job-related injuries and fatalities.
- Safer and healthier foods as a result of less microbial contamination, as well as fortification of foods with supplements and vitamins.
- Healthier mothers and babies, thanks to improved prenatal care and greater access to care.
- Better access to family planning information and greater use of contraceptives, which has improved the socioeconomic status of US citizens.
- Fluoride in drinking water, which reaches 144 million people safely and is an inexpensive method of preventing tooth decay independent of a person's socioeconomic status.

There has been a major effort by dental organizations, policymakers, and advocacy groups to address the issues of access to care for American citizens. The American Dental Association (ADA) held the first Access to Dental Care Summit in the summer of 2009. This summit drew together diverse oral health stakeholder groups in a forum that examined relevant issues of the past, present, and future, clarifying common ground and empowering members to take responsibility for collective action through focused initiatives. It laid the foundation for a common vision to begin to improve access to oral health care for underserved people. At the conclusion of the Summit, the participants identified the following eight areas on which to focus future efforts[18]:
- Workforce development strategies
- Reorganization of the dental delivery system
- Financing models
- Population-based prevention strategies and strengthening the public health infrastructure
- Improving oral health literacy through social marketing
- Collaboration between the medical and dental communities
- Developing metrics for measuring and defining access
- Building a sustainable infrastructure for communication and collaboration

Dental hygienists attended the ADA Access to Care Summit and are taking an active role in assessing and prioritizing dental health needs in the community. They have a responsibility to participate in the activities that will list community oral health practice as an important achievement in the twenty-first century. Social responsibility and the dental hygienist's commitment to the community are discussed further in Chapter 9.

The dental hygienists who have chosen careers as state dental directors or public health educators contribute to the advancement of dental public health, but much more needs to be accomplished by all members of the dental hygiene profession. The ADHA in 2005 adopted an updated version of the six roles of the dental hygienist, originally established in the 1980s. The most important change included positioning the role of the public health as an integral component of the other roles of clinician, educator, researcher, advocate, and administrator (see Chapter 2).

Common Goal

The goal of dental public health is optimal oral health for all citizens and universal access to comprehensive dental care. With this goal in mind, both dentists and dental hygienists have entered the field of public health by accepting employment within programs that include health promotion, community disease prevention, and provision of dental care to selected groups of people.

Dentists become recognized specialists in the field of dental public health through specialty certification with the American Board of Dental Public Health. In most states, dental hygienists have no required formal or specialty education to work within this field in the community, although some have pursued advanced degrees in public health or community health. Further education prepares the dental hygienist to work with underserved populations who continually face barriers to health care. These barriers, such as inadequate geographic and financial access, pose challenges to the dental and dental hygiene profession.

In an attempt to reach underserved populations (see Chapter 2), some states are permitting less restrictive dental hygiene supervision for dental hygienists working in the community and new workforce models are being established. For example, in 2004, the Arizona state legislature approved an affiliated practice relationship between dentists and dental hygienists. This new law provided an opportunity for children to receive preventive services offered by a dental hygienist without direct supervision or prior examination by a licensed dentist. Another example occurred when the California state legislature recognized the title, *Registered Dental Hygienist in Alternative Practice* (RDHAP). The purpose of this title is to qualify dental hygienists to practice the full scope of dental hygiene services with less supervision in underserved areas. The dental hygienist who has a concern for the improvement and protection of the oral health of the whole population can participate in community oral health practice at a level of professional choice.[19,20]

In June 2004, the ADHA House of Delegates, addressing the problem of access to health care, approved the creation of the Advanced Dental Hygiene Practitioner (ADHP) credential. This credential is designed to allow dental hygienists to provide diagnostic, restorative, and therapeutic services directly to the public. Those dental hygienists who receive the ADHP credential will have graduated from an accredited dental hygiene program and also completed the ADHA-approved advanced educational curriculum. This credential is being developed to improve and enhance the oral health care delivery system. Because dental supervision is not required of the ADHP, it will open doors for dental hygienists to work in places such as school systems, hospitals, and nursing homes and with underserved populations throughout the country.[20] The role of the mid-level provider and its development in dentistry is further discussed in Chapter 2.

SUMMARY

An understanding of people's health includes learning the basic terminology to define health, public health, and dental public health. People's health is the health of the public living within a community, state, or nation. Identifying public health problems and solutions provides dental hygienists with the knowledge to explore this field of health further and a means by which they might become involved. The government's role in people's health is mentioned briefly as an introduction to the programs to be discussed in more detail in future chapters. Comparison of private practice to community oral health practice demonstrates the similarities and prepares dental hygienists for the planning, implementation, and evaluation phases that constitute public health programs. As health care providers, with many roles and responsibilities, dental hygienists have a calling and a duty to serve the communities in which they live.

Applying Your Knowledge

1. Bring articles to class from the daily news or current magazines that present a public health issue and discuss what the problem is and how it is being addressed. (Use the seven characteristics described in this chapter to evaluate the issue.)
2. Choose a government public health program and further investigate its purpose and success in accomplishing this purpose.
3. Read and report on one of the Institute of Medicine Reports on oral health care in the US. (See www.iom.edu/Reports.aspx.)
4. Research and report on the creation of the mid-level provider. Select a state and report on the practice act that allows for improved access to dental care for underserved populations.
5. Go to www.oralhealthatlas.org and report on dental disease as a worldwide public health problem (use maps and charts in this atlas for comparison).

Dental Hygiene Competencies

Reading the material within this chapter and participating in the activities of Applying Your Knowledge will contribute to your ability to demonstrate the following competencies:

Health promotion and disease prevention
HP.1 Promote the values of oral health and general health and wellness to the public and organizations within and outside the profession.
HP.4 Identify individual and population risk factors and develop strategies that promote health-related quality of life.

Community Case

In your new position as the Oral Health Program Coordinator at the State Health Department, you are asked to conduct a statewide screening project to determine the oral health status of school-age children. After you collect and analyze the data from the statewide survey, you are to determine what oral health programs you would like to plan that will address the needs of children in your state.
1. Which core public health function is addressed through the screening project?
   a. Assurance
   b. Assessment
   c. Policy development
   d. Planning
2. If dental caries in school-age children is the problem you want to address, what public health solution would be best for this problem?
   a. School fluoride mouth rinse
   b. Grade-specific oral health education program

c. School sealant program

d. Community water fluoridation

3. Which one of the major agencies within the Department of Health and Human Services (DHHS) would have the most possibilities for funding the project you select to conduct?

a. PHS (Public Health Service)

b. ACF (Administration for Children and Families)

c. CMS (Centers for Medicare & Medicaid)

d. AOA (Administration on Aging)

4. The survey you conduct relates to which private practice function?

a. Diagnosis

b. Treatment

c. Examination

d. Evaluation

5. After your statewide screening project and data analysis, you examine solutions to the dental problems you have documented. If the program you select is to be an effective public health solution, it will have the all of the following characteristics except:

a. It is not hazardous to life or function.

b. It is easily and efficiently implemented.

c. It is attainable by those who can afford it.

d. It is effective immediately upon application.

References

1. Constitution of the World Health Organization. Geneva: World Health Organization; 1946.
2. Winslow CE. The untitled fields of public health. Mod Med 1920;2:183.
3. Block LE. Dental public health: An overview. In: Gluck GM, Morganstein WM, editors. Jong's Community Dental Health. 5th ed. St. Louis: Mosby; 2003.
4. Knutson JW. What is public health? In: Pelton WJ, Wisan JM, editors. Dentistry in Public Health. 2nd ed. Philadelphia: WB Saunders; 1955.
5. Kindig D, Stoddart G. What is population health? American Journal of Public Health 2003;93(3):380. Accessed Nov. 2009.
6. Burt BA, Ecklund SA. Dentistry, Dental Practice, and the Community. 6th ed. Philadelphia: Elsevier/Saunders; 2005.
7. Allukian M, Horowitz A. Effective community prevention programs for oral diseases. In: Gluck GM, Morganstein WM, editors. Jong's Community Dental Health. 5th ed. St. Louis: Mosby; 2003.
8. Oral Health in America. A report of the Surgeon General. Rockville, MD: US Department of Health and Human Services, National Institute of Dental and Craniofacial Research, National Institutes of Health; 2000.
9. Gluck GM, Morganstein WM, editors. Jong's Community Dental Health. 5th ed. St. Louis: Mosby; 2003.
10. Kuthy R, Odum JG. Local dental programs: A descriptive assessment of funding and activities. J Public Health Dent 1988;48:36.
11. Healthy People 2010. Understanding and Improving Health (Conference ed, 2 vols). Washington, DC: US Department of Health and Human Services; 2000.
12. A National Call To Action To Promote Oral Health. Rockville MD: US Department of Health and Human Services, Public Health Service, Centers for Disease Control and Prevention and the National Institutes of Health, National Institute of Dental and Craniofacial Research; NIH Publication No. 03-5303, May 2003.
13. US Department of Health and Human Services. Healthy People 2020: The Road Ahead. Washington, DC: November 2009. Available at www.healthypeople.gov/HP2020. Accessed August 8, 2010.
14. Institute of Medicine Committee for the Study of the Future of Public Health, Division of Health Care Services. A Vision of Public Health in America: An Attainable Ideal in the Future of Public Health. Washington, DC: National Academy Press; 1998.
15. Public Health in America. Washington, DC: Public Health Functions Steering Committee; 1994.
16. Corbin SB, Marten FR. Future of dental public health report—preparing dental public health to meet the challenges: Opportunities of the 21st century. J Public Health Dent 1994;54:80.

17. American Dental Hygienists' Association. Lifestyle, public health top ten. Access 1999;13:7.
18. American Dental Association Summit on Access. Summary Report. Available at www.ada.org. Accessed November 2009.
19. American Dental Association. Direct access settings expanded, Arizona. Access 2009;23:7.
20. American Dental Hygienists' Association. ADHP Resource Center. Available at www.adha.org/adhp/index.html. Accessed January 2010.

Additional Resources

Association of State & Territorial Dental Directors
   www.astdd.org
Healthy People 2020
   www.healthypeople.gov
Health Resources and Services Administration
   www.hrsa.gov
Office of the Surgeon General
   www.surgeongeneral.gov/library
Oral Health Atlas
   www.oralhealthatlas.org

Careers in Public Health for the Dental Hygienist

2

Sharon Logue, RDH, MPH
Kathy Voigt Geurink, RDH, MA

Objectives

Upon completion of this chapter, the student will be able to:
- Explain public health career options for dental hygienists.
- Discuss public health careers as a means of addressing the problem of access to oral health care.
- Define the mid-level provider role in addressing access to oral health care.
- Define skills and educational requirements for various roles in public health.
- Explain the relationship of private practice activities to public health activities.
- Identify specific careers, categorized by the American Dental Hygienists' Association (ADHA)-designated roles of the dental hygienist.

Key Terms

Alternative practice	General supervision	Legislation
Primary prevention	Follow-up/referral	Policy changes
Access to care	Health education	Technical assistance
Shortage areas	Networking	
Mid-level provider	Social marketing	

Opening Statements

Career Possibilities
- Public health hygienist at a local health department
- Statewide coordinator for a school-based fluoride varnish program
- Dental hygienist at a Veterans Affairs hospital
- Dental hygienist working with a state migrant farm worker program
- Dental hygienist at a state correctional facility
- State dental director in a state health department
- Dental hygienist with a university hospital department
- Dental health educator with a school system
- Dental hygienist on a dental sealant team
- Dental hygienist in the US Public Health Service (PHS)
- Dental hygienist contracting for service in a nursing home
- Consultant to a Head Start program

15

COMMUNITY ORAL HEALTH PRACTICE AS A CAREER

Dr. Alfred Fones is credited with initiating the development of the profession of dental hygiene and establishing the public health career for dental hygienists. In 1906, he trained the first dental hygienist, Irene Newman, and in 1913, he started the Fones School of Dental Hygiene in Bridgeport, Connecticut. Dr. Fones developed a curriculum for dental hygienists who began work within the Bridgeport Public School system. The first dental hygienists were trained to work in the community providing education and preventive services in their role as an advocate for dental public health.[1]

Public health careers for dental hygienists now run the gamut from high-level administrative posts to providing oral hygiene care for elderly residents in a nursing home or providing dental education for school-age children. In the public health field, some dental hygienists have an associate's degree or certificate, a bachelor's, a master's, or a doctoral degree. Many dental hygienists with advanced degrees working in public health began their public health careers with the minimum level of education. They chose to continue their education as their interests developed, their challenges expanded, and their desire grew to do more for the oral health of their community. A career in community oral health practice offers a variety of rewarding experiences that tend to feed the desire to make a difference in the oral health of all people.

A career chapter in the beginning of this text has been provided to allow you to make a connection with the role you might play in performing the functions discussed in the successive chapters. In private practice, the individual patient is your focus; in public health, the community is your patient. Your responsibilities will advance beyond individual clinical care, although in many positions, individual care still remains a very important duty. Public health takes you into the realm of program development, implementation, and evaluation and offers an opportunity to work with various populations, other professionals, agencies, financing mechanisms, and rules and regulations.

FUTURE TRENDS FOR DENTAL HYGIENISTS IN PUBLIC HEALTH

The Problem of Access to Oral Health Care

In a national report entitled *Oral Health in America,* the Surgeon General reviewed the profound disparities among specific population groups in oral health status and access to dental care.[2] Dental disease is a chronic problem among low-income populations.[3] Federal agencies and state governments are addressing these gaps in access to oral health care through legislation and policy development. Examples of some actions created through these processes are shown in the Guiding Principles box.[3,4] At the 2009 Access to Dental Care Summit, the American Dental Association (ADA) listed expansion and distribution of a well trained workforce with nationwide evaluation, standards, and regulations as a long-term strategy in improving access to dental care for underserved populations. Under this heading, the mid-level provider in dentistry was discussed and models are being developed and reviewed.[5] Summits and conferences on access such as this and the follow-up strategies and action plans will very likely increase the demand for dental hygienists working in community oral health practice.

GUIDING PRINCIPLES

Creating Access to Oral Health Care through Legislation and Policy Development[3,4]
- Allocating additional funds for dental services.
- Expanding treatment for special populations.
- Creating volunteers and donated dental services.
- Providing service programs.
- Additional dental benefits through existing public insurance programs.
- Extending educational loans and loan forgiveness for dental professionals.
- Creating tax credits for providers.
- Forming career ladders for dental providers.
- Increasing flexible licensure requirements.
- Increasing the scope of the dental hygienist's duties.
- Expanding coverage for provider services.

Alternative Practice Settings

Public health settings are categorized as **alternative practice** settings (i.e., providing oral hygiene services outside the private office in a "nontraditional" setting). Examples of the setting might be a community clinic, a mobile van, a school, a hospital, or a nursing home (**Figures 2-1 and 2-2**). The delivery of dental services offered in private practice does not reflect the need for services for those without means or without the capability of accessing care. In an alternative setting, dental care can be brought to people in need. Dental hygienists can provide preventive services in these settings, reaching large numbers of people who might not otherwise receive care.

Preventive services, or **primary prevention,** are more effective, less costly, and involve less technology than secondary or tertiary prevention (**Box 2-1**). Methods such as fluoride varnish or sealant programs, nutritional counseling, dental health education to community groups, and oral hygiene services and instruction are at the primary level. Often primary prevention strategies do not require a dentist.[6] Therefore, with less restrictive supervision, the dental hygienist can perform functions at this level and reach underserved populations.

Public Health Supervision

Regulatory Changes

Because of the need for services in places such as schools, nursing homes, and migrant health centers, dental hygienists are initiating oral health programs in these alternative settings. They are also filling positions beyond those connected with public health agencies. To create such positions, dental hygiene regulatory changes are being discussed and are under way throughout the United States. As a solution to the access problem, many states have changed restrictive dental practice acts that prevent the dental hygienist from practicing without the supervision of a dentist and that prevent dental hygienists from receiving direct reimbursement form third-party payers such as Medicaid or private dental insurers. To view which states allow direct **access to care** without the need for a dentist to examine or authorize the dental hygiene services see the map in **Figure 2-3**. To determine supervision levels for specific dental hygiene services by state, view the website www.adha.org/governmental_affairs/practice_issues.htm. Examples of changes in state regula-

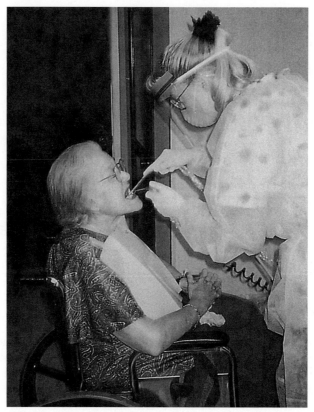

Figure 2-1 A dental hygienist provides oral hygiene care to a resident of a nursing home.

BOX 2-1 **Levels of Prevention**

- Primary prevention prevents the disease before it occurs. This level includes health education, disease prevention, and health protection. (Dental prophylaxis, sealants, and water fluoridation are examples.)
- Secondary prevention eliminates or reduces diseases in the early stages. (Restorations such as amalgams or composites are examples. This level requires more technology and is more costly than primary prevention.)
- Tertiary prevention limits disability from disease in later stages and requires rehabilitation and surgical procedures. (Dentures, implants, and bridge work are examples. This level is most costly and requires highly trained professionals to treat the disease.)

tions around the scope of practice for dental hygienists include New Mexico, where dental hygienists are allowed to practice in certain settings without the oversight of a dentist through a collaborative practice agreement with a dentist or group of consulting dentists, and Washington state, where dental hygienists may practice unsupervised in hospitals, nursing homes, home health agencies, group homes, state institutions, and public health facilities provided the hygienists refers to the dentist for treatment and meets a requirement of clinical experience. Colorado is one of

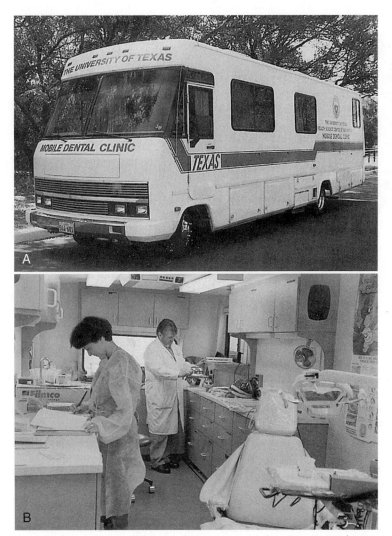

Figure 2-2 A, A mobile dental van is used as an alternative practice setting. **B,** Inside treatment area of a mobile dental van.

the states that allows dental hygienists to practice without supervision in all settings and allows licensed dental hygienists to own a dental hygiene practice. In a 2001 ADHA *Access to Care Position Paper,* the ADHA confirmed its position that dental hygienists who are graduates from an accredited dental hygiene program can be fully used in all public and private practice settings to deliver preventive and therapeutic oral health care safely and effectively. "Licensed dental hygienists, by virtue of their comprehensive education and clinical preparation, are well prepared to deliver preventive oral health care services to the public, safely and effectively, independent of dental supervision."[7]

In determining the necessity of regulatory changes, one must consider many factors such as the following:

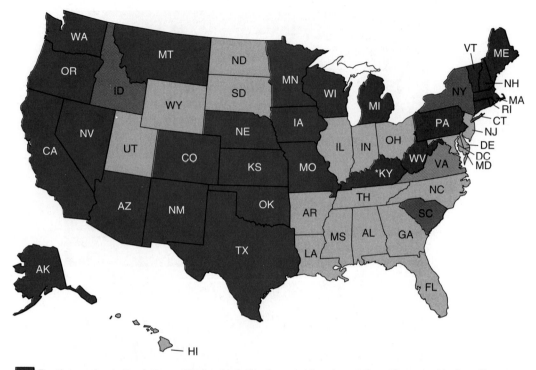

Dentist need not examine or authorize dental hygiene services in certain settings outside the office.

Dentist need not examine patient before hygienist performs services in certain settings outside the office.

Virginia Pilot Project seeks to assess the impact dental hygienists practicing in an expanded capacity have on increasing access to dental health care for underserved populations in three dental health professional shortage areas (Cumberland Plateau, Lenowisco, and Southside counties).

* Rules pending

Figure 2-3 Map of direct access.

1. The ratio of dentists to people
2. The number of dentists and dental hygienists in the state
3. The number of low-income adults and children who need dental care

These factors contribute to defining dental health professional **shortage areas.** Statistics compiled from Synopsis of State and Territorial Dental Health Programs provide information necessary in determining the available workforce of dental professionals and of community health departments and clinics.[8] The workforce numbers, compared with population size, are useful in determining professional shortage areas and the need for community oral health programs. Inadequate access to health care caused by professional shortages and geographic and financial barriers prevents people from attaining improved health status and improved quality of life. The dental profession, in realizing the need for reaching these underserved populations, is initiating preventive programs conducted by dental hygienists in many states.

It is interesting that some dental hygienists, initially volunteers, have found creative ways to be reimbursed for working in alternative settings. Writing grants, seeking school board funds, collecting Medicaid payments through an accepted provider, or contracting with a facility in states that allow it are a few of the innovative reimbursement plans currently being used. With less restrictive dental hygiene supervision and an increased number of dental hygienists seeking public health work, funding changes in the way of direct payment may be further explored in the future.

Mid-Level Provider

In the medical field, a **mid-level provider** is the term for a clinical medical professional who provides patient care under the supervision of a physician. Examples of mid-level providers include the nurse practitioner and the physician assistant. These professionals have advanced medical training but not on the level of the physician. It has been reported that physician assistants and nurse practitioners provide a majority of physician services for a much lower cost than the physician, thereby addressing the unmet need for medical services by providing quality care to more people at a lower cost. This concept applied to dentistry also addresses the problems of access to oral health care for underserved populations. Various models of workforce delivery are being developed to serve the populations who cannot easily access dental services as the result of problems of geographic location, poor financial resources, no dental insurance, and a lack of understanding about disease prevention measures. A shortage of dentists to meet the needs of the population and low dentist participation in Medicaid programs also affects access. The burden of oral disease is spread unevenly throughout the population (see Chapter 6), with minority children from low income families and the elderly population being most vulnerable. Models of delivery are provided in the next section, including the advanced dental hygiene practitioner (ADHP) defined in Chapter 1. Dental hygienists should develop an understanding of the necessity for new provider types in the existing health care system.

Dental Therapist

More than 50 countries worldwide have developed dental therapist programs to meet the dental needs of the people in their countries.[9] In 1921, a dental therapist program was first introduced in New Zealand. At that time, the dental therapist was called the *dental nurse.*

Services provided by the dental therapist vary by country, although most include basic restorative procedures, emergency treatment and preventive measures. The dental therapist in Alaska, called the *dental health aide therapist* (DHAT), completes 2 years of training and works under the **general supervision** of a dentist to provide preventive procedures, emergency care, and basic restorative procedures. DHATs provide services to the most isolated rural regions of Alaska in which little to no care was previously provided.

Community Dental Health Coordinator

In 2006, the ADA proposed the development of the community dental health coordinator (CDHC) to support the existing dental workforce in reaching out to underserved communities.[9] The CDHC works under the supervision of the dentist to promote oral health for communities and to assist patients in navigating through the health care system to establish a dental home. They would complete a 12-month training program and 6-month internship.

Advanced Dental Hygiene Practitioner

In June 2004, the ADHA House of Delegates, addressing the problem of access to health care, approved the creation of the ADHP credential. As stated in Chapter 1, this credential allows dental hygienists to provide diagnostic, preventive, restorative, and therapeutic services directly to the public.[9] Dental hygienists who receive the ADHP credential have graduated from an accredited dental hygiene program and also have completed an ADHA-approved advanced educational curriculum. This credential is designed to improve and enhance the oral health care delivery system. Because dental hygienists with the ADHP credential do not have to be supervised by a dentist, the door will open for them to work in school systems and nursing homes, as well as with underserved populations throughout the country.

Minnesota Dental Therapist and Advanced Dental Therapist[10]

The effort to establish a mid-level oral health provider went through a legislative process in Minnesota in 2008–2009. The result was the establishment of dental therapist (DT) and advanced dental therapist (ADT) programs. ADT trained at the University of Minnesota can provide basic preventive services, limited restorative services, extractions of primary teeth, and have limited prescriptive authority. A dentist is required to be present for the more complicated procedures, such as restorative procedures and extractions, but not required to be on site for preventive services. In the fall of 2009, the first dental hygienists entered a Master's program at Metropolitan State University based on the ADHP competencies developed by the ADHA. Graduation from this program provides the dental hygienist with a master's degree and the ADT title. The ADT will evaluate, assess, and plan treatment; perform nonsurgical extractions of permanent teeth; and administer all services of a DT without the requirement of onsite supervision. An ADT can also work in a collaborative management agreement with the dentist. The ADHA website (www.adha.org/governmental_affairs) posts the most current state legislative news on the ADHP and the DT and ADT programs, as well as other related legislative processes.

Table 2-1 describes the oral health current and proposed providers. See Additional Resources for more information on the oral health care workforce.

CAREERS IN PUBLIC HEALTH

Dental hygienists in public health positions use a variety of skills in implementing community oral health programs that have positive effects on their communities. In this chapter, the roles of the dental hygienist are further defined as they apply to specific career options (Figure 2-4). The ADHA has designated five dental hygiene roles, and public health is a component of each. Most public health jobs require a combination of skills defined in these multiple roles. Positions held by dental hygienists working in public health are included to inspire and illustrate the variety of career possibilities.

Clinician

In this familiar role, the public health dental hygienist provides clinical services to targeted populations, including assessment of oral health conditions and delivery of periodontal and preventive care. Often, the population served in a public health dental clinic has had limited access to dental

Table 2-1 Oral Health Care Workforce—Current and Proposed Providers

	Advanced Dental Hygiene Practitioner (ADHP)	Alaskan Dental Health Aide Therapist (DHAT)	Minnesota Dental Therapist/Advanced Dental Therapist (DT/ADT)	Community Dental Health Coordinator (CDHC)
Developed by	American Dental Hygienists' Association www.adha.org/adhp	Alaska Native Tribal Health Consortium (ANTHC) – Community Health Aide Program www.anthc.org	Minnesota State Statute and Rules www.dentalboard.state.mn.us	American Dental Association www.ada.org
Stage of Development	ADHP educational competencies were finalized in 2008. The first educational program based on ADHP competencies began in Fall 2009.	DHAT practice began in Alaska in 2004. The first graduates from the US-based DENTEX program began practice in 2008.	Educational programs for the DT (at the University of Minnesota School of Dentistry) and ADT (at Metropolitan State University) began in Fall 2009.	Curriculum complete and initial educational pilot program began in Winter 2009.
Education/Training	Master's level education at accredited institution; open to individuals currently licensed as dental hygienists who have a bachelor's degree	24 month program administered by ANTHC in partnership with the University of Washington DENTEX program	DT—minimum Baccalaureate degree ADT—Master's degree	Completion of 18 months of training.
Regulation/Licensure	Providers are already state licensed dental hygienists. ADHP is envisioned to be state licensed and regulated.	Providers are certified and regulated by Indian Health Service's Community Health Aide Program	Providers required to hold state license; can be dually licensed as a dental hygienist and administer dental hygiene scope.	Providers envisioned to be certificated; no formal state licensure
Proposed Setting	Community and public health settings, possibly private practice	Remote Alaskan villages	Settings that serve low-income and underserved patients, or are located in designated dental health professional shortage areas.	Community and public health settings
Proposed Supervision	Collaborative arrangement envisioned with strong communication and referral networks; presence of a dentist not required; use of teledentistry.	Remote/general supervision of a dentist; presence of a dentist not required; use of teledentistry	DT—General or indirect supervision depending on service ADT—Collaborative management agreement with dentist, presence of a dentist not required for most services	On site or general supervision, depending on service

Continued

Table 2-1 Oral Health Care Workforce—Current and Proposed Providers—cont'd

	Advanced Dental Hygiene Practitioner (ADHP)	Alaskan Dental Health Aide Therapist (DHAT)	Minnesota Dental Therapist/ Advanced Dental Therapist (DT/ADT)	Community Dental Health Coordinator (CDHC)
Preventive Scope	— Oral health and nutrition education — Full range of dental hygiene preventive services, including complete prophylaxis, sealant placement, fluoride treatments, caries risk assessment, oral cancer screenings — Expose radiographs — Advanced disease prevention and management therapies (e.g. chemotherapeutics)	— Oral health and nutrition education — Sealant placement — Fluoride treatments — Coronal polishing — Prophylaxis — Expose radiographs	— Oral health and nutrition education — Sealant placement — Fluoride varnishes — Coronal polishing — Oral cancer screenings — Caries risk assessment — Expose radiographs	— Oral health and nutrition education — Sealant placement — Fluoride treatments — Coronal polishing — Scaling for Type I Periodontal patients — Collection of diagnostic data
Periodontal Scope	— Provide non-surgical periodontal therapy.	— Provide non-surgical periodontal therapy	N/A	N/A
Restorative Scope	— Preparation and restoration of primary and permanent teeth — Placement of temporary restorations — Placement of pre-formed crowns — Temporary recementation of restorations — Pulp capping in primary and permanent teeth — Pulpotomies on primary teeth — Uncomplicated extractions of primary and permanent teeth — Place and remove sutures — Provide simple repairs and adjustments on removable prosthetic appliances	— Restorations of primary and permanent teeth — Placement of pre-formed crowns — Pulpotomies — Non-surgical extractions of primary and permanent teeth	— Restorations of primary and permanent teeth — Placement of pre-formed crowns — Placement of temporary crowns — Extractions of primary teeth — Nonsurgical extractions of permanent teeth (ADT only) — Direct /Indirect pulp capping — Pulpotomies on primary teeth — Atraumatic restorative therapy	— Palliative temporization (with hand instrumentation only) — Placement of temporary restorations

Professional Roles of the Dental Hygienist

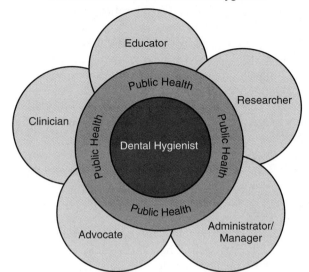

Figure 2-4 American Dental Hygienists' Association's (ADHA) roles of the dental hygienist.

care, has been excluded from dental benefits under employer insurance, and is often described as having lower socioeconomic status. Socioeconomic status includes factors such as income, education, and occupation. Populations of low socioeconomic status generally are at increased risk for dental disease.[11] These factors and different social and cultural values can influence use of dental services offered in public health clinics. Additional skills needed by the clinician include the ability to assess the perceived dental needs of the patient and to recognize the social and economic barriers to successful oral health outcomes. Examples of barriers to accessing dental services may include transportation problems, geographic distances, missed work hours, or lack of daycare services for children.[12] Immigrant families new to a community present language challenges and the need for cultural competency skills (see Chapter 10).

The clinician must utilize evidence-based preventive strategies for populations who are at high risk for dental caries. Topical and systemic fluorides, including fluoride varnish, and dental sealants are recognized as effective interventions for caries reduction in public health settings. The Association of State & Territorial Dental Directors (ASTDD) describes best practices on its website and highlights successful clinical community programs by state.

A public health clinician may see many types of patients during a given week providing care to infants, children, and adults. For example, a dental hygienist may place varnish on infants' teeth during a nutrition clinic. On another day, the same hygienist may provide periodontal treatment to pregnant women coming to the health department for prenatal care visits. Another part of the clinician's job may be to visit a nursing home on a monthly basis to provide clinical care to bedridden residents. Depending on the state's general supervision regulations, the dental hygienist may or may not be working from treatment plans previously determined by a dentist.

Clinicians in public health learn to be flexible with their dental environment. Clinical facilities may be in local health departments, in stationary school dental trailers, or in mobile dental vans that can be moved to multiple locations within a geographic area. Some states have school-based dental programs with dental teams using portable dental equipment instead of fixed operatories.

Clinical dental hygiene positions are available in many community settings, including hospitals, senior homes, and prison facilities. These locations offer the clinician additional challenges of complex medical histories and patients with physical or mental disabilities. Federal and state agencies have established clinical dental hygiene positions (e.g., the Indian Health Service, the National Health Service Corps, Community and Migrant Health Programs, or military bases). In addition, clinical care programs in communities may be supported by nonprofit volunteer or religious organizations. As local economies fluctuate, the number of "free" dental clinics can increase and public health clinicians may be involved with their operation. In nonprofit and in publicly funded programs, clinicians must be accountable with the most cost-effective way to provide quality dental services to the most people.

Public health dental hygienists may participate in the ongoing assessment of the prevalence of dental disease. Oral health surveys and clinical assessments are essential for public health program planning and evaluation. Clinical dental hygiene skills are used in both dental surveys and screenings for targeted populations. For example, ASTDD promotes the use of the Basic Screening Survey (BSS) tool to collect dental caries data in states (see Chapter 4). The dental hygienist may coordinate the supplies, the portable equipment, and infection control protocol to be used by the screening team. The clinician may communicate with school personnel and parents to create the screening schedules. Knowledge of dental indices, data collection, and reporting is essential. With any screening program, there must be a **follow-up/referral** component. The plan for action includes a system to provide prevention and treatment for the documented needs.

Oral health education would be a component of a clinical role just as it is in private practice. In some instances, the audience would be a group instead of individual instruction. This could require additional preparation by the dental hygienist, knowledge of instructional objectives, and familiarity with the target audience (see Chapter 6). For example, an oral health presentation might be given to parents in the waiting area of the immunization clinic.

Educational requirements for a public health clinical position may vary from an associate's degree to a bachelor's degree. If the public health job requires more administrative or management skills (see later section), an employer may require more work experience or a master's degree.

Educator

A dental hygienist in a faculty role may focus his or her career on teaching community dental health/public health courses to dental hygiene students. It is important for students to graduate and be aware of the segment of society that does not have access to dental care and to be knowledgeable of disparities in dental disease. This educator can familiarize students with new dental hygiene workforce models and encourage service learning in a dental hygiene curriculum (see Chapter 11). Service learning experiences for students improve education, promote civic engagement and benefit society. Community rotations can reinforce humanitarian ideals and build skills in cultural competency. An effective public health educator can influence dental hygiene graduates to see lower income patients in practice and volunteer with community projects. Educational requirements for dental hygiene faculty are generally a master's degree with clinical dental hygiene experience. Work experience in public health would be preferred for an educator responsible for community courses.

Another educator role in public health is an oral health educator in the community. **Health education** is the process in which the client is encouraged to become responsible for personal oral health and is informed of scientifically based methods for preventing dental diseases. In public health the client becomes the community. Beyond oral health education, though, is the promotion of total wellness. The community oral health educator must reinforce the relationship of oral health to total health. For example, early childhood caries may be the result of infant feeding practices that are related to nutritional issues. Improved dietary habits by adults may mean less risk of dental decay and less risk of other chronic diseases. The dental hygienist working at the community level always needs to consider the larger picture of wellness in creating education programs. For example, current research indicates a possible relationship among periodontal health, cardiovascular health and diabetes. Programs planned to intervene in these chronic diseases must be expanded to include oral health education.[13]

The team approach is always essential in public health. Oral health educators can network with other health professionals to share information about a common population.

A dental hygienist working with public health nutritionists or Early Head Start Program staff could enable implementation of a fluoride varnish program for infants and toddlers. School nurses, who have a unique perspective on the dental needs of schoolchildren, can share this information for oral health programs. **Networking** means that health data, resources for educational materials, and general community information are exchanged among dental, medical and social services professionals. As noted at a 2008 American Academy of Pediatrics Summit on Children's Oral Health,[14] "the lack of integration of oral health into overall health adds a significant barrier to improving children's health outcomes." All health professionals must understand the impact of oral disease on systemic health. The Bright Futures Project initiated by the Maternal and Child Health Bureau provides comprehensive oral health guidelines from pregnancy to adolescence for health professionals. Effective networking of dental hygienists with other health professionals increases the awareness and importance of the relationship of oral health to general health. Community education therefore can be designed to include several health messages for a target group. This team approach is comprehensive and cost-effective.

Public health education programs have built upon the success of commercial marketing techniques by means of **social marketing** to promote the adoption of a behavior to improve health. Social marketing refers to using the effective advertising tools from commercial marketing to influence a valued health behavior change. Dental hygienists can use social marketing concepts to develop a public awareness campaign, to create educational materials, or to improve dental services.

An effective oral health educator researches the target population to identify the community's needs and concerns about dental health. A town forum or smaller focus groups may be organized to learn about the community's ideas on dental issues. The dental hygienists must understand the community to develop and implement culturally appropriate oral health education programs. Mass media, the means of communication that reaches large numbers of people, can be a marketing tool. Skills in developing websites, writing newsletter articles, and developing public service announcements can be valuable assets in a public health education position. Oral health educators may work statewide on preventive programs or may work with the county or community level. Examples of oral health education programs include the following:

- A smokeless tobacco intervention program related to prevention of oral cancer
- Promotion of dental sealants for schoolchildren
- Education about prevention of early childhood caries for daycare providers
- Denture care classes for nursing home staff
- Promotion of mouth guards for athletes in a school district

The months of February (National Children's Dental Health Month) and October (Dental Hygiene Month) provide excellent opportunities for oral health educational activities. Health fairs are events that can reach the general public and provide information on numerous dental topics. The ADA in partnership with the Crest dental products company promotes their "Give Kids A Smile!" program during February, when on a specific day dental professionals can provide free dental care to the community. Oral health educators can also collaborate with local dental hygiene components on National Children's Dental Health Month plans.

The successful oral health education program is planned to target a specific dental need identified in a population. Oral health educators in the community need organizational skills, current scientific knowledge, excellent communication skills, creativity, and flexibility to meet the challenges of community health improvement (see Chapter 8). Educational requirements for health educator positions may vary from an associate's degree to a graduate degree, depending on specific job requirements.

Advocate

With the community considered to be a "patient," the public health dental hygienist assesses the dental needs and concerns of the population. After exploring the available dental resources, the dental hygienist also identifies any health disparities with access to health care (see Chapter 10). For example, an indigent group of older adults may lack finances to obtain dental care. The dental hygienist might represent these individuals in seeking community resources and in developing special programs. Once consumer issues are brought to the attention of local media or powerful citizens, changes can occur and access problems may be solved. The consumer advocate sees problems related to achieving optimal oral health and attempts to develop a solution.

As a dental professional, the hygienist can be a leader for the consumer and can be asked to be a vocal advocate for oral health. Dental hygienists who serve on state dental boards are evaluating skills of recent graduates, thus protecting the public and acting as a consumer advocate. The role of advocate may not be a full-time position but may be part of another role in the dental hygiene profession. Membership in the ADHA guarantees a platform to be an advocate for dental hygiene. A request for expert testimony on dental issues might come from state legislative bodies or boards of health. In this role, the dental hygienist is working to advance the health of the public through **legislation** and public **policy changes.** A public health dental hygienist may also provide **technical assistance** to nondental community groups interested in oral health issues. Some states have active oral health coalitions that have consumers ready to work on access to care issues. These coalitions welcome the participation of a dental hygienist. A dental hygienist can also provide guidance to community groups on the appropriateness of oral health educational materials.

An advocate dental hygienist could participate in legislative activity to change dental hygiene supervision laws; this is a task of the dental hygienist in the role of change agent. The ADHA cites restrictive supervision laws. As discussed earlier in this chapter, new dental hygiene workforce models are emerging that are the direct results of changing supervisory laws. Dental hygienists working under direct supervision (i.e., a dentist must be physically present during procedures performed by a hygienist) are limited in performing preventive services for segments of the population who do not have access to regular oral health care such as the poor, elderly, and physically challenged. Through the advocate role, dental hygienists have changed supervision from direct to general in many states. As a result of legislative involvement by dental hygienists in California, certification of the Registered Dental Hygienist in Alternative Practice (RDHAP) was initiated in 1998. The RDHAP is a licensed dental hygienist who provides unsupervised dental hygiene services in settings such as schools or institutions as prescribed by a dentist or physician.[15]

Dental hygienists who become advocates may have several years of experience in their profession and have the ability to visualize the "big picture." A specific educational degree beyond Registered Dental Hygienist may not be needed in this role. An effective advocate is current in scientific knowledge, confident, and eager for all citizens to have optimal oral health.

Researcher

As a researcher, a dental hygienist uses scientific methods and knowledge to identify and pursue a specific area of interest (see Chapter 7 for a discussion of the scientific method used in research). Dental hygienists employed in the research arena work in settings that vary from state health departments to universities to private industry.

In a state health department dental program, the epidemiology of dental diseases is a likely area of interest. Knowledge of dental indices to survey the prevalence of dental diseases is required, and biostatistical skills for analyzing data are important. Funding for state dental programs is becoming difficult to maintain, given the trend toward government downsizing in some states. Being accountable for public funds is an essential part of program evaluation. Dental data must be continually gathered to evaluate and demonstrate the effectiveness of public health programs in improving oral health and reducing barriers to oral health care.

In a research position, the dental hygienist could coordinate a statewide needs assessment. For a dental survey of this size, the dental hygienist must select a sample of appropriate size across the state and obtain permission to examine a specific population. If an oral health needs assessment involves the caries rates for children, the researcher may work through the school system to arrange for the children to be examined. Dental examiners are trained to use the dental indices through a calibration exercise to ensure that valid data have been obtained by the survey. Ultimately, the dental data analysis is important for future public health program planning. Epidemiologic research is crucial in maintaining existing oral health programs or in initiating new ones.

Research positions are available at many university or dental school settings. For example, a dental hygienist might be hired to participate in a periodontal research project to study the effectiveness of a new antimicrobial product, a microbiology department might seek dental hygienists as research associates, or a dental hygienist at a Veterans Affairs hospital might study therapeutic procedures for patients with head and neck cancer.

Certainly, dental product companies have ongoing research to scientifically determine the effectiveness of new methods and products to prevent and treat oral diseases. A dental hygienist working as a researcher has an appropriate background in basic sciences and dental sciences to join a research team. Dental hygienists choosing research positions may work part-time as a researcher, with the remainder of the job description being one of the previously discussed roles. Educational requirements for research positions may require a bachelor's degree. The specific background needed for research positions varies with the employer.

Administrator

The expanded coordination needed for community-wide oral health programs creates the need for a dental hygienist to be an administrator. In this role, the hygienist is an initiator who develops, organizes, and manages oral health programs to meet the needs of targeted groups of people. Planning skills may be required for local, state, or federal oral health programs. If the oral health program is implemented for a large population or within a large geographic area, supervision of other professional and technical staff may be required.

The type of oral health program managed depends on the needs of the population. For example, a hygienist may manage a statewide school-based fluoride mouth rinse program funded by state or federal funds. In this position the dental hygienist needs the following:

1. Knowledge of how systemic and topical fluorides work to prevent dental caries.
2. Good communication skills to establish a working relationship with school superintendents, principals, and teachers.
3. Organizational skills to plan a budget, to order supplies, and to keep records.
4. Knowledge of evaluation procedures to account for the cost versus the program effectiveness.

To assess the dental caries rate among participating schoolchildren, one ideally conducts a dental survey before and after initiating this preventive program. Writing skills are important for summarizing survey results and program successes and for soliciting for additional grant funds.

An administrator may often have additional roles, as previously discussed. The administrator may be required to provide some consulting, to become an advocate for changing public policy, or to be involved with social marketing for a new oral health initiative. Educational requirements of this administrative role are usually several years of experience and a bachelor's or master's degree in a related field such as public health or health administration.

DENTAL HYGIENIST MINI-PROFILE

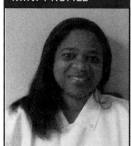

Clinician

Name: Ginger Melton, RDH, BS

Position and place of employment: Dental Hygienist/Director of Dental Administration, Healthy Smiles Dental Center of the Portsmouth Community Health Center, Portsmouth, Virginia

Qualifications and experience required for this position: Registered Dental Hygienist, Virginia Dental Hygiene License, minimum 2 years of work experience; community education experience preferred.

Main dental hygiene role filled in this position: Community Health Clinician

Duties performed in this position
Provide oral health education, preventive dental services, and administrative services for the department. Provide oral hygiene services and dental education to adults and children at school and community sites using the "Healthy Smile Mobile," which is a 40-foot, two-operatory, Mobile Dental Unit. Screen and refer children and adults to the appropriate program for dental care. Coordinate care for indigent adults at the Healthy Smiles Dental Center. Educate families about oral hygiene care. Supervise dental assistants and work closely with the Chief Dental Officer with management issues for the dental center.

Clinician—cont'd

Personal comment
As a community health dental hygienist, I face many challenges that are rewarding and motivating for me. In my clinical role, I provide much needed oral health education; preventive services, including fluoride and sealants; and some administrative services. With our changing economy and the discretionary dollar being scrutinized even more, it is great to know that patients are understanding the importance of keeping a healthy smile and are continuing to come to the Community Health Center for preventive dental services. This is very significant when you have a population that may see dental care as secondary. My challenge and reward is to get the community to understand the importance of oral health and the prevention of disease.

DENTAL HYGIENIST MINI-PROFILE

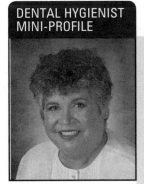

Clinician

Name: Leonor Ramos, RDH

Position and place of employment: Hospital Dentistry Dental Hygienist, Department of Defense, US Air Force, Wilford Hall Medical Center, Lackland Air Force Base, Texas

Qualifications and experience required for this position: Registered Dental Hygienist, graduated from an accredited school of dental hygiene. Broad-based knowledge of complex medical and pathologic conditions and their impact on overall health. Experienced in providing appropriate clinical techniques and instructions for oral care and able to perform complex functions that differ with the needs of each medically compromised patient. Exceptional judgment, organizational skills, and leadership qualities preferred.

Main dental hygiene role(s) fulfilled in this position: Educator, Clinician

Duties performed in this position

Educator
Educate hospitalized patients on oral hygiene care, provide numerous in-service presentations to medical professionals and various support groups on the oral management of medically compromised patients, and present continuing education programs in this area. In 1991, I initiated an affiliation with the University of Texas Health Science Center Department of Dental Hygiene; as adjunct faculty, I supervise dental hygiene students on a hospital rotation. In this rotation, students gain insight to state-of-the-art cancer treatment modalities such as intensity-modulated radiation therapy (IMRT), use of the hyperbaric chamber for osteoradionecrosis (ORN), acupuncture to provide moisture for patients with hyposalivation, psoralen + ultraviolet wave (PUVA) treatment for

Clinician—cont'd

patients with oral graft-versus-host disease (GVHD), and the use of i-CAT for head and neck imaging.

Clinician
Provide preoperative and postoperative preventive oral care and patient education in the Department of Defense's only allogeneic bone marrow transplant center. Autologous, syngeneic, umbilical cord stem cell, and nonrelated donor bank transplants are also done here. Patients undergoing head and neck radiation by means of conventional radiation or IMRT are also a large portion of my patient population. In addition, I treat patients who are medically compromised as the result of receiving organ transplants or major orthopedic joint replacements and those with autoimmune diseases, poorly controlled diabetes, or hematologic disorders. Long-term follow-up of the patients ranges from 5 years to a lifetime. The chronic sequelae of bone marrow transplantation sometimes necessitates the management of chronic GVHD for the life of the patient.

Personal comment
In my 37 years of providing oral care, I have had unusual opportunities for professional development through the military experience and training made available to me in my Air Force career and subsequently in federal civil service. Experiences in both environments provided me with the inspiration to initiate a yearly Dental Hygiene Symposium—now in its 24th year, which provides continuing education opportunities, and to promote the development of a monograph pertaining to the oral management of cancer patients. Now in its third revision, the *Oral Health in Cancer Therapy Monograph* is accessible at the website of the Dental Oncology Education Program of the Texas Cancer Council (www.doep.org). It is my hope that the future will provide many more opportunities for dental hygienists to network with medical professionals as an integral part of an interdisciplinary team providing comprehensive patient care.

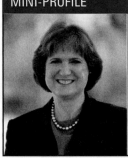

DENTAL HYGIENIST MINI-PROFILE

Advocate

Name: Diann Bomkamp, RDH, BSDH, CDHC

Position and place of employment: A 40+ year clinical dental hygienist who has worked in public health as a part-time consultant for the Missouri Department of Health and Senior Services and has advocated for optimal public health through various positions in the Missouri Dental Hygienists' Association (MDHA) and the American Dental Hygienists' Association (ADHA).

Qualifications and experience required for this position: A strong dedication to advocating for access to and improved oral health for the public; the ability to interpret research and translate it into

Advocate—cont'd

understandable information for policymakers and the public; tenacious energy and stamina; a consensus and relationship builder; an understanding of how public policy evolves; knowledge of dental hygiene accreditation standards and practice acts and how they affect the delivery of health care

Main dental hygiene role filled in this position: Advocate

Duties performed in this position
Researcher; communicator/educator; public health and dental hygiene advocate; public health policy strategist

Personal comment
I served as the 2008–2009 President of the ADHA. My interest in dental hygiene was triggered after working for my uncle, a dentist in St. Louis, when I was 16 years old. I have practiced as a dental hygienist more than 40 years since earning my bachelor's degree in dental hygiene from Marquette University in Milwaukee, Wisconsin.

Initially, I worked in general practice but have spent most of my years as a clinical dental hygienist in a periodontal practice. Additionally, I was the clinic coordinator and lead preclinical instructor at St. Louis Community College at Forest Park's Dental Hygiene Program.

My advocacy began in the early 1980s through involvement with the MDHA as the public health chairperson, and eventually I served as president of both the Greater St. Louis dental hygienists' association and the MDHA. I was also the editor of the *Curette Gazette*, the MDHA newsletter, and then a 17-year MDHA legislative chair, which gave me a perspective of how public policy is made and the importance of advocacy. In addition, my legislative activities led me to be more involved in politics so that MDHA formed the Missouri Dental Hygienists' Political Action Committee and I was elected as the first chairperson.

I served as a delegate/alternate delegate to ADHA for many years, and in 1998, I ran for ADHA District VIII Trustee and served the states of Iowa, Nebraska, Kansas, Illinois, and Missouri for 4 years.

Because of my interest in improving access to care and in public health, I earned a Community Dental Health Certificate (CDHC) at Northeast Wisconsin Technical College in 2006. Most recently, I worked with the Missouri Department of Health and Senior Services as an oral health consultant with four other dental hygienists to implement a Preventive Services Program (PSP), which is a K-12 oral health educational curriculum, along with several other educational programs (see: www.mohealthysmiles.com).

After recognizing the strong need for the dental profession to be involved in the political arena, I decided to run for Missouri state representative in 2002 and 2004 and lost by a very slim margin.

Later, I was elected as Vice President and then served as President of the ADHA. During my year as president, I had tremendous opportunities to work on the access to oral health care agenda, including the

Advocate—cont'd

implementation of the ADHP, which is the ADHA's proposal for a dental mid-level provider. I also worked on health care reform and had the chance to promote the utilization of dental hygienists to positively affect the public health infrastructure.

My career path shows the positive impact that a clinical dental hygienist can have in promoting better oral health in their own state and to the nation by active involvement in our professional organization.

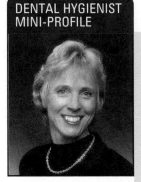

DENTAL HYGIENIST MINI-PROFILE

Researcher

Name: Kathy Phipps, RDH, MPH, DrPH

Position and place of employment: Associate Professor, Oregon Health & Science University, Portland, Oregon

Qualifications and experience required for this position: Doctoral degree with experience in research; postdoctoral research fellowship recommended. With research experience, candidate may be in the process of doctoral degree completion.

Main dental hygiene role(s) fulfilled in this position: Researcher

Duties performed in this position
Research is concerned with epidemiology, which is the study of disease trends in populations. With an RDH background, oral epidemiology is the area of research that is emphasized. For example, the present researcher is studying the impact of fluoride on skeletal health (osteoporosis).

Assisting local, state, and federal agencies in tracking the oral health status of people in their jurisdictions is also a function of the position.

Research interests may be expanded from dentistry to medicine. This researcher is a co-investigator for a major 7-year research project looking at risk factors for osteoporosis, cardiovascular disease, and prostate cancer in older men. Primary duties of the epidemiology aspect include writing grant proposals, developing research protocols, analyzing research data, and writing manuscripts. Research assistants actually work with the study participants and collect the data.

Personal comment
I am a graduate of the dental hygiene program at Oregon Health & Science University with a Bachelor of Science degree in Dental Hygiene. At the same time, I also attended classes at Portland State University and received a Bachelor of Science degree in general science with an emphasis in public health studies.

After receiving my bachelor's degrees, I practiced dental hygiene for about 1 year. I then applied to graduate school and received a scholarship to attend the Program in Dental Public Health, School of Public Health at the University of Michigan.

Researcher—cont'd

My emphasis during the master's program was in health care administration. I returned to the state of Oregon and worked as a health administrator and social service manager for an agency serving senior citizens.

I was away from dentistry for about 6 years and decided that it was time to return to the field. I applied for and received funding to complete my doctoral degree at the University of Michigan. I became interested in fluoride and started doing my research on fluoride and osteoporosis while still in graduate school.

Since that time, I have had three research projects funded by the National Institute of Dental and Craniofacial Research. The results of these projects have been published in the *Journal of Dental Research* and the *British Medical Journal.*

Although research may not sound glamorous or exciting, it has given me an opportunity to experience many different aspects of life. For example, I have done research in Russia and remote villages in Alaska, I have made presentations to dentists and hygienists in both the United States and the United Kingdom, and I am on several advisory panels for the National Institutes of Health and the Centers for Disease Control and Prevention.

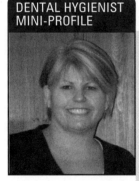

DENTAL HYGIENIST MINI-PROFILE

Administrator

Name: Lynn Bethel, RDH, MPH

Position and place of employment: Director of Oral Health, Massachusetts Department of Public Health

Qualifications and experience required for this position: Current license or eligibility as a dentist or dental hygienist under the Massachusetts Board of Registration in Dentistry. Graduate of an institution accredited by the ADA's Commission on Dental Accreditation. A minimum of 7 years clinical experience and at least 5 years of full-time supervisory or managerial experience in the particular specialty, as well as content knowledge and experience in implementing essential dental public health services and initiatives. Significant experience in developing and delivering creative and successful dental public health assessment and delivery systems, knowledge of survey methodology, oral health prevention strategies, and experience in implementing and evaluating community-based prevention programs, including school sealant programs and community water fluoridation. Knowledge and experience in coalition and consensus building, as well as knowledge of applicable laws, regulations, and policies.

Main dental hygiene role filled in this position: Administrator

Administrator—cont'd

Duties performed in this position
Surveillance, including assessing the oral health status of the state's residents; identifying risk factors and barriers to accessing dental care; planning, managing and evaluating statewide oral health prevention programs (i.e., water fluoridation, school sealant programs, and fluoride mouthrinse/varnish); grant and report writing; dental workforce initiatives; collaborating with stakeholders to identify policy changes to improve and promote oral health; fiscal accountability in managing program budgets; and staff supervision.

Personal comment
I knew in high school, after working one summer in a Head Start classroom, that I wanted to be a dental hygienist in public health, and I haven't regretted my decision a single minute. After dental hygiene school (Cape Cod Community College), I transferred to Old Dominion University to earn my bachelor's degree in Dental Hygiene. I also earned a minor in Sociology. When I returned home, I began working in a pediatric dental office and I remained working at this office (at times, just part-time) until the later part of 2009.

In 1995, while raising a family and attending graduate school (part-time), I earned my Master's degree in Public Health from Boston University's School of Public Health. During that time, I also worked in a community health center dental program in the City of Boston. In 2000, I began my full-time teaching career, developing the community dental health curriculum and the externship rotations for Mount Ida College's newly accredited Dental Hygiene Program. It was while teaching at Mount Ida that I developed my first school-based sealant program to be implemented by the second year dental hygiene students using portable equipment. That program is still in existence today and is part of a larger collaborative effort called *Smart Smiles* in Boston Public Schools. I am still an adjunct faculty member at Mount Ida College, and I continue to teach its community dental health course every fall.

The variety of experiences I have had (and still have) in my dental hygiene career serves as a foundation for the leadership I demonstrate as the Director of Oral Health. While public health offers me the chance to help people and improve the lives of many at one time, it also affords me the opportunity to work alongside different professional disciplines and be challenged each day. I truly enjoy my work.

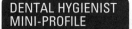

DENTAL HYGIENIST MINI-PROFILE

Clinician

Name: JoAnn W. Wells, RDH, BS

Position and place of employment: Human Service Program Coordinator-Regional Dental Hygienist, Virginia Department of Health, Division of Dental Health, Chesterfield/Crater Health District

Qualifications and experience required for the position: Undergraduate degree in dental hygiene and 1 to 2 years of clinical experience and health education

PREFERRED: Master's degree in an education area and/or strong emphasis in health education. Demonstrate community based and clinical dental hygiene service.

Personal Note: Currently, I am enrolled in the online Master's program in Dental Hygiene at Old Dominion University. The graduate program will provide me with the education I need in dental hygiene to be a successful clinician, and my emphasis in community health will help me provide dental hygiene clinical services and oral health education to underserved populations. In addition, through my distance learning at Old Dominion University, I have been able to establish partnerships with dental hygiene programs in Virginia.

Main dental hygiene roles filled in the position: My role in the clinician/educator position is one of comparison or control for a recent bill passed in Virginia (SB 1202 and HB2180 for the Practice of Dental Hygienists). This bill states that dental hygienists holding a license may provide educational and preventive dental care in health districts designated as Virginia Dental Health Professional Shortage Areas by the Virginia Department of Health. This bill was passed to improve access to preventive dental care for the underserved and increase career opportunities for dental hygienists in Virginia.

Duties performed in this position
My position as a Regional Dental Hygienist supports district-wide delivery of oral health clinical services and oral health education. I have the chief responsibility of planning and coordinating patient-based clinical services, community oral health educational activities and oral health promotion with Women, Infants and Children (WIC), pregnant women, school health services, and seniors.

In collaboration with local and state partners to increase the awareness of oral health to the citizens in these health districts, clinical services are provided to high-risk populations that include children aged 6 months to 5 years in WIC through screening, providing fluoride varnish, education, and referrals. In addition, dental hygiene clinical services are provided to pregnant women in their second trimester of pregnancy through the Chesterfield County Health Department's "Maternal Access to Dentally Related Risk Reduction Education and Services Program" (MADRES).

Clinician—cont'd

In collaboration with the Virginia Dental Association, Southside Dental Component, my duties include coordination of the "Give Kids a Smile Program" with the Chesterfield County Communities-In-Service Schools (CIS), in which high-risk school-age students are provided screenings, preventive services, and clinical services on Give Kids a Smile Day. Along with private practitioners who participate in Give Kids a Smile Day, we have specialists in pediatric dentistry, oral surgery, endodontics, and orthodontics who volunteer their time to provide care. In School Health Services, dental sealants are provided to second graders on the Virginia Department of Health's Mobile Dental Van in the Crater Health District.

Finally, oral health education is provided to seniors in our community through a Senior Smiles Grant we received from the Alliance of the ADA.

Personal comment

My role as a public health dental hygienist has changed over the past 20 years, and I find my current position very rewarding, as well as challenging. My position as the comparison or control for dental hygienists to work in underserved areas under general supervision will provide data needed to expand the dental hygiene scope of practice in the state of Virginia.

DENTAL HYGIENIST MINI-PROFILE

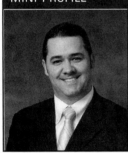

Administrator

Name: Matt Crespin, RDH, MPH

Position and place of employment: Oral Health Project Manager, Children's Health Alliance of Wisconsin/Children's Hospital of Wisconsin, Inc.

Qualifications and experience required for this position: Current Wisconsin licensure and a bachelor's degree in dental hygiene if preferred, with 3 to 5 years of clinical experience preferred, as is any work in the field of dental public health.

Main dental hygiene role filled in this position: Project Manager

Duties performed in this position

Managing the Wisconsin school-based dental sealant program, Seal-A-Smile, in collaboration with the Wisconsin Division of Public Health. Currently, $600,000 is available annually for technical assistance, grant monitoring, and administration. Lead and manage the Wisconsin Oral Health Coalition comprised of more than 140 individuals and organizations working together to improve oral health access to low-income children and families. Manage other local and statewide initiatives dealing with oral health access. Participate on several local, state, and national advisory boards and work groups.

Administrator—cont'd

Personal comment

I knew in high school that I wanted to go to dental school; after I arrived at Marquette University and spent a year as a biology major, I knew I wanted to begin working in the dental field sooner. I transferred into the dental hygiene program and really enjoyed the integrated program that Marquette provided because it allowed me to begin my work in the field of oral health almost immediately.

Upon graduation from Marquette University's dental hygiene program in 2002, I worked in private practice in a suburb of Milwaukee for about 4 years. This was what I thought I was trained to do and did not think any differently. Over time, I began to think about my training as a dental hygienist and my commitment to serving low-income populations, which was one of the cornerstones of my Marquette education: service to others. Working in the suburbs with mostly affluent children, families, and adults, I felt as though there was more I could be doing to give back to my community. After all, for 2½ years, the majority of the population I saw in my dental chair was either uninsured or underinsured.

I began exploring options outside of private practice and came across an advertisement for my current position. I was not completely clear on my responsibilities but after speaking to my now supervisor, I knew this was the job for me. Planning local events for kids with little or no access to care, meeting with legislators to discuss policy change, and working at the grassroots level in improving access was right up my alley.

In 2006, I became the Oral Health Project Manager for the Children's Health Alliance of Wisconsin, which is part of Children's Hospital of Wisconsin. After taking some time to figure out how to navigate the world of dental public health, I have developed a true passion for this line of work. Improving the oral health of children, especially those with limited or no access to dental care, is my goal. I enjoy working with local programs and providing assistance with program development or improvement of efficiencies. Planning and organizing coalition activities that drive policy change and raise awareness of the issue is very exciting to me.

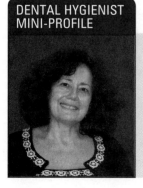

DENTAL HYGIENIST MINI-PROFILE

Educator

Name: Kathy Lituri, RDH, MPH

Position and place of employment: Oral Health Promotion Director, Clinical Instructor, Division of Community Health Programs, Department of Health Policy and Health Services Research, Boston University Henry M. Goldman School of Dental Medicine, and Adjunct Faculty, Forsyth School of Dental Hygiene, Massachusetts College of Pharmacy and Health Sciences.

Educator—cont'd

Qualifications and experience required for this position: Current license as a dental hygienist under the Massachusetts Board of Registration in Dentistry. Graduate of an institution accredited by the ADA's Commission on Dental Accreditation. Graduate of an institution accredited by the Association of Schools of Public Health. A minimum of 5 years clinical experience and a minimum of 5 years experience in community oral health promotion and health education.

Main dental hygiene role filled in this position: Clinician, Health Educator/Wellness Promoter, Oral Health Advocate and Instructor

Duties performed in this position
Provide a variety of community-based oral health education and promotion activities, including screenings and fluoride varnish applications, to a wide range of vulnerable populations in and around the Boston area. Provide experiential opportunities for both dental and dental hygiene students to learn firsthand about the oral health needs of low-income families, high risk pregnant women, and homeless veterans. Lecture in predoctoral and postdoctoral courses in preventive dentistry, teach community health to dental hygiene students, and oversee a public health project requirement of fourth year dental students.

Personal comment
My first job out of hygiene school was in a pediatric dental practice where most families paid out-of-pocket for dental services for their children. Although my professors urged me not to work in pediatrics full time (because I might forget how to scale), I believe that doing so is what launched my career into public health and working with the underserved of all ages. After 8 years and a short break from dental hygiene, I worked at Children's Hospital in Boston for 11 years and provided pediatric clinical dental hygiene services to medically, physically, mentally, emotionally, and socially compromised patients, while also serving as Dental Outreach Coordinator, Dental Rehabilitation Coordinator, and Extramural Dental Hygiene Clinical Instructor. During this time, I also started a family and earned a Bachelor of Science Degree in Management. In 1999, I joined the Division of Community Health Programs at Boston University and helped expand the range of community-based oral health promotional activities and events, including school-based sealant programs, and programs designed for the elderly and preschool children and nondental providers. During this time, I completed a master's degree in Public Health, was elected as an officer in the Oral Health Section of the American Public Health Association, and began my teaching career as a lecturer in various courses at the dental school and as an adjunct faculty at Forsyth, where I teach a course in community health. My job is quite varied and can be a challenge at times, but it enables me to interact with and establish relationships with people from different walks of life, as well as both dental and dental hygiene students and health providers from other disciplines, all in an effort to promote oral health and overall well-being.

SUMMARY

Various career options exist for dental hygienists in the public health arena. The public health career options offer many challenges and opportunities for the dental hygienist to become actively involved in providing optimal oral health for the community. The trend of less restrictive dental hygiene regulation to facilitate the dental hygienist's desire to provide preventive treatment to underserved populations is explored. Data collected on population numbers related to dental manpower and community programs are mentioned and can be located at the website for the ASTDD (www.astdd.org).

Public health career options and public health positions for dental hygienists are available in a variety of settings. Within the primary setting of your dental hygiene career, you may choose to develop public health skills working as a clinician, educator, advocate, researcher, or administrator. The skills and education necessary to fulfill these roles are delineated in the chapter. Workforce models are defined, and these models, such as the ADHP, may be an advanced career path that students can take to address the problems of access to oral health for underserved populations.

Applying Your Knowledge

1. Check with your state health department to determine whether public health or community dental hygiene positions are available in your community. Obtain a job description and evaluate the skills needed for this position using the dental hygiene roles described in the chapter.
2. Research all available dental resources in your community for older adults who are unable to afford or travel to private dental offices. Whom would you contact to find out the location of these dental services? Write a job description for yourself to treat elderly residents unable to have access to care in private offices.
3. Review dental supervision laws in your state, and determine whether there is a need for change. Which populations might benefit from a change? How might you be involved in initiating a change?
4. Participate in a community rotation/service project that is considered an alternative practice setting.
5. Report on the progress of the oral health mid-level providers in addressing the oral health needs of the underserved. Review the reports listed in Additional Resources.

Dental Hygiene Competencies

Reading the material in this chapter and participating in the activities of Applying Your Knowledge will contribute to the student's ability to demonstrate the following competencies:

Core competencies
C.8 Communicate effectively with individuals and groups from diverse populations verbally and in writing.

Community involvement
CM.3 Provide community oral health services in a variety of settings.

Professional growth and development
PGD.1 Identify alternative career options within health care, industry, education, and research, and evaluate the feasibility of pursuing dental hygiene opportunities.

PGD.2 Develop management and marketing strategies to be used in nontraditional health care settings.

PGD.3 Access professional and social networks and resources to assist entrepreneurial initiative.

Community Case

In your position as the oral health program coordinator for the Division of Dental Health, State Health Department, you are assigned the task of developing an educational campaign promoting oral health as part of overall health. You also are in charge of setting up a dental sealant program in an area of the state with a dental health professional shortage. You will be selecting schools to participate in the dental sealant program, and you will be organizing the project, including all planning meetings, ordering supplies, supervising personnel, and arranging the schedule.

1. One of the first steps in planning your educational campaign would be:
   a. Use your public health directory to contact each health division
   b. Define the target population for your educational campaign
   c. Develop the educational materials yourself and distribute to focus groups
   d. Develop strategies other than mass media because of the expense
2. You decide to set up a committee to help develop the "healthy mouth, healthy body" campaign and invite a public health nurse, nutritionist, and chronic disease health educator to join. This step is an example of:
   a. Networking to pool resources and skills
   b. Taking steps toward policy changes
   c. A dental hygienist working under general supervision
   d. Secondary prevention strategies
3. Your role with the school-based sealant program would be categorized as:
   a. Clinician
   b. Researcher
   c. Administrator
   d. Educator
4. You will be reviewing all of the following factors in determining the location for the sealant program in the state except:
   a. The ratio of dentists to people
   b. The number of low income adults and children who need care
   c. The number of high schools in the area
   d. The number of dentists and dental hygienists
5. The educational campaign would be categorized as a primary prevention measure. The sealant program would be a secondary method of prevention.
   a. The first sentence is correct, and the second sentence is false.
   b. Both sentences are true.
   c. Both sentences are false.
   d. The first sentence is false, and the second sentence is true.

References

1. Burt BA, Ecklund SA. Dentistry, Dental Practice, and the Community. 6th ed. Philadelphia: Elsevier/Saunders; 2005.
2. Oral Health in America. A Report of the Surgeon General. Rockville, MD: US Department of Health and Human Services, National Institute of Dental and Craniofacial Research, National Institutes of Health; 2000.
3. Oral Health. Dental Disease Is a Chronic Problem Among Low-Income Populations. Washington, DC: US General Accounting Office; 2000.

 4. State of the States. Overview of 1999 State Legislation on Access to Oral Health. Washington, DC: Center for Policy Alternatives; 1999.
 5. American Dental Association Access to Dental Care Summit. Summary Report. Available at www.ada.org. Accessed January 2010.
 6. Warren RC. Oral Health for All: Policy for Available, Accessible and Acceptable Care. Washington, DC: Center for Policy Alternatives; 1999.
 7. Access to Care Position Paper 2001. American Dental Hygienists' Association; 2001. Available at www.adha.org/profissues/access_to_care.htm.
 8. Synopsis of State and Territorial Dental Public Health Programs. Association of State & Territorial Dental Directors (ASTDD) Home Page, 2009. Available at www.astdd.org. Accessed August 6, 2010.
 9. The Pew Center on the States, W.K. Kellogg Foundation, National Academy for Health Policy. Help Wanted, A Policy Maker's Guide to New Dental Providers. May 2009. Available at www.pewcenteronthestates.org/report_detail.aspx?id=52478. Accessed October 2010.
10. American Dental Hygienist's Association. ADHP Resource Center: The History of Introducing a New Provider in Minnesota. Available at www.adha.org/downloads/mn_mid-level_history_and_timeline.pdf. Accessed January 2010.
11. Brick P. Working in public health. Access 1993;7:12.
12. Capilouto E. Improving the oral health of at-risk children. J Health Care Poor Underserved 1991;2:132.
13. Berthold M. Profiles in public health: Dental hygienists reach out. Access 1998;12:13.
14. Results of the American Academy of Pediatrics 2008 National Summit on Children's Oral Health. Available at www.aap.org/commpeds/dochs/oralhealth/summit/index.cfm. Accessed January 2010.
15. American Dental Hygienists' Association, Division of Governmental Affairs, Stateline. Access 2000;12:32.

Additional Resources

Information on the Advanced Dental Hygiene Practitioner
   www.adha.org
Training new dental providers in the US. Burt Edelstein DDS, MPH. December 2009
   www.wkkf.org
Supervision levels for dental hygiene services by state
   www.adha.org/governmental_affairs/practice_issues.htm
Sufficiency of the US Oral Health Workforce in the coming decade: A Workshop
   www.iom.edu/Reports/2009/oralhealthworkforce.aspx

3

Assessment in the Community

Jane E. M. Steffensen, RDH, BS, MPH, CHES

Objectives

Upon completion of this chapter, the student will be able to:

- Explain the importance of assessment as a core public health function.
- Describe the roles of public health professionals in assessment.
- Discuss the basic terms and concepts of epidemiology.
- Describe the conceptual models that illustrate the determinants of health.
- Identify the determinants of health that affect the health of individuals and communities.
- Identify the specific stages of a planning cycle.
- Discuss a community oral health improvement process.
- Describe the main steps followed and key activities undertaken in a community oral health assessment.
- Compare and contrast the different methods of data collection that can be used in community health assessments.

Key Terms

Assessment
Epidemiology
Host factors
Agent factors
Environmental factors
Determinants of health
Mandala of health
Determinants of oral health

Planning cycle
Assess
Plan
Implement
Evaluate
Community health
    improvement process

Community oral health
    assessment
Community profile
Data collection
Quantitative data
Qualitative data

Opening Statements

National Leading Health Indicators

Indicators

- Access to health insurance

- Access to personal health care

- Prenatal care

Related Statistic*

- 17% of children and adults (younger than 65 years) do not have health insurance (2008)
- 4% of children and adults do not have a source of ongoing primary health care (2008)
- 16% of pregnant women have not received prenatal care during the first trimester (2002)

*Statistics from *Healthy People 2010 Database.* Available at http://wonder.cdc.gov/data2010/. Accessed February 2010.

- Child immunizations

- Physical activity

- Overweight and obesity
- Tobacco use
- Substance abuse

- Environmental quality

- Adult immunizations

- 81% of young children (aged 19 to 35 months) are fully immunized (2006)
- 67% of adults are not physically active on a regular basis (2008)
- 33% of adults are obese (2006)
- 21% of adults smoke cigarettes (2008)
- 20% of adolescents have used alcohol or illicit drugs during the past month (2007)
- 39% of Americans are exposed to harmful air pollutants (2004)
- 67% of high risk older adults (65 years and older) not living in institutions are fully immunized for influenza and pneumonia (2008)

PUBLIC HEALTH PRACTICE

Professional work in community health is dynamic because the environment changes continuously. Community health is affected by social, demographic, political, economic, and technologic changes. In this milieu, public health practitioners perform a broad array of duties focused on entire populations, with the overarching goal that people are healthy and live in healthy communities.[1,2] The mission of public health is to "fulfill society's interest in assuring the conditions in which people can be healthy."[3,4] Public health carries out this mission through organized, interdisciplinary efforts that address health problems in communities. Its mission is achieved through the application of health promotion and disease prevention and control efforts designed to improve health and enhance quality of life.[1-4]

Public health services incorporate the roles of a myriad of public health professionals in various sectors and from diverse disciplines that form the public health workforce in the United States.[4,5] Public health professionals can belong to many professional disciplines, including oral health, nursing, nutrition, social work, health promotion, laboratory science, environmental health, administration, and epidemiology. Public health professionals have expertise in diverse public health practices.[5] Several organizations and agencies have called for an increase in the visibility of public health and the core workforce that forms its foundation.[1,2]

As a result, collaborative efforts have been undertaken to enhance the recognition of the public health professions by measuring and improving the competency and consistency of public health workers nationwide. In 2005, the National Board of Public Health Examiners (NBPHE) was established to ensure that graduates from schools and programs of public health accredited by the Council on Education for Public Health (CEPH) have mastered the knowledge and skills relevant to contemporary public health.[1] The NBPHE has developed and now administers an examination for the credential, Certified in Public Health (CPH).[1] The national examination covers the five core areas of knowledge offered in CEPH–accredited schools and programs, as well as interdisciplinary cross-cutting areas relevant to contemporary public health. The core areas include biostatistics, environmental health sciences, epidemiology, health policy and management, and social and behavioral sciences.[1,2] The cross-cutting areas are communication and informatics, diversity and culture, leadership, public health biology, professionalism, programs planning, and systems thinking.[1,2]

BOX 3-1 **Core Competencies for Public Health Professionals Developed by the Council on Linkages between Academia and Public Health Practice**

- Analytical/assessment skills
- Policy development/program planning skills
- Communication skills
- Cultural competency skills
- Community dimensions of practice skills
- Basic public health sciences skills
- Financial planning and management skills
- Leadership and systems thinking skills

In addition, the Council on Linkages Between Academia and Public Health Practice has developed a set of core competencies for public health professionals to help strengthen public health workforce development.[1,2] The competencies guide academic institutions and training providers to develop curricula and course content and to evaluate public health education and training programs. The competencies are used in practice settings as a framework for hiring and evaluating staff and assessing organization-wide gaps in skills and knowledge. The competencies are divided into the eight domains outlined in **Box 3-1**. Skills and knowledge are outlined within each domain, linked with important attitudes relevant to the practice of public health. This effort of the Council focuses on core competencies as they apply to three different categories of professional positions: front line staff, senior level staff, and supervisory and management staff.

The core competencies were crafted to transcend the boundaries of specific disciplines and to help unify the public health profession. The list has been cross-walked with the Essential Public Health Services to ensure that the competencies help build the skills necessary for assuring the provision of these services. Academic institutions and health departments nationwide, as well as the Centers for Disease Control and Prevention (CDC), the Centers for Public Health Preparedness (CPHP), and the Health Resources and Services Administration (HRSA)-funded Public Health Training Centers, have used the core competencies to extend capacity and to ensure that public health professionals have expertise in key public health services.

Successful provision of public health services requires collaboration among public, nonprofit, and private partners within a given community and across various levels of government.[4] To fulfill these goals, partnerships must have broad-based representation of constituency and stakeholder groups, including private, voluntary, nonprofit, and public agencies or organizations involved in health, mental health, substance abuse, environmental health protection, and public health.[6] Examples of organizations and agencies that can be engaged in coalitions and collaborative partnerships to improve health in communities are presented in Appendix C.

ASSESSMENT: A CORE PUBLIC HEALTH FUNCTION

The contemporary principles of public health practice and science have been highlighted in several national reports.[3-5] These consensus reports, published by the Institute of Medicine (IOM), detail past contributions and identify challenges to public health. They outline recommendations to improve the nation's public health system and to ensure universal access to necessary public health services.

The *Future of Public Health* report specified three core public health functions that shape the basic practice of public health at the federal, state, and local levels.[3] Health agencies and health departments must perform these functions to protect and promote health, wellness, and quality of life and to prevent disease, injury, disability, and death. These functions (as noted in Chapter 1) are (1) assessment, (2) policy development, and (3) assurance.[3] This chapter emphasizes the core public health function of assessment in the community.

The IOM report called for public health agencies to promote, to facilitate, and—when necessary and appropriate—to perform community health assessments and to monitor change in key measures to evaluate performance. **Assessment** is defined as the regular and systematic collection, assemblage, analysis, and communication on the health of the community.[3] The IOM report stated that assessment includes statistics on health status, community health needs, and epidemiologic and other studies of health problems.[3]

ROLES OF PUBLIC HEALTH PROFESSIONALS IN ASSESSMENT

The effective use of information in the twenty-first century is crucial to ensure that healthy children and adults are living in healthy communities. Technologies available to public health professionals influence the capacity and ability to generate and collect a vast amount of information.[1,2] In addition, evidence-based decision making is shaping the development of public health policies, programs, and practices.[4] Therefore it is essential for public health practitioners to have skills in collecting, analyzing, disseminating, and effectively using data and information.[5] Public health professionals must have the knowledge, skills, and values to do the following[5,7]:

- Work with communities to form partnerships
- Gather health-related data
- Identify health issues and resources
- Determine priority health concerns
- Implement solutions to address community health problems
- Use data and evaluate outcomes of public health policies and interventions[8]

Public health dental hygienists are expected to play a leadership role in community oral health assessments.[9,10] As agencies and organizations take on greater responsibility in conducting periodic assessments, public health dental hygienists will be involved in evaluating assets, needs, problems, and resources of the populations they serve in the community. Dental public health professionals working at the national, state, and local levels will be responsible for community oral health assessment.[9] Essential public health services for oral health were developed to describe community oral health assessment (see Chapter 6 and Guiding Principles box).

GUIDING PRINCIPLES

Essential Public Health Services for Oral Health Related to Assessment and Evaluation[9]
- Assess oral health status and needs so that problems can be identified and addressed.
- Analyze determinants of identified oral health needs, including resources.
- Assess the fluoridation status of water systems and other sources of fluoride.
- Implement an oral health surveillance system to identify, investigate, and monitor oral health problems and health hazards.
- Evaluate the effectiveness, accessibility, and quality of population-based and personal oral health services.
- Conduct research and support demonstration projects to gain new insights and applications of innovative solutions to oral health problems.

BOX 3-2 **Examples of Roles of Public Health Dental Hygienists in Assessment**

- Public health dental hygienist serves on a committee with the state oral health coalition. The committee collaborates with the state health oral program to develop a comprehensive document describing the burden of oral disease. The report includes chapters on the prevalence of disease and unmet needs, oral health disparities, and the societal impact of oral disease.
- Oral health program director evaluates the State Oral Health Plan by assessing the attainment of goals and specific objectives related to oral health promotion, disease prevention and control, and specific risk factors.
- Oral health policy analyst determines the number and geographic distribution of dentists statewide who participate in the Medicaid and state Children's Health Insurance Program (CHIP) programs and provide oral health care to children in infancy, early childhood, middle childhood, and adolescence.
- Oral health program administrator with a city health department assesses the oral health assets, needs, and resources of a metropolitan area.
- Oral health educator assesses the knowledge, attitudes, and opinions of a community about community water fluoridation to develop an oral health promotion campaign.
- Public health dental hygienist from a county health department assesses dental sealants in third-grade children in schools throughout the county.
- Oral health program manager evaluates the quality and outcomes of clinical preventive services in a school-based oral health program.
- Oral health service provider monitors oral health indicators in the neighborhood surrounding a community health center.
- A dental hygienist, appointed to a state oral health advisory committee, evaluates the performance measures in a work plan to implement state level programs for community water fluoridation and school-based dental sealants.

Dental hygienists working within the public, private, or nonprofit sectors must have skills to assess community oral health problems, as well as evaluate outcomes of oral health population-based and personal oral health services. Dental hygienists working in community settings generally participate in a variety of assessment and evaluation activities. Examples of some of these roles and potential activities are shown in **Box 3-2**.

OVERVIEW OF EPIDEMIOLOGY: POPULATION-BASED STUDY OF HEALTH

Public health dental hygienists involved in assessment and evaluation should become well versed in the basic concepts of epidemiology, which is a core science of community health. This section provides a broad overview of epidemiology. **Table 3-1** provides the definitions of terms used in epidemiology and community health assessments.

Epidemiology is the study of the distribution and determinants of health-related states and events in specified populations and the application of this study to the prevention and control of health problems.[11] Epidemiologists consider the interactions and relationships among the multiple factors that influence health status and health problems.[12] Methods used in epidemiology and research are combined to focus on comparisons between groups or defined populations. Epidemiologists make comparisons by examining the occurrences of the health events, locations,

Table 3-1   Common Terms Used in Epidemiology

Term	Definition
Acute	Referring to a health effect, brief exposure of high intensity
Case	Epidemiologic study that compares persons with a disease or condition ("cases") with another group of people from the same population without the disease or condition ("controls"). The study is used to identify risks and trends, suggest some possible causes for disease, or for particular outcomes.
Chronic	Referring to a health-related state lasting a long time.
Cohort study	The method of epidemiologic study in which subsets of a defined population can be identified and observed for a sufficient number of person-years to generate reliable incidence or mortality rates in the population subsets; usually a large population, study for a prolonged period (years), or both. (*Synonym:* concurrent, follow-up, incidence, longitudinal, prospective study.)
Cross-sectional study	A study that examines the relationship between diseases (or other health-related characteristics) and other variables of interest as they exist in a defined population at one particular time.
Dichotomous scale	A measurement scale that arranges items into either of two mutually exclusive categories.
Ecoepidemiology	Conceptual approach that unifies molecular, social, and population-based epidemiology in a multilevel application of methods aimed at identifying causes, categorizing risks, and controlling public health problems.
Ecologic study	Epidemiologic study in which the units of analysis are populations or groups of people rather than individuals.
Endemic disease	The constant presence of a disease or infectious agent within a given geographic area or population group.
Epidemic	Occurrence in a community or region of cases of an illness, specific health-related behavior, or other health-related events clearly in excess of normal expectancy. (From Greek *epi* [upon], *demos* [people].)
Eradication (of disease)	Termination of all transmission of infection by extermination of the infectious agent through surveillance and containment.
Etiology	Science of causes, causality; in common use, cause
Incidence	Number of instances of illness commencing, or of persons falling ill, during a given period in a specified population; more generally, the number of new events (e.g., new cases of a disease in a defined population) within a specified period of time. (*Synonym:* incident number.)
Index	In epidemiology and related sciences, usually refers to a rating scale or a set of numbers derived from a series of observations of specified variables (e.g., health status index, scoring systems for severity or stage of cancer, heart murmurs, mental retardation).
Monitoring	Intermittent performance and analysis of routine measurements aimed at detecting changes in the environment or health status of populations; not to be confused with surveillance, which is a continuous process.
Morbidity	Any departure, subjective or objective, from a state of physiologic or psychologic well-being; in this sense, sickness, illness, and morbid condition are similarly defined and synonymous.
Mortality	Related to death.

Continued

Table 3-1   Common Terms Used in Epidemiology—cont'd

Term	Definition
Multifactorial etiology	Referring to the concept that a given disease or other outcome may have more than one cause; a combination of causes or alternative combinations of causes may be required to produce the effect.
Occurrence	In epidemiology, a general term describing the frequency of a disease or other attribute or event in a population without distinguishing between incidence and prevalence.
Pandemic	An epidemic occurring over a very wide area and usually affecting a large proportion of the population.
Prevalence	Number of instances of a given disease or other condition in a given population at a designated time; when used without qualification, term usually refers to the situation at a specified point in time (point prevalence).
Prospective	A research design used that looks forward.
Retrospective	A research design that uses a review of past events.
Sensitivity	Proportion of truly diseased persons as identified by the screening test; the measure of the probability of a correct diagnosis or the probability that any given case will be identified by the test. (*Synonym:* true-positive rate).
Specificity	Proportion of truly nondiseased persons identified by the screening test; a measure of the probability of correctly identifying a nondiseased person with a screening test. (*Synonym:* true-negative rate.)
Surveillance	Ongoing systematic collection, analysis, interpretation of health data essential to planning, implementation, and evaluation of public health practice. Generally using methods distinguished by their practicability, uniformity, and rapidity. Closely integrated with the timely dissemination of health information to responsible parties. Application of data in public health decision making and use of data to prevent and control diseases and conditions. Surveillance is the essential feature of epidemiology.
Surveillance system	Functional capacity for data collection, analysis, and dissemination linked to public health programs.
Trend	A long-term movement in an ordered series (e.g., a time series); an essential feature is that the movement, while possibly irregular in the short term, shows movement consistently in the same direction over a long term.

Adapted from Porta M, editor. A Dictionary of Epidemiology. 5th ed. New York: Oxford University Press; 2008.

times, and variations to assess the distribution and determinants of health events.[13] The principal factors analyzed in epidemiology are as follows:

- Distribution
- Population dynamics
- Occurrences
- Affected population
- Place characteristics
- Time
- Determinants

Epidemiology is based on a multifactorial perspective, with consideration given to the interacting relationships among host factors, agent factors, and environmental factors.[12,14]

Host Factors

The host may be a person, an animal, or a plant. **Host factors** relate primarily to susceptibility and resistance to disease through biologic immunity, knowledge and cognition, behavior modification, screening, and personal power. Age, gender, socioeconomic status, race, ethnicity, culture, genetic endowment, behavior, physiologic and nutritional state, previous exposure, and other factors influence susceptibility and resistance.

Agent Factors

Agent factors are the biologic or mechanical means of causing disease, illness, injury, or disability, such as microbial, parasitic, viral, or bacterial pathogens or vectors; physical or mechanical irritants; chemicals; drugs; trauma; and radiation. Biology, marketing, engineering, regulations, and legislation can influence agent factors.

Environmental Factors

Environmental factors include physical, sociocultural, sociopolitical, and economic components. The media, beliefs, occupation, food sources, geography, climate, housing, social roles, technology, and other factors can influence environmental conditions.

The "epidemiologic triangle" depicts disease as the outcome of the interactions among host, agent, and environmental factors.[12] For example, the development and progression of dental caries is attributed to multiple factors.[15,16] **Figure 3-1** portrays the epidemiologic triangle, with dental caries shown as a multifactorial disease influenced by host, agent, and environmental factors.

Uses of Epidemiology

Health represents a general balance among host, agent, and environmental factors; health problems occur when the balance is threatened by changes in host, agent, or environment.[14] Prevention is concerned with maintaining or initiating a balance of these factors. Disease or health status depends on multiple factors such as exposure to a specific agent, strength of the agent, susceptibility of the host, and environmental conditions.[12]

Epidemiology can be used to provide different types of data and information.[17] Epidemiologists in public health agencies are responsible for surveillance, investigation, analysis, and evaluation.[12,14] The various uses of epidemiology are illustrated in **Box 3-3**. The three classifications of epidemiologic studies are outlined in the Guiding Principles box.

GUIDING PRINCIPLES

Classification of Studies in Epidemiology
- *Descriptive studies* involve description, documentation, analysis, and interpretation of data to evaluate a current event or situation
- *Analytic studies* identify the cause of diseases, disabilities, injuries, and deaths; determine that a causal relationship exists between a factor and a disease or condition
- *Experimental studies* are used when the etiologic mechanism of the disease is established and the investigator determines the effectiveness of altering factors; applying or withholding the supposed cause of a condition and observing the results

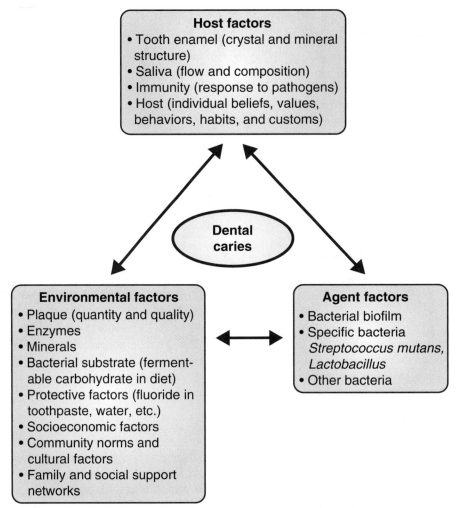

Figure 3-1 Epidemiologic triangle: Dental caries is a multifactorial oral disease.

CHANGING PERSPECTIVES OF HEALTH

During the twentieth century, major transformations took place in the concepts of health and the understanding of the determinants of diseases, disabilities, and injuries. Many historic developments contributed to these expanded visions and had a profound effect on the health of individuals and populations.[1,2,18] These developments contributed to changes in clinical health care and public health practice. **Box 3-4** outlines broad trends that influenced the conceptions of health in the twentieth century.

Reports from studies have identified many factors that influence the health of individuals and populations.[4,19-23,25-31] Several of these factors are generally recognized as broader determinants of health (e.g., employment; education; environment; income; shelter; food; social justice and equity; family, friends, and social supports; peace and safety; culture and race relations).[14,22-24,31-33] Other

BOX 3-3 Uses of Epidemiology

- Describe patterns among groups.
- Describe normal biologic processes.
- Elucidate mechanisms of disease transmission.
- Describe the natural histories of acute and chronic diseases.
- Test hypotheses for prevention and control of diseases, injuries, disabilities, and deaths through special studies in populations.
- Evaluate services (e.g., community preventive services, population-based health promotion services, and clinical health services).
- Study nondisease health and social problems such as occurrences of intentional and unintentional injuries.
- Measure the distribution of health status, diseases, injuries, disabilities, births, and deaths in populations.
- Identify determinants (e.g., protective and risk factors) for death or acquiring diseases, injuries, and disabilities.
- Evaluate interventions and strategies to prevent and control diseases, disabilities, injuries, and deaths.
- Predict trends of diseases, disabilities, injuries, and deaths.
- Identify health assets, gaps, needs, problems, resources, solutions, and partnerships within the context of a community assessment.

BOX 3-4 Trends Shaping the Perceptions of Health in the Twentieth Century

- Changes in social conditions and mores, professional ethos, and social institutions
- Shifts in views of civil and human rights
- Population growth, demographic change, and migration
- Recognition of environmental health and ecology
- Technologic changes influencing work, home, and life in communities (e.g., transportation, telecommunications, computing)
- Advancements in the biologic, physical, quantitative, social, and behavioral sciences
- Acknowledgment of the impact of globalization on population health

factors (e.g., language, learning, meaningful work, recreation, self-esteem, personal control) are considered contributors to well-being. These factors may also be classified as follows[14]:

1. Inherited determinants are factors that are inborn or genetically determined.
2. Acquired determinants, which influence health and are obtained after birth and throughout life, include multiple factors such as infections, trauma, cultural characteristics, and spiritual values.

There has been a broadening of the concepts of health promotion and disease prevention from an individual focus toward a human ecologic perspective.[17] Health became much more than just the absence of disability and disease. In 1948, The World Health Organization (WHO) Constitution defined health as "a state of complete physical, social and mental well-being, and not merely the absence of disease or infirmity." The fundamental conditions and resources for health were described in 1986 by the Ottawa Charter for Health Promotion (**Box 3-5**). Improvement in health requires a secure foundation in these basic prerequisites.

BOX 3-5 **Prerequisites for Health**

Ottawa Charter for Health Promotion, 1986
- Peace
- Shelter
- Education
- Food
- Income
- A stable ecosystem
- Sustainable resources
- Social justice and equity

Health promotion was discussed as the process of enabling people to increase control over and to improve their health. To reach a state of complete physical, mental, and social well-being, an individual or group must be able to identify and realize aspirations, satisfy needs, and change or cope with the environment. Health was therefore seen as a resource for everyday life not the objective of living. Health was a positive concept emphasizing social and personal resources, as well as physical capacities. Therefore health promotion is not just the responsibility of the health sector but goes beyond healthy lifestyles to well-being.

CONCEPTUAL MODELS OF THE DETERMINANTS OF HEALTH

Many models describing the multiple factors that influence the broader dimensions of health in individuals and populations were developed in the second half of the twentieth century.[4] Multicausal perspectives of health and disease began to take precedence over monocausal models.[12] The epidemiologic triangle model waned as the emphasis on infectious diseases diminished in the later part of the century. The concept of a "web of causation" emerged as multifactorial perspectives grew, with attention focused on the various determinants of chronic diseases, disabilities, and injuries. Health status and differences in health status were shown to be affected by genetic, environmental, social, and economic factors related to personal and family circumstances, income, education, where people live and work, and to a relatively limited extent, health care services.

Hancock, proposing a comprehensive framework to better understand the **determinants of health,** described the **mandala of health,**[22] a model of the human ecosystem (**Figure 3-2**). Its circular pattern symbolizes symmetry and wholeness. The confluent circles represent the multiple determinants of health. The center illustrates an individual whose total health and well-being are represented by the integration of mind, body, and spirit but not in isolation from other conditions. Within the global community of the biosphere, the individual is presented as only an element interdependent on larger systems. These larger systems include the family and the community within society. All domains depicted in the model are surrounded and affected by ubiquitous cultural influences. Also incorporated into the model are four groups of factors that influence the health of individuals, families, and communities:
- Psychosocioeconomic environment
- Physical environment
- Human biology
- Personal behavior

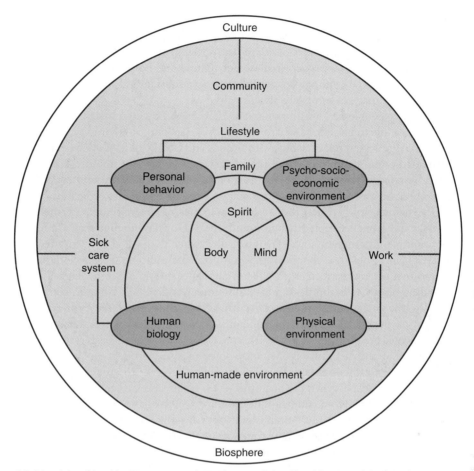

Culture

Community

Lifestyle

Personal behavior

Psycho-socio-economic environment

Family

Spirit

Body   Mind

Sick care system

Work

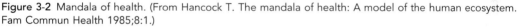

Human biology

Physical environment

Human-made environment

Biosphere

Figure 3-2 Mandala of health. (From Hancock T. The mandala of health: A model of the human ecosystem. Fam Commun Health 1985;8:1.)

A broader and more comprehensive view of health has become recognized as the importance of the determinants of health have been reported in the scientific literature and an emphasis has been directed toward improving health among populations. International reports have described the determinants of health as having a great influence on collective and personal well-being with a profound effect on the health of individuals, families, communities, nations, and thus the world.[6,23,24] *Health determinants* are the range of personal, social, economic, and environmental factors that determine the health status of individuals or populations. The determinants of health include the following:

- Individual biology and genetics
- Individual behavior
- Physical environment
- Social environment
- Access to quality health services

Health determinants are embedded in the social and physical environments. To improve health in the future, plans, policies, and programs should target reductions in adverse social and physical determinants. *Social determinants* include family, community, income, education, gender, race/

ethnicity, place of residence, and access to health care, among others. People who lack social and economic resources are likely to be less healthy, which may both result in and result from discrimination. Frequently, issues of equity and social justice are involved in the social determinants of health. *Physical determinants* include our natural and built environments. Exposure to natural toxins (e.g., coal tar), human-made pollutants, or substandard housing are examples of physical determinants that can adversely affect health.

Whether people are healthy or not is determined by circumstances and environment. To a large extent, factors, such as where people live, the state of environment, genetics, income, and education levels, and relationships with friends and family, all have considerable impacts on health, whereas the more commonly considered factors, such as access and use of health care services, often have less of an impact. The context of people's lives determine their health. Individuals are unlikely to be able to directly control many of the determinants of health.

The boundaries between the specific categories of determinants are indistinct because they interact and influence each other continuously.[1,14] During different stages of human development, the multiple determinants act synergistically, rather than separately, to affect health. No single determinant of health is the most important because multiple factors work in combination. Thus causation is often described as multifactorial; that is, multiple factors determine health conditions, including diseases, disabilities, and injuries among individuals living in communities.

Also, the social determinants of health have become the targets for refocused strategies for population health. The social determinants of health have been described as the conditions in which people are born, grow, live, work, and age, including the health system. These circumstances are shaped by the distribution of money, power, and resources at global, national, state, and local levels, which are themselves influenced by policy choices. The social determinants of health are mostly responsible for health inequities—the unfair and avoidable differences in health status seen within and between countries. Responding to increasing concern about these persisting and widening inequities, WHO established the Commission on Social Determinants of Health (CSDH) to provide advice on how to reduce the social determinants of health. The Commission's final report released in 2008 outlined the following three overarching recommendations:

- Improve daily living conditions
- Tackle the inequitable distribution of power, money, and resources
- Measure and understand the problem and assess the impact of action

A contemporary movement in public health called "Healthy Cities/Healthy Communities" has promoted a broader multidimensional perspective of health.[19] WHO has promoted this concept, which focuses on the root determinants of health.[19] Nations and communities around the world have adopted community health approaches based on this perspective. "Healthy Communities" groups ascribe to key principles.

DETERMINANTS OF ORAL HEALTH IN INDIVIDUALS AND POPULATIONS

Multiple **determinants of oral health** have been described in the literature.[16,31-34] **Figure 3-3** highlights multiple influences on people's oral health. Also, the figure shows that many of the determinants of oral health are common to other significant health conditions such as cancer, obesity, cardiovascular disease, diabetes, respiratory diseases, mental illness, and trauma.

Health promotion theory has moved toward a complex, holistic, interactive approach, with a systems orientation focused on healthy people living in healthy communities.[19] Health promotion approaches are embracing the principles of population health, social ecology and epidemiology,

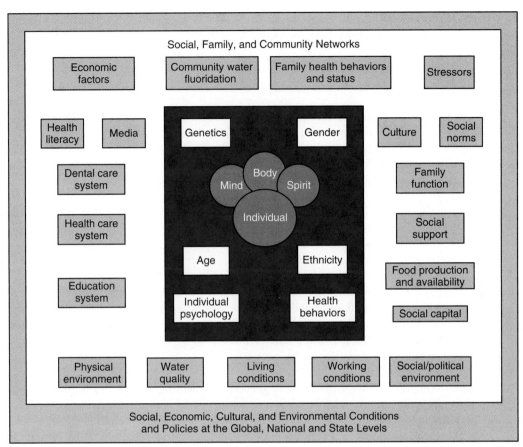

Figure 3-3 Framework for determinants of oral health.

and community participation.[17,19-21] These transformations about the meanings of health, wellness, and quality of life, as well as health problems within communities are continuing to evolve in the twenty-first century. By adopting a holistic approach to improving oral health and through collaborative work with partner agencies and organizations dental public health professionals can achieve the aim of improving both the oral health and general health of populations.

GUIDING PRINCIPLES

Healthy Communities: Perspective of Health[19]
- Broad definition of health
- Broad definition of community
- Shared vision from community values
- Quality of life addressed for everyone
- Diverse citizen participation and widespread community ownership
- "Systems change" emphasized
- Capacity built with the use of local assets and resources
- Progress and outcomes benchmarked and measured

The next section is an overview of assessment as a key component within a comprehensive process that communities can adopt to improve health.

THE PLANNING CYCLE

The **planning cycle** is a model commonly used in public health practice; it provides a basic flow-chart of steps in a process to (1) **assess,** (2) **plan,** (3) **implement,** and (4) **evaluate. Figure 3-4** shows a basic planning cycle. The planning cycle can be used to develop an oral health plan and measure oral health outcomes at a population level. Also, the planning cycle can serve as the framework to develop a dental public health intervention and measure the performance of a program.

The planning cycle is continuous[2]; each stage can be further subdivided into detailed steps for a long-term health improvement process in the community. The **community health improvement process** has been described as a comprehensive approach for communities to achieve sustained improvements in community health.[23]

Embedded into the basic planning cycle is a framework for a community oral health improvement process (**Figure 3-5**). Because of the dynamics in community health, it is important to understand the necessity of flexibility in public health plans. If new circumstances arise, activities outlined initially in a plan may not be followed as sequentially ordered, and work would need to be adjusted. However, it is important to include all of the steps for a community oral health improvement process.

Following such a planning cycle allows a systematic approach of assessing different factors, considering options for action, planning, and implementing policies or programs, and evaluating their outcomes. This process can allow for coordinated community efforts in assessment, planning, implementation, and evaluation. When these efforts are institutionalized over time into the community fabric, long-term oral health benefits are likely to be achieved by the community.

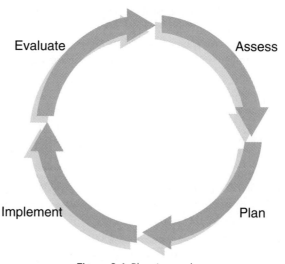

Figure 3-4 Planning cycle.

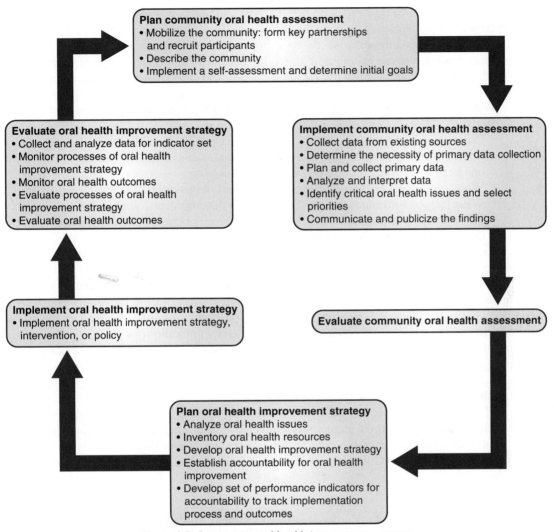

Figure 3-5 Community oral health improvement process.

ASSESSMENT OF ORAL HEALTH IN COMMUNITIES

This section reviews community oral health assessment, which is one component of a community oral health improvement process. It describes the steps undertaken and the indicators that can be included in an assessment.

A **community oral health assessment** is a multifaceted process that is community-oriented and community-directed. It focuses on population health, and it can concentrate on the entire population or a specific segment of the population in a community.

An oral health assessment considers assets, gaps, needs, problems, resources, solutions, and partnerships within the context of the community. Its purpose is to identify factors that affect the oral health of a population and to determine the availability of resources and interventions that affect these factors. Communities are better served and improved outcomes are more sustainable when assets-oriented assessment methods are used, in contrast to deficiency-based approaches that focus on needs and problems. By engaging and fostering the community in a community-building process, one can gain insight about the specific factors in the community that influence health. Through a participatory framework for action and capacity development, a better understanding of opportunities for health enhancements can emerge over time.

With information gleaned from a broad-based assessment process, a community can begin to answer the following questions about oral health:

- What community strengths, assets, and resources influence oral health in the community?
- What capacities, resources, and interventions are available within the community to promote oral health?
- What are the oral health problems, concerns, and obstacles faced by the community?
- What factors contribute to these community oral health gaps and needs?
- What are the potential solutions? What partnerships in the community can support strategies to ensure future oral health improvements?

Answers to these questions assist in final determination of critical oral health issues and priorities.

Assessment is the first and an essential step in the development of a community oral health improvement plan. The findings from the assessment can lead to the formation of oral health goals, objectives, plans, policies, interventions, and programs to solve oral health problems. Oral health programs best serve communities and address community oral health problems when priorities and actions are determined by current information and are grounded in evidence-based public health practices and contemporary principles. Several resources with models are available to guide collaborative health planning in communities. Examples of these resources community health assessment models are shown in **Box 3-6**.

Many ways exist to collect information that can be used to evaluate the determinants of health for a population and a community. Numerous resources are available to describe methods and to offer guidance for community health assessments. Use of these resources can assist in a methodic approach to the assessment process in communities (see References and Assessment Resources).

BOX 3-6 Examples of Community Health Assessment Models

- Mobilizing for Action through Planning and Partnerships (MAPP) developed by the National Association of County and City Health Officials in collaboration with the Centers for Disease Control and Prevention (CDC)[4]
- Community Tool Box Framework for Collaborative Action
- Association for Community Health Improvement (ACHI) Community Health Assessment Toolkit
- AssessNow Assessment Toolkit in Washington state
- New York State Community Health Assessment (CHA) Clearinghouse How-To Guide: 10-Step Assessment Process
- Minnesota Community Health Assessment and Action Planning (CHAAP)
- North Carolina Community Health Assessment Guide
- Community Health Improvement Process (CHIP) reviewed in an *Institute of Medicine* (IOM) report[23]

One resource, developed by the Association of State & Territorial Dental Directors (ASTDD), is the *Assessing Oral Health Needs: ASTDD Seven-Step Model*. This publication provides a step-by-step guide for planning, implementing, and evaluating an oral health assessment.[10] This comprehensive guidebook outlines the main steps of a systematic and effective oral health assessment and reviews a broad array of alternatives that can be adapted for an oral health assessment. The ASTDD has additional resources available to support oral health assessment initiatives. Also, the American Association for Community Dental Programs (AACDP) has publications that discuss oral health assessments as part of a model framework and guide for developing and enhancing community oral health programs (see References and Assessment Resources at the end of this chapter).

The Division of Oral Health at the CDC has also developed *Infrastructure Development Tools*. These materials provide "how-to" guides for planning and implementing assessment activities using logic models for guidance. These publications focus on standards and priorities of the CDC for surveillance, monitoring, and evaluation. The purpose of these tools is to assist programs in the planning, designing, implementation, and use of practical and increasingly comprehensive evaluation of oral health promotion and disease prevention efforts. The Internet-based materials are a resource for dental public health professionals responsible for program planning and evaluation activities to demonstrate accountability to diverse stakeholders (see References and Assessment Resources).

No single formula exists for conducting a community oral health assessment. However, the ASTDD outlines a useful model. A community oral health assessment should be developed on the basis of the specific aims and available resources, special circumstances, and expertise in the community. The essential components should be included in all community oral health assessments (**Figure 3-6**). The essential elements are reviewed in more detail in the following section.

Planning a Community Oral Health Assessment

The first step in any assessment process is the planning stage. During this stage, it is important to methodically consider the overall purpose, potential partners, resources, and alternatives for conducting a community oral health assessment.

Mobilizing the Community: Forming Key Partnerships and Recruiting Participants

Community involvement is crucial in identifying oral health concerns and actions to resolve oral health problems. Collaborative partnerships and community coalitions are prominent strategies for community health improvement.[4,35-37] Mobilization of community partnerships to identify and solve oral health problems has been identified as a key public health service to improve oral health in communities.[9] Community action and community-building efforts that engage and empower communities can have positive outcomes when they are sustained over time.[7,35] Contemporary public health practices and principles encourage multisectoral collaboration and broad community engagement to improve health-related conditions, outcomes, and well-being of entire communities.[4,23,24,30]

At the beginning and throughout a community assessment process, it is essential to involve diverse partnering agencies, organizations, associations, and individuals to collaborate in partnerships.[38] Looking to the public, private, and nonprofit sectors may offer opportunities for potential champions of the assessment mission and process. Partners can broaden the scope, approaches, and perspectives in the process and provide community input, data sources, resources, expertise,

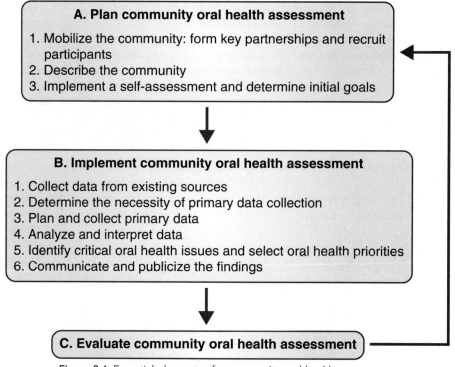

A. Plan community oral health assessment

1. Mobilize the community: form key partnerships and recruit participants
2. Describe the community
3. Implement a self-assessment and determine initial goals

B. Implement community oral health assessment

1. Collect data from existing sources
2. Determine the necessity of primary data collection
3. Plan and collect primary data
4. Analyze and interpret data
5. Identify critical oral health issues and select oral health priorities
6. Communicate and publicize the findings

C. Evaluate community oral health assessment

Figure 3-6 Essential elements of a community oral health assessment.

and sponsorship. Partners can also lend support to collaborative community efforts that develop from the assessment outcomes. This may include support for communication of the findings and promotion of the strategies identified by the assessment. Engaging the community in the assessment process is key to building support for community oral health improvements. Involvement and support of partnering agencies and organizations throughout the assessment process can have a positive influence on the attainment of mutual missions and goals.

Potential partners should include a cross-section of the community such as technical staff, program managers, and leaders from business, media, religious, civic, philanthropic, community, and political realms.[27,39,40] Appendix C outlines partners that can be supportive in community-based efforts, including an assessment. The partners should represent a broad spectrum of the community and involve a wide variety of constituents and stakeholders from health and social service groups, organizations, and associations; governmental agencies and programs; community organizations; education-related groups (schools, colleges, and universities); advocacy organizations; nonprofit, charitable, and service groups; media; and business organizations.[27,38-40] The partners involved in an assessment may vary according to the overall focus of the assessment process.[38]

Mechanisms for community participation, input, and dialog must be incorporated throughout the assessment process.[38] It is imperative to a successful community oral health assessment that the community be mobilized and actively involved throughout the process.[7] Broad-based community partnerships should be engaged and participants enlisted to reflect the cultural, racial, ethnic, gender, economic, and linguistic diversities of the community.[38] Procedures should be in place to ensure opportunities for communication with and feedback to the community, sustaining support throughout the process, and evaluation of the assessment.

It is important to consider ways of identifying and recruiting partners in the development of an inclusive and empowering process. Resource materials can be helpful by offering innovative ideas about building effective collaborative partnerships and community coalitions.[35] Many of these resources discuss in-depth ways to initiate and sustain vitality of collaborative relationships. Specific factors and conditions that are conducive to effective collaborative partnerships should be supported and nurtured for measurable and lasting results (see References and Assessment Resources).

Describing the Community

An important task of the assessment is to provide a description of the community, which must be clearly defined at the onset of the process.[13,27] Communities are a collection of peoples, places, and systems that define how people and places interact on an ongoing basis.[4,7] The Guiding Principles can be used to provide an understanding and a description of a community.

GUIDING PRINCIPLES

Factors to Use in Understanding and Describing a Community[7]
- People (socioeconomics and demographics, health status, risk profiles, cultural and ethnic characteristics)
- Location (geographic boundaries)
- Connectors (shared values, interests, motivating factors)
- Power relationships (communication patterns, social and political networks, formal and informal lines of authority and influence, stakeholder relationships, resource flows)

Initially, the description can include a general overview of the community but not detailed statistics at this point. More comprehensive, detailed community data should be compiled during the data collection phase. This information should be incorporated into the **community profile,** which is a comprehensive description of the community.[13,20,27] Examples of information in a community profile are presented in Appendix D.

Implementing a Self-Assessment and Determining Initial Goals

During the initiation of an oral health assessment process, it is worthwhile to conduct a self-assessment.[10] At this step of self-reflection, it is useful to conduct an internal assessment to evaluate your organization and to consider its role. It is important to make an external assessment by exploring the missions and roles of other organizations in the community. Organizational capacity, power structures, strategic plans, commitment, and resources should be considered during this phase.

The next step is to determine the goals of the assessment. The goals should come from the self-assessment and through a group consensus process among the partnering organizations. Before embarking on an oral health assessment process, partners must understand why the community is conducting an assessment and what the community hopes to achieve from it. It is important to clarify the scope and size of the assessment. The objectives and activities undertaken to achieve the goals of the assessment must be refined continually as information is collected and in light of available resources.

Implementing a Community Oral Health Assessment

Collecting Data from Existing Sources

Data collection is the gathering of information that the community can use to make decisions and to set priorities. Different types, sources, and levels of information are needed for a comprehensive assessment.[41-49] For a community health assessment, it is vital to collect information and evaluate data related to the current status of assets, gaps, needs, problems, resources, solutions, and partnerships in the community.[47-49]

A standard element of an assessment is the compilation and synthesis of existing data and information from secondary sources.[10] After existing information is assessed, a decision should be made about the collection of new information from primary sources.

What data sources are available?

Multiple resources of information are widely available to the general public. The sources of data used in an oral health assessment should be diverse to ensure a broad portrayal of the factors influencing oral health in the community.[10,16,40-44] A variety of data resources should be tapped to compile and review information during the data collection process.[46-49] Government agencies and private and nonprofit organizations produce and compile excellent reports on the various determinants of health and oral health. Sources of local information include local reports, literature reviews, magazines, newspapers, newsletters, maps, and marketing data. It is also important to review previous assessments that have been conducted in the community. **Table 3-2** outlines examples of various sources of information for community health assessments. Examples of government resources for health data are provided in Appendix D.

During data collection, it is important to systematically conduct a broad search of available information and to organize an inventory of this information. It is essential to carefully compile the information from secondary sources and to establish a system to record, process, and organize the data and information.

What types of information should be included?

Different types of information are necessary to ensure that a complete assessment accurately describes the factors influencing health in the community.[7,12,14,46] Community health assessment efforts can accomplish the following[46]:

1. Evaluate determinants of health.
2. Assess needs and assets.
3. Quantify disparities and inequities among population groups.
4. Measure preventable disease, injury, disability, and death.

The following two main classes of data are used to describe a community and to characterize dimensions of health within the community:

1. **Quantitative data** refer to information that is objective and measurable. The data can be expressed in a quantity or amount (e.g., the percentage of children with dental sealants, percentage of children or adults with untreated tooth decay).[6,10,16,41] These data numerically represent the size of a problem and determine its statistical significance. Data may include demographic information and vital statistics such as numbers of births or deaths, incidence or prevalence rates of disease, number of schools in a county, and employment statistics.

Table 3-2 **Sources of Information**

Potential Source	Example
Federal, state, and local government agencies (see Appendix D)	Health department, human services department, and social services department; department of aging; department of disabilities and special needs; highway safety department; police departments (documents, reports, surveys, statistics)
	Population surveys
	National, state, and local health surveys
	Surveillance system; reports and records
	Population-based registries
	Health agency records and reports of participants enrolled in programs
	Agency records and reports of health professionals; health professional shortage areas; community health centers
	State or local child protection agency records
	Environmental agency records and reports
Private and public (community) health, health care (clinical or personal health care), social, and human service programs	Hospitals; health plans (health insurance claims data); health care systems (health charts and dental records, pathology reports); professional associations; trade groups; community advisory committees; community collaborative groups and coalitions (community surveys); health and social service groups; organizations; societies; associations (documents; reports, surveys, statistics)
Philanthropic, nonprofit, and charitable organizations	Religious organizations and groups; voluntary agencies; civic organizations; service and voluntary groups; community organizations; advocacy groups (documents, reports, surveys, and statistics, local information and referral service inventories)
Schools and colleges	School districts; school boards; school campuses; colleges; universities (student statistics, school health reports, school entry records)
Businesses, employers, and business organizations	Major employers or chambers of commerce; marketing data and survey data (e.g., Nielsen Claritas); economic statistics and financial records; corporate annual reports (e.g., sales of drugs, foods, tobacco)
Media	Media sources (newspapers, magazines, newsletters, radio, television, Internet, social media)

2. **Qualitative data** refer to information that cannot be numerically measured or analyzed but reflects the quality or nature of factors influencing a health problem.[43] Qualitative data add meaning to the numbers and help to answer the question of why a problem exists in a community. Data may include information gleaned from personal interviews, descriptions of traditions and the history of a community, and information gathered from participant observations or focus groups.*

The types of data to be collected and the selection of a data collection method and instrument to use depends on the aims of an assessment and the resources available for the assessment.[10,13] Various data collection methods and instruments are indicated for specific types of assessments. Each method has advantages and limitations.[10,43] Appendix D summarizes the diverse data collection methods, instruments, and applications used in community assessments.

*References 10, 16, 27, 40, 42-45, and 47.

A spectrum of health indicators can be used to profile the health of a community.[46] Data collected for a "snapshot" in a community health assessment can describe:
- Population characteristics
- Summary measures of health status in the community
- Leading causes of death
- Measures of birth and death
- Measures of disease, injury, and disability
- Vulnerable populations
- Environmental health
- Use of community preventive services and personal health services
- Protective factors and risk factors for disease, injury, disability, and death
- Access to public health (e.g., community preventive services), personal health care, and social service system in the community

A tool, the Leading Health Indicators, was used to monitor national health along with *Healthy People 2010*, the health goals for the decade in the United States.[6] These first-ever Leading Health Indicators include 10 focus areas, based upon the *Healthy People 2010* objectives. These measures allow Americans to assess the overall health of the nation and their communities to make comparisons and improvements over time. The topic areas of the Leading Health Indicators are described in **Box 3-7**. The Leading Health Indicators are supported by 21 specific measurable objectives that reflect the influence of behavioral and environmental factors and community health interventions. These objectives can be assessed by states and communities to assess current status and to monitor changes over time. Examples of information for a community health assessment are presented in Appendix D.

Chapter 4 reviews specific measures that can be used in an assessment of oral health in a community and details the *Healthy People 2010* and *2020* initiatives.

Determining the Necessity of Primary Data Collection

A key step in the assessment process is determining the need for additional data and information.[10] This decision should be made based on the following:
1. A reevaluation and possible refinement of the assessment goals
2. An analysis of the findings from the existing data sources
3. Available resources to support future assessment activities

BOX 3-7 Topics of Leading Health Indicators

- Physical activity
- Overweight and obesity
- Tobacco use
- Substance abuse
- Mental health
- Injury and violence
- Environmental quality
- Immunizations
- Responsible sexual behavior
- Access to personal health care

The partners determine and prioritize information needs and evaluate alternative methods of data collection. One option might be the integration of specific measures into ongoing surveys and assessments. Sometimes, it may be necessary to collect original data.

During this phase, it is crucial to study the many alternative ways by which data can be collected for community health assessments. It is essential to consider both the advantages and disadvantages of the data collection options that are available to the group. After this analysis, the group strategically determines the final goals according to identified priorities and resources.

Planning and Collecting Primary Data

When it is necessary to collect original data, the partners develop a work plan that outlines the objectives, activities, roles, responsibilities, budget, and timetable.[10] Once the scope of the assessment is determined, methods can be selected and criteria defined in preparation for the primary data collection phase. Examples of tasks that should be considered for conducting primary data collection are listed in Appendix D.

Analyzing and Interpreting Data

Analysis and interpretation of data often require knowledge and experience, and this is where the backgrounds and experience of community members, representatives of partnering organizations, and professionals in the community are invaluable. Partners can call on local community members to enlist their expertise and assistance in validating impressions and interpretations of the data examined for the assessment.

To analyze and interpret both primary and secondary data, numerous steps are necessary. The initial step is to synthesize the information and summarize the findings. Data collected must be analyzed to determine meaning and significance.[10] A critique of each data source is required to assess its trustworthiness. The partners must consider the limitations of the data and data sources by checking for potential errors or biases. It is important to consider the sampling technique such as type of sample, sample size, participation of population segments, and generalization of findings to population groups based on the sample.

Because potential errors can be made in collecting, recording, and analyzing data, it is essential to review the data collection process to check that protocols have been followed to ensure standardization and to reduce the potential of bias or variation. The partners should evaluate that methods and techniques were in place to collect information consistently, record and compile information accurately, and analyze data completely and appropriately. Information should be reviewed carefully to consider the possibility of misinterpretation, errors in coding and groupings, erroneous instructions, or typographic errors.

When the data have been determined to be reasonably free of errors, they should be compared with other data. The partners ensure that the data being compared are alike as possible. Data of a community can be compared with those of surrounding communities, other counties, the region, the state, or the nation. It may be worthwhile to compare data with those of a baseline source such as the *Healthy People 2010* and *2020* objectives (see Chapter 5). Analysis of trends can be included by comparison of new data in one time period with data from previous years. This comparison may show changes in the community over a specific time period. Also, data showing changes among communities over time can be very useful for planning purposes.

The group determines whether there are opportunities to analyze existing data sets further. If existing data sets are available and additional analysis will generate new information, this alternative may result in more insight. In addition, the group might add or integrate the collection of new types of data into ongoing data collection efforts.

The group assesses the significance of the data collected; the term *significance* means that the information truly reflects a problem existing in a community. Studying the data for significance means that possible misleading findings are identified before conclusions are drawn from the findings. An abundance of data combining different data types allows for an easier determination of the significance of the findings.

Numeric calculations are made through statistical analysis for data collected by means of quantitative methods. A mathematical method is used to calculate relationships among quantitative variables to determine statistical significance. The calculations show whether the observed relationships among the variables happened by chance or not by chance (see Chapter 7 for an explanation of data analysis in research).

The relationships among data collected by qualitative methods are not calculated through statistical analysis. Textual data collected from transcripts of interviews or focus groups or field notes of observations are explored with the use of contextual analysis.[43] Steps in qualitative data analysis include familiarization, identifying a thematic framework, indexing, charting, mapping, and interpreting.[45] With the use of specific methods, data in contextual form are indexed to assess common or unique themes and to generate analytic categories and theoretic explanations.

The following questions are answered:
- Does this information reflect relationships?
- Does this information describe a pattern of key themes and explain a social phenomena?

The partners with expertise and experience can provide feedback on the findings. Partners can consider the implications of the data by evaluating the meaning of the data within the context and expectations of the community.

The findings from quantitative and qualitative data can provide direction for future actions to build on community assets. With potential strategies indicated, this step may move the assessment phase toward the planning stage of a community oral health improvement process. At the same time, additional questions may arise that may direct the process toward the need for more information and supplementary assessment activities.

Identifying Critical Oral Health Issues and Selecting Priorities

In conjunction with the community, it is essential to identify critical oral health issues. During this stage, it is important to consider the identified assets, gaps, needs, problems, resources, solutions, and partnerships in the community. During the assessment process, community partners should evaluate the community's assets and resources to create a shared vision of change.[47] This encourages greater creativity when community partners are engaged in building capacity to address problems and obstacles.

Community partners should be actively involved in all aspects of determining and prioritizing the critical issues. Based on all the evidence, it is crucial to analyze the situation and to determine the priority of oral health problems to be addressed in the future. Through a deliberative process, the community partners must reach a consensus about long-term and short-term solutions to address the identified oral health problems. Key steps that can be followed to determine and prioritize community oral health issues are outlined in **Box 3-8**.

BOX 3-8 Key Steps to Determine and Prioritize Community Oral Health Issues

1. Develop a prioritization process. Community input is vital in this process.
2. Ensure clear determination of oral health priorities in conjunction with the community.
3. Determine the community's capacity to address oral health priorities. Consider the assets and resources that were identified during the assessment process. How can the wide array of community assets and resources be expanded and maximized to address the oral health issues?
4. Consider how amenable each oral health priority is to change. What realistic degree of change can the community achieve in a specific time period?
5. Assess the economic, social, and political issues that influence the community's ability to address the priority oral health issues. When formulating oral health improvement strategies to address public health priorities, be cognizant of economic, social, and political factors that can affect plans and strategies.
6. Identify community programs currently addressing oral health priorities that were identified through the assessment efforts. Consider expanding partnerships and building upon effective strategies. This may allow for more effective and efficient use of limited resources.
7. Identify best practices to determine effective approaches to guide future planning, development, implementation, and evaluation of policies and programs.

Communicating and Publicizing the Findings

It is essential to establish a plan to communicate and disseminate the findings. The partners present the findings from the data collection and analysis and share information about the overall assessment quest. These findings should be publicized and distributed widely to various community members with the use of the diverse channels of communication available such as public forums, news conferences, publications, electronic media, and social media.[50,51] Components of a report can include a statement of the purpose, materials and methods used, results, a discussion, conclusions, a summary, and an abstract. An executive summary and a full report may be useful to communicate the findings.

The outcomes should be communicated in a straightforward manner. It is important to summarize the findings by highlighting key findings and by including the outcomes of the inventory of community assets and resources to emphasize the availability of resources and to note the limitations of existing resources in the community. It is helpful to illustrate the findings through charts, graphs, tables, and maps. In addition, partners can provide the audience with a frame of reference to show how the community data compare with similar data from other local, state, or national figures. Also, it is vital to explain the limitations of the data.

Chapter 8 describes contemporary strategies for promoting community oral health and communicating oral health findings.

Evaluating the Assessment Process

As with any process, it is important to incorporate evaluation. Throughout the oral health assessment process, the collaborating partners should, on a systematic basis, step back and evaluate the process.[10] Allowing time for evaluation along the way can provide opportunity to implement changes and to improve the process. Recording a critique of the assessment at the end of the process can allow a feedback loop in which lessons can be learned for future health assessments in the community.[10]

NEXT STEPS: DEVELOPING AND IMPLEMENTING AN IMPROVEMENT PLAN

With the published report of the assessment disseminated and the priorities identified, it is time to move to the next phase of the community oral health improvement process. At this stage oral health improvement strategies can be developed to address the prioritized oral health issues outlined in the oral health assessment. Concrete goals, objectives, policies, and programs can be planned and implemented based on the findings, evidence, best practices, and priorities from the oral health assessment.

A community oral health assessment is virtually useless unless the information is used to develop and implement evidence-based oral health strategies. *Healthy People 2010* and *2020* (see Chapter 4) can provide guidance in the development of an oral health improvement plan.

SUMMARY

Assessment is a core public health function, and dental hygienists involved in public health practice must be proficient in the various aspects of oral health assessment. Assessment is an integral component of a community oral health improvement process. Information gained from a community assessment can be used to plan, implement, and evaluate oral health improvement strategies.

Community health assessment efforts are applied to evaluate assets, gaps, problems, resources, solutions, and partnerships in the community. This allows a community to assess the determinants of health, evaluate needs, quantify disparities and inequities among population groups, and measure preventable disease, injury, disability, and death. A systematic approach is crucial to accomplish a comprehensive community oral health assessment. This chapter has reviewed the key elements necessary when a community undertakes an assessment. Data collection methods and instruments are varied, and their application depends on the overall aims of the assessment and resources available in the community.

This chapter reviewed how epidemiology involves a multifactorial perspective to analyze the interacting relationships among host factors, agent factors, and environmental factors that contribute to health in populations. As information about the determinants of oral health grows, it will be essential for dental public health professionals to have the knowledge, values, and skills to assess oral health at global, national, state, and local levels.

Applying Your Knowledge

1. Illustrate the determinants of oral health for the following groups and situations:
    a. Dental injuries among schoolchildren in a neighborhood
    b. Dental caries among adolescents in a city without fluoridated drinking water
    c. Oral cancer among older adults in a county
    d. Adults without access to annual dental visits in a rural county
    e. Periodontal disease among disabled young adults in a region of a state
    f. Early childhood caries among preschool children in a state

     g. Edentulism among adults in a region of the country and comparisons between multiple states

     h. Dental caries among children across nations on a global level

2. Group discussion: Read over the following situations and discuss your answers within small groups.

     A: The social worker from the County Agency on Aging calls you to discuss the dental problems of the senior citizens attending local nutrition sites near your community health center. The state health department has recently distributed the State Oral Health Improvement Plan, which notes a high rate of oral cancer among older men and a low rate of dental attendance for older edentulous adults. How would you maximize these "windows of opportunity" to initiate a community oral health assessment? Whom would you contact? What steps would you take? Do you think these efforts could advance the development and implementation of a community oral health improvement plan?

     B: At a local child care conference, a prominent speaker describes the high rate of early childhood caries among preschool children attending Head Start programs in the city. Also, during the conference, the new Director for the Supplemental Food Program for Women, Infants and Children (WIC) from the local health department highlights the need to improve the nutrition, health, and dental education for families enrolled in WIC. After the conference, the Community Coalition for Healthy Children (CCHC) asks you to join as a representative of the local component of the American Dental Hygienists' Association. How would you maximize this opportunity to focus on oral health and young children? Whom would you contact? What steps would you take to initiate a community oral health assessment? How might the CCHC evaluate the assets, gaps, needs, problems, resources, solutions, and partnerships within the context of your community? How might this assessment promote the development and implementation of a community oral health improvement plan?

Dental Hygiene Competencies

Reading the material in this chapter and participating in the activities of Applying Your Knowledge will contribute to the student's ability to demonstrate the following competencies:

Community involvement
CM.1 Assess the oral health needs of the community and the quality and availability of resources and services.
CM.6 Evaluate the outcomes of community-based programs and plan for future activities.

Health promotion and disease prevention
HP.4 Identify individual and population risk factors and develop strategies that promote health-related quality of life.
HP.5 Evaluate factors that can be used to promote patient adherence to disease prevention and health maintenance strategies.

Community Case

You are a dental hygienist serving on a health team at a community health center. The Executive Director has called a meeting about the need to plan a community health assessment in the surrounding neighborhood served by the community health center. This community health assessment is an essential component of the center's application to receive continued funding. Your role as a member of the planning committee is to provide input on the components of the community health assessment.

1. What would be the first step the committee should take for the community health assessment?
   a. Collect data from existing resources.
   b. Identify critical health issues and select health priorities.
   c. Mobilize the community by forming key partnerships and recruiting participants to collaborate in the community health assessment.
   d. Plan and collect primary health data in the community.
2. During the data collection phase of the community health assessment, all of the following are government resources for health data that the committee could use except one. Which one is not a government resource?
   a. Population surveys from the Bureau of the Census
   b. State health surveys
   c. Health and dental records from a private hospital
   d. CDC Cancer Registry
3. What is the initial description and general overview of the community called?
   a. Community asset map
   b. Community profile
   c. Primary data collection
   d. Plan for the community assessment
4. The data collection method that would be the most costly and time-consuming would be which of the following?
   a. Windshield tour
   b. Mailed survey
   c. Person-to-person interview
   d. Telephone interview
5. Both qualitative and quantitative data can be used to describe the health of the community. Qualitative data are expressed in a quantity or amount.
   a. The first statement is true and the second statement is false.
   b. The second statement is true and the first statement is false.
   c. Both statements are true.
   d. Both statements are false.

References

1. Scutchfield FD, Keck CW. Principles of Public Health Practice. 3rd ed. Clifton Park, NY: Delmar Cengage Learning; 2009.
2. Turnock BJ. Public Health: What It Is and How It Works. 3rd ed. Sudbury, MA: Jones and Bartlett; 2009.
3. Institute of Medicine, Committee for the Study of the Future of Public Health. The Future of Public Health. Washington, DC: National Academies Press; 1988.
4. Institute of Medicine, Committee on Assuring the Health of the Public in the 21st Century. The Future of the Public's Health in the 21st Century. Washington, DC: National Academies Press; 2003.
5. Institute of Medicine, Committee on Educating Public Health Professionals for the 21st Century. Who Will Keep the Public Healthy? Educating Public Health Professionals in the 21st Century. Washington, DC: National Academies Press; 2003.
6. US Department of Health and Human Services. Healthy People 2010: Understanding and Improving Health. 2nd ed. Washington, DC: US Government Printing Office; 2000.
7. Centers for Disease Control and Prevention. Principles of Community Engagement. Atlanta: Public Health Practice Program; 1997.
8. Centers for Disease Control and Prevention. Framework for program evaluation in public health. MMWR Morb Mortal Wkly Rep 1999;48(RR11):1.
9. Association of State & Territorial Dental Directors. Guidelines for State and Territorial Oral Health Programs. Jefferson City, MO: 2007.

10. Kuthy RA, Siegal MA, Phipps K. Assessing Oral Health Needs: ASTDD Seven-Step Model. Jefferson City, MO: Association of State & Territorial Dental Directors; 2003.
11. Porta M, editor. A Dictionary of Epidemiology. 5th ed. New York: Oxford University Press; 2008.
12. Timmreck TC. An Introduction to Epidemiology. 4th ed. Boston: Jones & Bartlett; 2002.
13. Abramson JH, Abramson ZH. Survey Methods in Community Medicine. 5th ed. New York: Churchill Livingstone; 1999.
14. Last JM. Public Health and Human Ecology. 2nd ed. Stamford, CT: Appleton & Lange; 1998.
15. Pitts NB, editor. Detection, Assessment, Diagnosis and Monitoring of Caries. Monogr Oral Sci. Basel: Karger; 2009.
16. Cohen LK, Gift HC, editors. Disease Prevention and Oral Health Promotion: Socio-dental Sciences in Action. Copenhagen: Munksgaard; 1995.
17. Green LW, Ottoson JM. Community and Population Health. 8th ed. Boston: McGraw-Hill; 1999.
18. Starr P. The Social Transformation of American Medicine. New York: Basic Books; 1982.
19. Lee PR. Focus on healthy communities: Healthy communities—a young movement that can revolutionize public health. Public Health Rep 2000;115:114.
20. Huff RM, Kline MV. Promoting Health in Multicultural Populations: A Handbook for Practitioners. Thousand Oaks, CA: Sage Publications; 1999.
21. Airhihenbuwa CO. Health and Culture: Beyond the Western Paradigm. Thousand Oaks, CA: Sage Publications; 1995.
22. Hancock T. The mandala of health: A model of the human ecosystem. Fam Commun Health 1985;8:1.
23. Institute of Medicine. Improving Health in the Community. Washington, DC: National Academies Press; 1997.
24. Institute of Medicine. Healthy Communities: New Partnerships for the Future of Public Health. Washington, DC: National Academies Press; 1996.
25. Spector RE. Cultural Diversity in Health and Illness. 5th ed. Upper Saddle River, NJ: Prentice Hall; 2000.
26. Hahn RA. Anthropology in Public Health: Bridging Differences in Culture and Society. New York: Oxford University Press; 1999.
27. Aspen Reference Group. Community Health Education and Promotion: A Guide to Program Design and Evaluation. Gaithersburg, MD: Aspen; 1997.
28. Waxler-Morrison N, Anderson J, Richardson E. Cross-cultural Caring. Vancouver, BC: University of British Columbia Press; 1990.
29. Mechanic D. Medical Sociology. 2nd ed. New York: The Free Press; 1978.
30. Amick BC, Levine S, Tarlow AL, et al, editors. Society and Health. New York: Oxford University Press; 1995.
31. US Department of Health and Human Services. Oral Health in America: A Report of the Surgeon General. Rockville, MD: US Department of Health and Human Services, National Institute of Dental and Craniofacial Research, National Institutes of Health; 2000.
32. Sanders AE. Social Determinants of Oral Health: Conditions Linked to Socioeconomic Inequalities in Oral Health and in the Australian Population, Population Oral Health Series. Canberra: Australia: Australian Institute of Health and Welfare; Number 7, 2007.
33. Fisher-Owens SA, Gansky SA, Platt LJ, et al. Influences on children's oral health: A conceptual model. Pediatrics 2007;120:510.
34. Patrick DL, Lee RS, Nucci M, et al. Reducing oral health disparities: A focus on social and cultural determinants. BMC Oral Health 2006;15(6 Suppl. 1):S4.
35. Roussos ST, Fawcett SB. A review of collaborative partnerships as a strategy for improving community health. Annu Rev Public Health 2000;21:369.
36. Berkowitz W, Wolff T. The Spirit of the Coalition. Washington, DC: American Public Health Association; 1999.
37. Kaye G, Wolff T. From the Ground Up (companion workbook to The Spirit of Coalition). Washington, DC: American Public Health Association; 1995.
38. Community Roots for Oral Health. Guidelines for Successful Coalitions. Olympia, WA: Washington Department of Health, Community and Family Health; 2000.
39. Kretzmann JP, McKnight JL. Building Communities from the Inside Out. Chicago: ACTA Publications; 1993.
40. McKnight JL, Pandak CA. New Community Tools for Improving Child Health: A Pediatrician's Guide to Local Associations. National CATCH Meeting, American Academy of Pediatrics, Community Access to Child Health (CATCH) Program and Asset-Based Community Development Institute, Institute for Policy Research, Northwestern University, CATCH 2000, Elk Grove Village, IL: April 15-16, 1999.

41. Weintraub JA, Douglass CW, Gillings DB. Biostats: Data Analysis for Dental Health Care Professionals. Chapel Hill, NC: CAVCO; 1984.

42. Blinkhorn AS. Qualitative research: Does it have a place in dental public health? J Public Health Dent 2000;60:3.

43. Bailey KD. Methods of Social Research. 4th ed. New York: The Free Press; 1994.

44. Marshall C, Rossman GB. Designing Qualitative Research. 2nd ed. Thousand Oaks, CA: Sage Publications; 1995.

45. Pope C, Mays N. Qualitative Research in Health Care. 2nd ed. London: BMJ Books; 1999.

46. Health Resources and Services Administration, Community Health Status Indicators Project (CHSI), Community Health Status Report: Data Sources, Definitions, and Notes. Washington, DC: US Department of Health and Human Services; 2000.

47. Sharpe PA, Greaney ML, Lee PR, et al. Assets-oriented community assessment. Public Health Rep 2000;115:114.

48. Minkler M. Community Organizing and Community Building for Health. New Brunswick, NJ: Rutgers University Press; 1998.

49. Anderson E, McFarlane J. Community as Partner: Theory and Practice in Nursing. 2nd ed. Philadelphia: JB Lippincott; 1996.

50. Schiavo R. Health Communication: From Theory to Practice. San Francisco: John Wiley & Sons; 2007.

51. Neslon DE, Hesse BW, Croyle RT. Making Data Talk: Communicating Public Health Data to the Public, Policy Makers, and the Press. New York: Oxford University Press; 2009.

Additional Resources

American Association for Community Dental Programs (AACDP)
A Model Framework for Community Oral Health Programs Based upon the Ten Essential Public Health Services
A Guide for Developing and Enhancing Community Oral Health Programs
   www.aacdp.com/index.html
American Public Health Association
   www.apha.org
Association for Community Health Improvement
   www.communityhlth.org/
Association of State & Territorial Dental Directors
Assessing Oral Health Needs: ASTDD Seven-Step Model
Basic Screening Survey
Proven and Promising Best Practices for State and Community Oral Health Programs
   www.astdd.org
Community Toolbox
   http://ctb.ukans.edu
Health Resources and Services Administration (HRSA)
   www.hrsa.gov/
HRSA Data Warehouse
   http://datawarehouse.hrsa.gov/
Data Resource Center for Child and Adolescent Health (DRC)
   http://childhealthdata.org/content/Default.aspx
Healthy Cities and Healthy Cities Resources
Healthy Communities Institute
   www.healthycommunitiesinstitute.com/index.html
International Healthy Cities Foundation
   www.healthycommunitiesinstitute.com/ihcf.html
Healthy City
   www.healthycities.org
National Association of County and City Health Officials
   www.naccho.org
Mobilizing for Action through Planning and Partnerships (MAPP) (Part of the Assessment Protocol for Excellence in Public Health [APEXPH] project)
   www.naccho.org/topics/infrastructure/MAPP/index.cfm
National Institute of Dental and Craniofacial Research (NIDCR)
   www.nidcr.nih.gov
NIDCR Healthy People 2010 Oral Health Toolkit
   www.nidcr.nih.gov/EducationalResources/DentalHealthProf/HealthyPeople2010/

Dental, Oral, and Craniofacial Data Resource Center (DRC) [cosponsored by the National Institute of Dental and Craniofacial Research (NIDCR) and the Centers for Disease Control and Prevention's (CDC) Division of Oral Health]
   http://drc.hhs.gov/
National Maternal and Child Oral Health Resource Center
   www.mchoralhealth.org/
Office of Disease Prevention and Health Promotion, US Department of Health and Human Services
Healthy People 2010
   www.health.gov/healthypeople
Healthy People 2020
   www.healthypeople.gov/HP2020/
Public Health Foundation
   www.phf.org/
US Department of Health and Human Services, Centers for Disease Control and Prevention (CDC)
Tracking Healthy People 2010
   www.cdc.gov/nchs/healthy_people/hp2010/hp2010_thp.htm
Centers for Disease Control and Prevention, Data 2010: The Healthy People 2010 Database
   http://wonder.cdc.gov/data2010
Centers for Disease Control and Prevention, Division of Oral Health and Association of State & Territorial Dental Directors
National Oral Health Surveillance Systems (NOHSS)
   www.cdc.gov/nohss/
Centers for Disease Control and Prevention, Division of Oral Health
Oral Health Infrastructure Development Tools and State Oral Health Plans
   www.cdc.gov/OralHealth/state_programs/infrastructure/index.htm
   www.cdc.gov/OralHealth/state_programs/OH_plans/index.htm
   www.cdc.gov/OralHealth/state_programs/states/index.htm
Centers for Disease Control and Prevention, National Center for Chronic Disease, Prevention and Health Promotion (NCCDPHP)
   www.cdc.gov/chronicdisease/about/index.htm
Centers for Disease Control and Prevention, Healthy Communities Program
   www.cdc.gov/HealthyCommunitiesProgram/
Centers for Disease Control and Prevention, Office of the Director, Office of Chief of Public Health Practice (OCPHP)
Public Health Systems Performance Program (PHSPP)
National Public Health Performance Standards Program (NPHPSP)
   http://cdc.gov/od/ocphp/
   www.phppo.cdc.gov/nphpsp/index.asp
World Dental Federation—FDI
   www.fdiworldental.org/
Beaglehole R, Benzian H, Crail J, et al. Oral Health Atlas: Mapping a Neglected Global Health Issue. Brighton, UK: Myriad Editions for FDI World Dental Federation; 2009
   www.oralhealthatlas.org/Read.html
World Health Organization (WHO), Oral Health
   www.who.int/oral_health/en/
WHO Oral Health Databases
   www.who.int/oral_health/databases/en/index.html

4

Measuring Progress in Oral Health

Jane E. M. Steffensen, RDH, BS, MPH, CHES

Objectives

Upon completion of this chapter, the student will be able to:
- Discuss the national Healthy People initiatives.
- Describe the oral health objectives of *Healthy People 2010* and *2020*.
- Discuss measures used to assess oral health in populations.
- Compare and contrast the procedures and methods used in oral health surveys.

Key Terms

Healthy People 2010
Healthy People 2020
Health equity
Health disparity
Association of State &
   Territorial Dental Directors
   (ASTDD)
Basic Screening Survey (BSS)
Index
Decayed, missing, and filled
   teeth (DMFT)
Decayed, missing, and filled
   surfaces (DMFS)

National Health and Nutrition
   Examination Survey
   (NHANES)
World Health Organization
   (WHO) WHO Basic
   Methods for Oral Health
   Surveys
Community Periodontal Index
   (CPI)
Behavioral Risk Factor
   Surveillance Survey
   (BRFSS)

National Health Interview
   Survey (NHIS)
Water Fluoridation Reporting
   System (WFRS)
Medical Expenditure Panel
   Survey (MEPS)
Quality of life
Health–related quality of life
   (HRQOL)
Oral health–related quality of
   life (OHRQOL)

Opening Statement

National 2010 Objectives for Leading Health Indicators*

- Increase access to health insurance

- Increase access to personal health care

- Increase access to prenatal care

- Immunizations

- 100% of children and adults (younger than 65 years) have health insurance
- 96% of children and adults have a source of ongoing primary health care
- 90% of pregnant women receive prenatal care during the first trimester
- 80% of young children (aged 19 to 35 months) are fully immunized

*Statistics from *Healthy People 2010 Database*. Available at http://wonder.cdc.gov/data2010/. Accessed April 2010.
HIV, Human immunodeficiency virus; *AIDS*, acquired immunodeficiency syndrome.

- Increase physical activity

- Decrease obesity
- Decrease tobacco use
- Decrease substance abuse

- Increase access to mental health services

- Reduce deaths caused by motor vehicle crashes
- Improve environmental quality

- Increase responsible sexual behavior

- 50% of adults are physically active on a regular basis
- 15% of adults are obese
- 12% of adults smoke cigarettes
- 89% of adolescents do not use alcohol or illicit drugs during the past month
- 50% of adults with recognized depression receive treatment
- 9.2 deaths per 100,000 population due to motor vehicle crashes
- 0% of Americans are exposed to harmful air pollutants
- 0.7 deaths per 100,000 population due to HIV/AIDS

ORAL HEALTH ASSESSMENT: ESSENTIAL IN MONITORING COMMUNITY HEALTH

To ensure that a comprehensive profile of a community's health is depicted, oral health should be included in a community health assessment. When the health of a community is assessed, oral health is often found to be an important concern for children, adults, and the elderly.[1,2] Common oral and craniofacial diseases and conditions that can be assessed include the following:

- Dental caries
- Periodontal diseases
- Edentulism (complete tooth loss)
- Oral and pharyngeal cancer
- Soft tissue lesions
- Craniofacial anomalies, including cleft lip and palate
- Malocclusion
- Orofacial injuries
- Temporomandibular dysfunction (TMD)

Multiple determinants influence oral health in populations.[1,3] The etiology and pathogenesis of diseases and disorders affecting craniofacial structures are multifactorial and complex. They involve the interplay among social, cultural, behavioral, environmental, and biologic dimensions.[1,3] These factors contribute to the development and progression of oral diseases, conditions, and injuries.[1,3] In addition, various factors affect the access of population groups to community preventive services (e.g., community water fluoridation) and clinical dental services. Community preventive services can prevent oral diseases at a community level and improve population oral health. Clinical preventive dental services can prevent oral problems among individuals with access to dental clinics or dental offices. Also, oral health practices and healthy behaviors by individuals can impact oral health outcomes. In a community oral health assessment, it is important to evaluate key determinants that influence oral health status and access to services. Appendix E outlines oral conditions and factors influencing oral health that have been assessed in oral health surveys. The national health objectives outlined in *Healthy People* provide an important framework for the development of oral health assessments at the state and local levels.

HEALTHY PEOPLE

Health promotion and disease prevention are important concepts in the United States. Therefore the nation has developed plans for the prevention of diseases and the promotion of health, embodied in the initiative known as *Healthy People*.[4] These national health objectives shape the health agenda in the United States and guide health improvements. Each decade since 1980, the US Department of Health and Human Services (DHHS) has released a comprehensive set of national public health objectives.[4,5] *Healthy People* provides national 10-year health targets aimed at improving the health of all Americans. It is grounded in the notion that establishing objectives and providing benchmarks to track and monitor progress over time can motivate, guide, and focus action.

The *Healthy People* initiative has been the nation's blueprint for disease prevention and health promotion beginning in the 1980s.[5] The initiative originated in a 1979 report by the Surgeon General that established the precedent for setting national health objectives and monitoring progress over an interval of a decade.[4,5] *Healthy People 2000* and **Healthy People 2010** set measurable national targets to be achieved by the years 2000 and 2010, respectively.[4,5] **Healthy People 2020**, the fourth generation of national benchmarks, was launched in 2010 and established national objectives to be reached by the year 2020.[4]

Healthy People 2020 is the outcome of an extensive collaborative process that has relied on input from a diverse array of individuals and organizations, both within and outside the federal government, with a common interest in improving the nation's health.[4,6]

The Secretary of Health and Human Services' Advisory Committee on National Health Promotion and Disease Prevention Objectives for 2020 and the Federal Interagency Workgroup (FIW) on *Healthy People 2020* guided the development of *Healthy People 2020*.[4,6] The *Healthy People 2020* FIW oversaw and managed the development of *Healthy People 2020*, using input from the Secretary's Advisory Committee on National Health Promotion and Disease Prevention Objectives for 2020 and other Healthy People stakeholders. Representatives from agencies within the DHHS served on the FIW. Federal agencies outside of DHHS also served on the FIW, in support of the *Healthy People 2020* framework, which embraces the social determinants of health approach to advanced health improvements.

In addition, the Healthy People initiatives were developed through the involvement of the Healthy People Consortium, a public-private alliance of national organizations and state, territorial, and tribal public health, mental health, substance abuse, and environmental agencies.[4,5] These national efforts have brought together national, state, and local agencies; nonprofit, voluntary, and professional organizations; businesses; communities; and individuals to focus on improvements in the health of all Americans. Organizations with an interest in improving oral health have participated actively in the Healthy People Consortium and advocated for oral health to be integrated into the Healthy People initiative.

The national objectives have served as a basis for the development of state and community plans to improve health for three decades.[4] Many states and localities have used the Healthy People frameworks to guide the development of health improvement plans and performance standards. Several resources based on the national health objectives have been developed to guide these planning initiatives (see Additional Resources in Chapter 3 and Appendix E).

HEALTHY PEOPLE 2020 FRAMEWORK

The *Healthy People 2020* framework consists of a vision statement, mission statement, overarching goals, and graphic model[4] (**Box 4-1**). The framework embraces the determinants of health as an approach to health improvement and promotes the integration of policies that advance health. Also, the framework is informed by a perspective of risk factors as a guide to improvements in health and builds on past iterations of Healthy People. The vision, mission, and overarching goals provide structure and guidance for achieving the *Healthy People 2020* objectives. Although the framework is general in nature, it offers a specific focus on important areas of emphasis in which action must be taken if the United States is to achieve better health by the year 2020. The framework provides the foundation for explicit objectives and strategies to attain them. The development process culminated in 2010 with the launch of the national health objectives for 2020 that outlined baseline measures and targets to be reached by 2020. Developed under the leadership of a FIW, the *Healthy People 2020* framework is the product of a collaborative process among the DHHS and other Federal agencies, public stakeholders, and the Secretary's Advisory Committee on Health Promotion and Disease Prevention Objectives for 2020.[4]

The *Healthy People 2020* initiative includes a vision of a society in which all people live long, healthy lives.[4] The *Healthy People 2020* vision statement outlines the focus for the overall initiative. The mission statement—a framework element that has not been included in previous iterations of Healthy People—is meant to summarize what *Healthy People 2020* does for the nation and how the public can use it. It reflects the view that *Healthy People 2020* offers practical guidance

BOX 4-1 *Healthy People 2020* **Framework**

Vision
A society in which all people live long, healthy lives.

Mission
Healthy People 2020 strives to:
- Identify nationwide health improvement priorities.
- Increase public awareness and understanding of the determinants of health, disease, and disability and the opportunities for progress.
- Provide measurable objectives and goals that are applicable at the national, state, and local levels.
- Engage multiple sectors to take actions to strengthen policies and improve practices that are driven by the best available evidence and knowledge.
- Identify critical research, evaluation, and data collection needs.

Overarching Goals
- Attain high quality, longer lives free of preventable disease, disability, injury, and premature death.
- Achieve health equity, eliminate disparities, and improve the health of all groups.
- Create social and physical environments that promote good health for all.
- Promote quality of life, healthy development, and healthy behaviors across all life stages.

Continued

BOX 4-1 *Healthy People 2020* Framework—cont'd

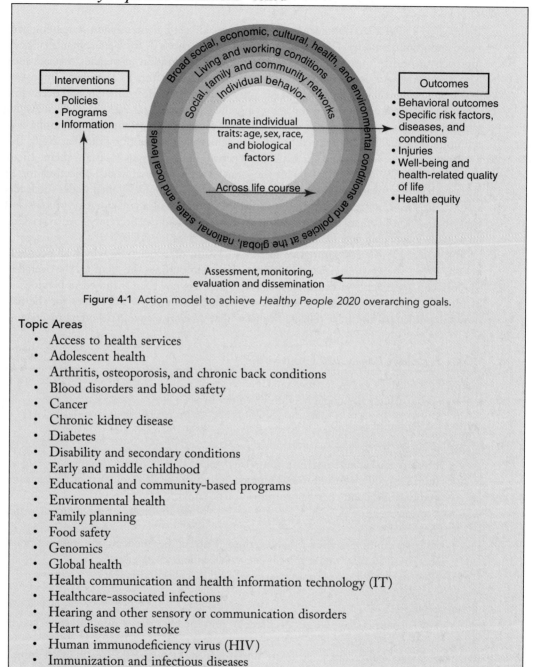

Figure 4-1 Action model to achieve *Healthy People 2020* overarching goals.

Topic Areas
- Access to health services
- Adolescent health
- Arthritis, osteoporosis, and chronic back conditions
- Blood disorders and blood safety
- Cancer
- Chronic kidney disease
- Diabetes
- Disability and secondary conditions
- Early and middle childhood
- Educational and community-based programs
- Environmental health
- Family planning
- Food safety
- Genomics
- Global health
- Health communication and health information technology (IT)
- Healthcare-associated infections
- Hearing and other sensory or communication disorders
- Heart disease and stroke
- Human immunodeficiency virus (HIV)
- Immunization and infectious diseases
- Injury and violence prevention
- Maternal, infant, and child health
- Medical product safety
- Mental health and mental disorders

BOX 4-1 *Healthy People 2020* **Framework—cont'd**

- Nutrition and weight status
- Occupational safety and health
- Older adults
- Oral health
- Physical activity and fitness
- Public health infrastructure
- Quality of life and well-being
- Respiratory diseases
- Sexually transmitted diseases
- Social determinants of health
- Substance abuse
- Tobacco use
- Vision

Adapted from The Secretary's Advisory Committee on National Health Promotion and Disease Prevention Objectives for 2020. Phase I Report Recommendations for the Framework and Format of Healthy People 2020. Washington, DC. October 28, 2008.

on using data and knowledge, as well as education and other actions to improve population health in communities.

The overarching goals for *Healthy People 2020* provide a general direction for the development of a set of objectives that will measure progress in population health within a specified time period.[4] These overarching goals continue the tradition of earlier Healthy People initiatives by advocating for improvements in the health of every person in the country. They address the environmental factors that contribute to collective health and illness by calling for healthy places and supportive public policies, placing particular emphasis on the determinants of health.

The overarching goals reflect that *Healthy People 2020* has been designed to redirect attention from health care to health determinants. Health determinants need to be a primary focus of *Healthy People 2020,* and health care is a secondary focus. *Health determinants* are the range of personal, social, economic, and environmental factors that determine the health status of individuals or populations. They are embedded in the social and physical environments. To improve health in the coming decade, *Healthy People 2020* targets reductions in adverse social and physical determinants as important areas for assessment and intervention.

The Action Model to Achieve *Healthy People 2020* Goals is graphically displayed in Box 4-1. The figure shows a feedback loop of intervention, assessment, and dissemination that would enable achievement of the *Healthy People 2020* overarching goals.[4] Also, this figure illustrates the Institute of Medicine's (IOM) model of the multiple determinants of health. The model is represented by an inner circle and four outer circles. Within the innermost circle are innate individual traits: age, sex, race, and biologic factors related to the biology of health and disease. The first circle outside the center circle represents individual behavior; the next circle represents social, family, and community networks; and the next circle represents living and working conditions. The figure defines living and working conditions as including psychosocial factors, employment status and occupational factors, socioeconomic status (e.g., income, education, occupation, etc.), the natural and built environments, public health services, and health care services. The built environment includes transportation systems, water and sanitation systems, housing, and other dimensions of community planning. The outermost circle represents broad social, economic, cultural, health, and environmental conditions and policies at the global, national, state, and local levels. Social conditions include economic inequality, urbanization, mobility, cultural values, attitudes, and policies related to discrimination and intolerance on the basis of race, gender, and other differences. Other conditions at the national level include major sociopolitical shifts such as recession, war, and governmental collapse.

The figure displays an action model showing the impact of interventions (e.g., policies, programs, and information) on the determinants of health at multiple levels across the lifespan to achieve the overarching goals of *Healthy People 2020*.[4] Results of such interventions are demonstrated through assessment, monitoring, and evaluation. Through application of evidence-based practices, the findings can be used to inform intervention planning and implementation of effective strategies.

HEALTHY PEOPLE 2020 FOCUSES ON ELIMINATING HEALTH DISPARITIES AND PROMOTING HEALTH EQUITY

Eliminating health disparities and promoting health equity is a focus of *Healthy People 2020* and requires actions to address all important determinants of health disparities that can be influenced by institutional policies and practices.[4] Disparities can include disparities in health care but also in other health determinants, such as living and working conditions, as well as social, economic, cultural, community, and environmental conditions that are needed for health. Social policies related to education, income, transportation, and housing are powerful influences on health because they affect factors such as the types of foods that can be purchased, the quality of the housing and neighborhoods in which individuals can live, and access to quality education and health care.

The concepts of **health equity** and **health disparity** are inseparable in their practical implementation. Policies and practices aimed at promoting the goal of health equity do not immediately eliminate all health disparities, but they can provide a foundation for moving closer to that goal. There are a variety of definitions of health disparity and health equity. The Advisory Committee on National Health Promotion and Disease Prevention Objectives for 2020 defined theses terms for the purposes of *Healthy People 2020*.[4]

The general public usually understands the term *health disparity* as referring to any difference in health. However, in the public health community and as defined by the Advisory Committee, the term refers to a particular type of health difference between individuals or groups that is unfair because it is caused by social or economic disadvantage. A health disparity is a particular type of health difference that is closely linked with social or economic disadvantage. Health disparities adversely affect groups of people who have systematically experienced greater social or economic obstacles to health based on their racial or ethnic group, religion, socioeconomic status, gender, mental health, cognitive, sensory or physical disability, sexual orientation, geographic location, or other characteristics historically linked to discrimination or exclusion.[4]

Health equity is a desirable goal and standard that entails special efforts to improve the health of those who have experienced social or economic disadvantage.[4] The Advisory Committee on National Health Promotion and Disease Prevention Objectives for 2020 states the following requirements are needed for health equity: (1) continuous efforts focused on elimination of health disparities, including disparities in health care and in the living and working conditions that influence health, and (2) continuous efforts to maintain a desired state of equity after particular health disparities are eliminated.[4] Health equity is oriented toward achieving the highest level of health possible for all groups. The Advisory Committee on National Health Promotion and Disease Prevention Objectives for 2020 recommended the following short- and long-term actions to achieve health equity:

- Particular attention to groups that have experienced major obstacles to health associated with being socially or economically disadvantaged.
- Promotion of equal opportunities for all people to be healthy and to seek the highest level of health possible.
- Distribution of the social and economic resources needed to be healthy in a manner that progressively reduces health disparities and improves health for all.
- Attention to the root causes of health disparities, specifically health determinants, a principal focus of *Healthy People 2020*.

NATIONAL OBJECTIVES FOR IMPROVING HEALTH

The national health objectives developed for Healthy People over the years have called for action to promote healthy behaviors and healthy and safe communities; improve systems for personal health and public health; and prevent diseases, injuries, disabilities, and disorders.[4-6] *Healthy People 2010* contained 467 objectives, grouped in 28 focus areas; each focus area had a specific overall goal.[5] Also, ten Leading Health Indicators were designated in *Healthy People 2010* as key measures for national report cards on population health.[5]

Healthy People 2020 continues the mechanisms for monitoring and tracking health status, health risks, protective factors, and use of services.[4,6] The *Healthy People 2020* Health Objectives integrate the determinants of health that encompass the combined effects of individual and community physical and social environments. Also, the objectives consider policies and interventions used to promote health; prevent diseases, injuries, and disabilities; and ensure access to effective personal and public health services. The ultimate measure of success in any health improvement effort will be gains in health status of specific populations.

Thirty-eight topic areas have been proposed for *Healthy People 2020*.[6] The proposed *Healthy People 2020* National Health Objectives were developed by Topic Area Workgroups led by various agencies within the Federal government.[6] They were reviewed by the FIW on *Healthy People 2020*.[6] The final set of *Healthy People 2020* objectives were developed with input from public comments collected at public meetings and in writing via a public comment website.[6] Also, the final national health objectives for 2020 were refined through further deliberations of the Topic Area Workgroups, FIW on *Healthy People 2020,* and Secretary's Advisory Committee on National Health Promotion and Disease Prevention Objectives for 2020.

NATIONAL ORAL HEALTH OBJECTIVES

The national oral health objectives have defined the nation's oral health agenda and served as a road map for national benchmarks since the early 1980s. Oral health is a specific topic area in

Healthy People 2020.[4] Also, oral health is integrated into other topic areas in the *Healthy People 2020* Objectives for the nation.

Table 4-1 summarizes the topics included in *Healthy People 2010* Oral Health Objectives and the proposed *Healthy People 2020* Oral Health Objectives. **Table 4-2** outlines selected health objectives with related oral health topics from those proposed in *Healthy People 2020*. Also, Appendix D provides additional information about measure used to monitor the objectives and the key data sources.

The *Healthy People 2020* Oral Health Objectives are based on the latest research and scientific evidence related to oral health. They combine current information with contemporary public health principles to benefit the largest number of people in the United States. The oral health objectives inform decision making and resource allocation by driving action at national, state, and local levels toward the achievement of common oral health improvement goals. States, territories, tribes, and localities can use the framework to guide health plans for oral health improvements. The oral health objectives can shape the development and implementation of policies, interventions, programs, and practices tailored for specific population groups. The objectives identify significant opportunities to improve oral health for all Americans by providing a focus for efforts in the public, private, and nonprofit sectors. These objectives provide a framework for measuring oral health indicators and progress toward achievement of targets.

ORAL HEALTH SURVEILLANCE SYSTEMS

A comprehensive public health surveillance system integrates oral health and is essential for programmatic activities to improve oral health. Several agencies and national organizations have stressed the importance of oral health surveillance systems to routinely collect data on oral health outcomes, risk factors, and intervention strategies for the whole population or representative samples of the population.[7,8] Oral health surveillance systems are not only oral health data collection systems but also involve timely communication of oral health findings to responsible parties and to the public. Also, it involves using oral health data to initiate and evaluate public health measures to prevent and control oral diseases.[7,8] An oral health surveillance system should contain at a minimum a core set of oral health measures that describe the status of important oral health conditions to serve as benchmarks for assessing progress in achieving oral health improvements.

Steps have been taken in the United States at the national, state, and local levels to formulate a systematic approach for oral health data collection and reporting. The focus of these collaborative efforts among organizations and agencies was to promote oral health assessment and monitoring that could be applied in a wide range of environments. These efforts also stressed the importance of oral health program evaluation in light of contemporary public health principles. An important aim of these efforts has been the dissemination of procedures for collecting comparable data to assess oral health. A long-term goal includes an approach for continuous monitoring of oral health at the national, state, and community levels, as well as an expansion of indicators in oral health surveillance systems. Results of these endeavors included the development of standard ways to monitor the national oral health objectives, an oral health needs assessment model, and documentation of uniform methods to measure community oral health.[7-13] Several resources have been developed to provide guidance to national, state, territorial, tribal, and local oral health programs in planning and implementing oral health surveillance systems.

Table 4-1   *Healthy People 2010* **and** *2020:* **Oral Health Objectives**

Healthy People 2010 oral health goal: To prevent and control oral and craniofacial diseases, conditions, and injuries and improve access to related services.

Healthy People 2010 *National Health Objective Number (*Healthy People 2020 *Proposed National Health Objective Number)**	*Topic of* Healthy People 2020 *Proposed National Health Objective*†
HP2010–21-1 (OH HP2020–6)	Reduce dental caries experience
HP2010–21-2 (OH HP2020–7)	Reduce untreated dental decay
HP2010–21-3 and HP2010–21-4 (OH HP2020–8)	Reduce permanent tooth loss and complete tooth loss
HP2010–21-5a	Reduce periodontal disease: Gingivitis (2010 objective achieved not included in *Healthy People 2010*)
HP2010–21-5b (OH HP2020–9)	Reduce periodontal disease: Destructive periodontal disease
HP2010–21-6 (OH HP2020–1)	Early detection of oral and pharyngeal cancers
HP2010–21-7 (OH HP2020–16)	Increase annual examinations for oral and pharyngeal cancer
HP2010–21-8 (OH HP2020–10)	Increase dental sealants
HP2010–21-9 (OH HP2020–2)	Increase community water fluoridation
HP2010–21-10 (OH HP2020–3)	Increase use of oral health care system
HP2010–21-11 (OH HP2020–11)	Increase use of oral health care system by residents in long-term care facilities
HP2010–21-12 (OH HP2020–4)	Increase dental services for low-income children
HP2010–21-13 (OH HP2020–12)	Increase school-based health centers with oral health component
HP2010–21-14 (OH HP2020–13)	Increase local health departments and Federally Qualified Health Centers (FQHCs) with an oral health component
HP2010–21-15 (OH HP2020–14)	Increase number of states and the District of Columbia with a system for recording and referring infants and children with cleft lips and cleft palates to craniofacial anomaly rehabilitative teams
HP2010–21-16 (OH HP2020–5)	Increase number of states and the District of Columbia with an oral and craniofacial health surveillance system
HP2010–21-17 (OH HP2020–15)	Increase the number of health agencies that have a public dental health program directed by a dental professional with public health training
Newly proposed *Healthy People 2020* oral health objective (OH HP2020–17)	Increase patients that receive oral health services at Federally Qualified Health Centers each year

*Numbers refer to the chapter and objective as referenced in *Healthy People 2010*. For example, 21-12 is Chapter 21, Objective 12. Numbers in parentheses refer to objective as referenced in Proposed Oral Health Objectives for *Healthy People 2020*. For example, OH HP2020-14 is Chapter 1, Proposed Objective 14 in the oral health chapter in *Healthy People 2020*.
†The *Healthy People 2020* health objectives were proposed; see the *Healthy People 2020* website for the final objectives to be achieved by 2020.
Adapted from Department of Health and Human Services (DHHS). Healthy People 2020: Public Meetings 2009 Draft Objectives. Washington, DC: DHHS; 2009. Healthy People 2010: Understanding and Improving Health. 2nd ed. Washington, DC: DHHS; 2000.

Table 4-2   *Healthy People 2010* and *2020:* Selected Health Objectives Related to Oral Health

Healthy People 2010 *National Health Objective Number (*Healthy People 2020 *Proposed National Health Objective Number)**	Topic of Healthy People 2020 *Proposed National Health Objective*†
Access to Quality Health Services: HP2010–1-6 (Access to Health Services: AHS HP2020–7)	Reduce individuals experiencing difficulties or delays in obtaining necessary medical care, dental care, or prescription medicines
Access to Quality Health Services: HP2010–1-8 (Public Health Infrastructure: PHI HP2020–11)	Increase degrees awarded in the health professions to members of underrepresented racial and ethnic groups, including dentistry
Cancer: HP2010–03-6 (Cancer: C HP2020–6)	Reduce oropharyngeal cancer deaths
Cancer: HP2010–3-10 a, b, c (Tobacco Use: TU HP2020–17)	Increase tobacco cessation counseling in health care settings, including in dental care settings
Newly Proposed *Healthy People 2020* Health Objective Tobacco Use: TU HP2020–19	Increase tobacco screening in health care settings, including dental care settings
Diabetes: HP2010–05-15 (Diabetes: D HP2020–9)	Increase annual dental examination for persons with diabetes
Newly Proposed *Healthy People 2020* Health Objective Educational and Community-Based Programs: ECBP HP2020–12	Increase number of preschools and Head Start programs that provide health education to prevent health problems, including unintentional injury; violence; tobacco use and addiction; alcohol and drug use, unhealthy dietary patterns; and inadequate physical activity, dental health, and safety
Newly Proposed *Healthy People 2020* Health Objective: Older Adults: OA HP2020–6	Increase health care workforce with geriatric certification, including dentists

*Numbers refer to the chapter and objective as referenced in *Healthy People 2010.* For example, 03-6 is Cancer Chapter 3, Objective 6. Numbers in parentheses refer to objective as referenced in Proposed Oral Health Objectives for *Healthy People 2020.* For example, Cancer: C HP2020–6 is Cancer Chapter 6 and Proposed Objective 6 for *Healthy People 2020.*
†The *Healthy People 2020* health objectives were proposed; see the *Healthy People 2020* website for the final objectives to be achieved by 2020.
Adapted from Department of Health and Human Services (DHHS): Healthy People 2020: Public Meetings 2009 Draft Objectives. Washington, DC: DHHS; 2009. Healthy People 2010: Understanding and Improving Health. 2nd ed. Washington, DC: DHHS; 2000.[4]

The **Association of State & Territorial Dental Directors (ASTDD)** has developed and updated several resources that provide guidance on oral health surveillance. The ASTDD has developed a best practices report that provides a review of oral health assessment measures, methods, and standards.[8] **The Basic Screening Survey (BSS)** has established standards for oral health screenings for preschool and school children.[9] The ASTDD has also developed the BSS for assessing oral health among adults and elderly individuals.

The National Oral Health Surveillance System (NOHSS) is an important oral health data system. NOHSS is a collaborative effort between the Centers for Disease Control and Prevention (CDC), Division of Oral Health, and the ASTDD. It is designed to help public health programs monitor the burden of oral disease, use of the oral health care delivery system, and status of community water fluoridation on both a state and a national level. NOHSS includes indicators of oral health from national and state data sources, information on state oral health programs, and links to sources of oral health information. NOHSS has been developed to track basic oral health

BOX 4-2 Oral Health Indicators in National Oral Health Surveillance System (NOHSS)

Oral Health Indicator	Assessment
Dental visit	Adults aged 18+ who have visited a dentist or dental clinic in the past year
Teeth cleaning	Adults aged 18+ who have had their teeth cleaned in the past year (among adults with natural teeth who have ever visited a dentist or dental clinic)
Complete tooth loss	Adults aged 65+ who have lost all of their natural teeth due to tooth decay or gum disease
Lost six or more teeth	Adults aged 65+ who have lost six or more teeth due to tooth decay or gum disease
Fluoridation status	Percentage of people served by public water systems who receive fluoridated water
Dental sealants	Percentage of third-grade students with dental sealants on at least one permanent molar tooth
Caries experience	Percentage of third-grade students with caries experience, including treated and untreated tooth decay
Untreated tooth decay	Percentage of third-grade students with untreated tooth decay
Cancer of the oral cavity and pharynx	Incidence and mortality of oral and pharyngeal cancer

From Centers for Disease Control and Prevention (CDC), Division of Oral Health, and the Association of State & Territorial Dental Directors (ATSDD). National Oral Health Surveillance System (NOHSS). Atlanta: CDC and ASTDD; 2006.

indicators.[8] NOHSS includes a minimal set of standard oral health indicators, to be expanded in the future, based on data sources and surveillance capacity available to most states. A functioning state oral health surveillance system should enable the state to submit data for inclusion in the NOHSS. **Box 4-2** outlines the indicators currently included in NOHSS.[8]

Also, data from several sources are presented in interactive web-based oral health maps that present state and/or county level data. For the oral health maps, the adult indicators come from the Behavioral Risk Factor Surveillance System (BRFSS) and the child indicators come from state oral health screenings for states that choose to provide the results of the surveys. The water fluoridation indicators come from the Water Fluoridation Reporting System (WFRS), and these indicators reflect the most recent data entered into WFRS by states. Also, historic data are available for years in which the CDC prepared fluoridation status reports.

The Dental, Oral, and Craniofacial Data Resource Center (DRC) is another important source of information for oral health surveillance and oral health assessments. The DRC is cosponsored by the National Institute for Dental and Craniofacial Research (NIDCR), National Institutes for Health (NIH), and the Division of Oral Health, CDC. The DRC serves as a resource on dental, oral, and craniofacial data for oral health educators, researchers, clinical practitioners, public health planners, policymakers, advocates, and the general public. Key resources related to oral health assessment are available from the DRC and include the (1) *Catalog of Oral Health Surveys and Archive of Procedures Related to Oral Health* and (2) *Oral Health Survey Questions: A Compilation of Dental and Oral Health Questions Included on National Health Surveys.* Appendix D includes information on the NOHSS, DRC, and other oral health data systems and data sources.

MEASURING ORAL HEALTH AND ITS DETERMINANTS IN POPULATIONS

This chapter focuses on measurements of oral health used in population-based oral health surveillance systems and oral health surveys. The text highlights common measures used to assess population oral health, specifies oral health indicators included in *Healthy People 2010* and *2020*, and provides an overview of clinical and nonclinical data collection methods related to oral health assessment. Measures and methods used for assessment of individual patients in clinical settings or in clinical studies (including clinical trials) are not emphasized in this chapter. Other books review clinical evaluation techniques or clinical research methods.[14]

Selection of a data collection method for a community oral health assessment should be based on the following:

1. Information of interest (e.g., types of conditions and factors to be assessed)
2. Social and demographics of the population and community
3. Purpose of the assessment (e.g., how data collected are to be used after assessment)

Common nonclinical measures include face-to-face personal interviews, telephone interviews, a self-administered questionnaire, and a computer-assisted personal interview, although other nonclinical methods can be used to assess different factors influencing oral health.[11] The topics of oral health questions that can be used in oral health surveys are outlined in Appendix E.

Clinical methods include basic screenings and epidemiologic examinations.[9,11,12,15,16] Basic screenings involve the use of direct observation techniques established for visual detection and identification of gross dental and oral lesions in the oral cavity with a tongue blade, a dental mirror, and appropriate lighting. Epidemiologic examinations entail the use of detailed visual-tactile assessment of the oral cavity with dental instruments and a light source in an oral health survey.

Basic screenings and epidemiologic examinations do not constitute a thorough clinical examination[9,11]; they do not involve making a clinical diagnosis that would result in a treatment plan. Surveys are cross-sectional when they look at a population at a point in time. Surveys are descriptive because they allow for oral health determinants to be ascertained and oral health status to be estimated for a defined population.

Common dental indexes are used for clinical measures in oral health surveys. A dental **index** is an abbreviated measurement of the amount or condition of oral disease in a population. An index is based on a graduated numeric scale with defined upper and lower limits. It is an aid in data collection, allowing for comparisons among population groups that are classified by the same criteria and methods. The attributes of a good index are reviewed in **Box 4-3**.

BOX 4-3 **Attributes of a Good Index**

- Valid
- Reliable
- Clear, simple, and objective
- Sensitive to shifts in disease
- Acceptable to the participants involved
- Amenable to statistical analysis

From Burt BA, Eklund SA. Dentistry, Dental Practice and the Community. 6th ed. Philadelphia: WB Saunders; 2005.

TYPES OF MEASUREMENTS

Measurements of Dental Caries

Permanent Dentition

Dental caries (tooth decay) is an infectious disease that results in demineralization and ultimately, cavitation of the tooth surface if the process is not controlled or if the tooth is not remineralized. This bacterial infection is influenced by a variety of factors in the host, agent, and environment. Unless dental caries is arrested early, the process is irreversible.

Dental caries can occur in primary or permanent teeth. General types of tooth decay include coronal (occurring on the crowns of teeth) and root surface (occurring on the roots of teeth). In surveys of populations, coronal and root surface caries can be assessed by a systematic evaluation through epidemiologic examination or screening procedures.[9,12,15-20] The status of **decayed, missing, and filled teeth (DMFT)** or **decayed, missing, and filled surfaces (DMFS)** is commonly recorded by a basic screening or oral epidemiologic examination.[9,12,15,16]

The conventional decayed, missing, and filled (DMF) Indexes are used to count coronal caries of permanent teeth (DMFT) or surfaces (DMFS). Although the DMF Index has been used extensively in oral health surveys and has been a standard measurement in many countries, it is limited in its ability to measure thoroughly the characteristics of dental caries.[15,16] As patterns of dental caries change, technology develops, and the goals of oral health surveys shift toward more situational analyses in communities, different approaches for the measurement of dental caries may emerge in the future.[9,11,20]

For the DMF Index, each tooth space is scored as to whether it is sound or is diseased and whether there is evidence of treated or untreated clinical caries.[18,19] The DMF Index can be based on 28 or 32 permanent teeth in surveys of population. If ever diseased, the tooth must show one of three conditions:

1. Untreated, frank cavitation (decayed = D).
2. Evidence of restorative treatment resulting from caries (filled = F).
3. Evidence of a lost tooth caused by caries or periodontal disease (missing = M).

The DMF Index for an individual is the sum of either teeth (DMFT) or surfaces (DMFS) having these three conditions. The DMF Index is considered irreversible because it indicates the cumulative, lifetime caries experience and is used to measure past and present caries experiences.

The ASTDD's BSS assesses untreated dental caries and dental caries experience on a per-person basis.[9] Dichotomous measures (e.g., yes or no) are used during the screening of each individual to record the absence or presence of untreated dental caries and experience of dental caries (at least one decayed tooth, restored tooth, or missing tooth). Dental caries experience is defined as the presence of dental decay, dental fillings or other types of dental restorations, or missing teeth because of prior exposure to tooth decay. Population measures are formulated to indicate the percentage of the population with untreated dental caries and dental caries experience. Appendix D summarizes the ways dental caries have been monitored for *Healthy People 2010* and key data sources.

In oral health surveys, the terms *caries-free* and *caries experience* are commonly used to describe the status of population groups. When the DMFT score is equal to or more than 1, the person is considered to have experienced dental caries (at present, D; at some time in the past, M or F). When the DMFT equals 0, the person is considered to be caries-free. Population measures are used to indicate the percentage of the population with dental caries experience and its complementary measurement, the percentage of the population that is caries-free. For example, a survey can show that 52% of children in the population have experienced dental caries and the other 48% are caries-free.

In the United States, oral health surveys typically have used a dichotomous scale for the diagnosis of coronal caries. Dental caries is scored by the presence or absence of a cavitated lesion based on established diagnostic criteria. According to the ASTDD BSS methods, untreated dental caries is generally detected by visual inspection only—explorers are usually not used—and recorded by the screener.[9] A tooth is considered to have untreated decay when the screener can readily observe breakdown of the enamel surface. In other words, for the ASTDD BSS, only cavitated lesions are considered to be untreated decay. This applies to pits and fissures, as well as smooth tooth surfaces.

Some health jurisdictions have collected information for indicators relating to disease severity.[9] Although these indicators are not included in the NOHSS and have not been standardized for surveys, the ASTDD BSS manual outlines two approaches to assessing severity related to dental caries. These include (1) rampant decay: an individual has seven or more teeth with untreated and/or treated decay (no or yes) and (2) number of quadrants with untreated decay: record the number of quadrants with untreated decay (e.g., 0, 1, 2, 3, or 4).[9]

Intraoral epidemiologic examinations can be used to assess the occurrence of root surface caries in oral health surveys.[15,18] Assessments of each tooth (and surface) present can be evaluated by scoring,[15] as follows:

- Sound root
- Decayed root
- Filled root but with decay
- Filled root without decay
- Unexposed root (no gingival recession beyond the cementoenamel junction [CEJ])
- Bridge abutment/implant

The measurement of root surface caries in populations is generally based on the number of exposed root surfaces decayed or filled, with consideration given to the number of surfaces present in the mouth and at risk for dental caries.

Other surveys have used intraoral epidemiologic examinations and used a dichotomous scale for assessing root caries.[18] The examiner scores the status of the survey participant's whole mouth for the following variables[18]:

- Root caries detected/root caries not detected/cannot be assessed
- Root restoration detected/root restoration not detected/cannot be assessed

Additional measurements of dental caries have been developed to reflect treatment needs and to provide a broader profile of the impact of dental caries in population groups.[15] A measure of selected restoration and tooth conditions was developed to supplement the DMF Index and to characterize the prevalence and severity of physical and biologic conditions that result from dental caries. The Restorations and Tooth Conditions Assessment (RTCA) was measured in the third **National Health and Nutrition Examination Survey (NHANES** III).[15]

Primary Dentition

The DMF Index can be modified for primary teeth in children.[18,21] Indexes commonly used for assessing the primary dentition include the df index or dmf index. The df index is the sum of decayed (d) and filled (f) primary tooth surfaces (dfs) or teeth (dft). It does not include missing teeth because of the difficulty in distinguishing primary tooth loss as a result of dental caries from those lost by natural exfoliation.

NOTE: Upper case letters (e.g., DMFT) signify permanent teeth; lower case letters (e.g., dft) signify primary teeth.

For use in children before the age of exfoliation (<5 years), the dmf index can indicate the number of teeth or surfaces with history of decay: *d* denotes decayed teeth, *m* denotes missing teeth resulting from caries, and *f* denotes teeth that have been previously filled.

For preschool-age children, the assessment of early childhood caries has been used in population-based surveys. To assess the early childhood caries pattern, an examiner evaluates a young child's six maxillary anterior teeth and determines whether one or more of the teeth are decayed, filled, or missing because of dental caries.[9] Missing front teeth for preschool children are most likely a result of caries or traumatic injury. Therefore the cause of missing anterior teeth must be identified by questioning the parent or guardian, if present, during the screening or must include a question on the consent form. The ASTDD BSS includes methods for assessing early childhood caries and is only used for preschool children because this indicator is not used for children in kindergarten or higher grades.

Future Directions for Assessing Dental Caries

Numerous reports have acknowledged changes in both the pattern and distribution of dental caries and recommended evidence-based approaches to better detect, assess, diagnose, prevent, and monitor dental caries. During the past decade, there has been an increased concern about the dental caries status among vulnerable population groups that have not shown improvements in comparison to other groups. As more attention is focused on the prevention of dental caries, discussions are emerging about case definitions, diagnostic criteria, and stages of progression related to dental caries in clinical practice, clinical research, and population-based assessments.[20]

In light of these points, the International Caries Detection and Assessment System (ICDAS) was developed as a clinical scoring system and integrated into use within dental education, clinical practice, clinical research, epidemiology, and public health.[20] ICDAS was designed to lead to better quality information to inform decisions about appropriate diagnosis, prognosis, and clinical management at both the individual and public health levels. The ICDAS provides a framework to support and enable personalized oral health care for improved long-term health outcomes.

The ICDAS assesses coronal and root surfaces with criteria that extend the diagnostic criteria and definitions to evaluate specific stages of dental caries progression by including enamel carious lesions and dentinal carious lesions.[20] The system is based on standardized approaches to evaluate changes in the stages of the caries processes and integrates assessments of risks, measurement of caries activity (e.g., progressing, arrested, or regressing) and is linked with oral health care options.[20] Findings from assessments integrating ICDAS in population surveys would provide greater details about caries and be useful in monitoring dental caries to target prevention programs at the earliest stages of dental caries progression for individuals, groups, and communities.

Measurement of Dental Treatment Need

The **World Health Organization (WHO)** has established **Basic Methods for Oral Health Surveys** in its "Pathfinder" approach.[16] WHO includes the assessment of treatment needs. During the epidemiologic examination, the examiner records a treatment need for each tooth separately, and the treatment needs can be tabulated for population groups. Treatment categories include the following[16]:

- No treatment
- Preventive or caries-arresting care
- Sealant
- Restoration(s) (one or two or more surfaces)
- Crown for any reason
- Veneer or laminate
- Pulp care and restoration
- Indication for extraction
- Other treatment

For each person examined, the current status of a prosthesis and need for a prosthesis can be recorded by assessing the type of prosthesis needed and the arch in need.[15,16] It is also common to assess need for dental care and referral.

The assessment of treatment needs may be a problem because it is difficult to standardize clinical judgments for the most appropriate treatment required based on the treatment needs of the average person in the community. Findings of treatment needs can be useful for planning and monitoring purposes. They can be helpful in estimating personnel and service requirements, with demand levels for these services taken into consideration.

Summary assessments that record overall need for dental care (e.g., treatment urgency) are also used in oral health surveys. The ASTDD BSS methods use three categories of urgency evaluated during a screening to assess need and referral for dental care.[9] The categories of urgency outlined by the ASTDD are shown in **Box 4-4**.

Measurement of Dental Sealants

Dental sealants are traditionally assessed in populations through a basic screening or epidemiologic examination procedure.[9,18] Tooth surfaces and teeth can be evaluated for the presence or absence of dental sealants in the pits and fissures of erupted primary or permanent teeth. Sometimes, oral health survey protocols limit measurements for dental sealants to selected tooth surfaces or teeth (e.g., permanent molars).[9] The screener can assess for the presence of dental

BOX 4-4 Categories of Urgency According to ASTDD Basic Screening Survey (BSS) Methods

Category	Recommendation for Next Dental Visit	Criteria
Urgent need for dental care	As soon as possible	Signs or symptoms that include pain, infection, or swelling
Early dental care needed	Within several weeks	Caries without accompanying signs or symptoms or individuals with other oral health problems requiring care before their next routine dental visit
No obvious problems	Next regular checkup	Any patient without above problems

From Association of State & Territorial Dental Directors (ATSDD). Basic Screening Surveys: An Approach to Monitoring Community Oral Health—Preschool and School Children. Sparks, NV: ATSDD; 2008.

sealants on a per-person basis with the use of the ASTDD BSS methods.[9] The ASTDD protocol evaluates sealants on permanent molars, and this measure is collected only for elementary, middle, and high school children. During the screening a dichotomous measure is used to assess for the presence or absence of dental sealants. Children are coded as having sealants if they have at least one sealant on a permanent molar tooth, whether the sealant covers all or part of the pits or fissures or is partially lost. The ASTDD survey methods do not record sealants on primary teeth.

When a tooth is scored for treatment need in an oral health survey, the examiner can record the need for sealant or other preventive and caries-arresting care.[16] This measurement is included in the WHO Pathfinder methodology. This measure can be a problem because criteria for dental sealant need and caries-arresting care have not been standardized for oral epidemiologic surveys. Appendix D summarizes how dental sealants has been monitored for *Healthy People 2010* and key data sources.

Measurement of Periodontal Disease

Gingivitis is characterized by localized inflammation, swelling, and bleeding of the soft tissues surrounding a tooth without loss of connective tissue or bone support. The condition results in swelling and bleeding of the gums. Gingivitis usually is reversible with proper daily oral hygiene, and its presence or absence serves as a crude measure of a person's self-care practices (e.g., toothbrushing).[22] Although not all occurrences of gingivitis progress to periodontal disease, all periodontal disease starts as gingivitis.[22] Destructive periodontal disease is manifested by the loss of the connective tissue and bone that support the teeth.[22] Destructive periodontal disease places a person at risk for eventual tooth loss unless appropriate treatment commences.

Contemporary indexes to assess the health of periodontal tissues in population-based surveys reflect current theories of the pathogenesis of periodontal diseases.[17,22,23] A disaggregated approach is taken to evaluate and record clinical signs of disease. Each measure usually is scored separately. Typical clinical signs that can be measured to assess periodontal status include the following[17,18]:

- Gingival bleeding
- Loss of supporting structure as a measure of past disease (recession or loss of periodontal attachment)
- Pocket formation
- Calculus as a contributing risk factor

For the oral epidemiologic examination procedures, explicit protocols and criteria were outlined for assessments of periodontal status.[17,18,22-24] In an epidemiologic examination the examiner measured gingivitis with the use of the gingival bleeding index by "walking" the probe inside the gingival sulcus to determine the number of sites of gingival bleeding. In addition, periodontal pocket depth on probing, calculus (supragingival or subgingival), and furcations were assessed in the epidemiologic examination. The measurements allowed for the calculation of recession and loss of attachment. The loss of clinical periodontal attachment is defined as the distance in millimeters between the CEJ and the bottom of the sulcus (e.g., periodontal depth minus the distance from the CEJ to the free gingival margin). The extent and severity of destructive periodontal disease are often measured by loss of periodontal attachment, pocket-probing depth, and furcation involvement. The periodontal assessments for NHANES during specific years has included measures to determine loss of attachment and to identify bleeding on probing.[17,18,23-24] Appendix D summarizes how periodontal disease has been monitored for *Healthy People 2010* and key data sources.

The presence of at least one bleeding site has been used to define gingivitis in populations and is used to measure progress in *Healthy People 2010*.[13] The occurrence of destructive periodontal disease is often measured by loss of periodontal attachment. The presence of one or more sites with loss of periodontal attachment of 4 mm or greater has been used to delineate destructive periodontal disease in a population. This measure has been used to monitor achievement of targets for the national oral health objectives, and it has allowed the monitoring of changes in destructive periodontal disease over time, distinguishing the status of one population from that of another.

A method of assessing periodontal health status, the **Community Periodontal Index (CPI)**, has been developed by WHO and is included in the WHO basic methods for oral health surveys.[16] It is a modification of the Community Periodontal Index of Treatment Needs (CPITN). The CPI allows for a rapid assessment of periodontal status of a population according to various grades of periodontal health.

The CPI divides the teeth into sextants for measurement. The severest measurement of the sextant is scored during an epidemiologic examination. The CPI provides a measurement of the following:

- Healthy gingiva
- Presence or absence of gingival bleeding
- Supragingival or subgingival calculus
- Periodontal pockets (shallow, 4 to 5 mm, and deep, 6 mm or more)

Loss of periodontal attachment is measured, and the highest score is recorded by sextant. The treatment need codes for observed conditions were eliminated from the original CPITN because they did not reflect contemporary theories of periodontal diseases. The CPI calls for a specially designed lightweight probe with a 0.5-mm ball at its tip and bearing specific millimeter markings. In the United States, a modified version of the CPI, the Periodontal Screening Record (PSR), is used for screening in the clinical setting.[14]

Sometimes, to increase efficiency, to lower cost, and to decrease time spent on the epidemiologic examination, partial-mouth periodontal measurements are made to assess periodontal health. Historically, the Periodontal Disease Index (PDI) included specific index teeth to be measured, dubbed the "Ramfjord teeth."[17] The CPI identifies specific index teeth for different age groups.[16] Two quadrants (one maxillary and one mandibular) were randomly selected, and specific tooth sites were measured for the periodontal examination in the NHANES.[18,22]

Future Directions for Assessing Periodontal Disease

Current methods of periodontal disease surveillance in the population have traditionally required clinically based periodontal examinations, which are resource intensive and costly.[17,22,24] Thus the capacity to monitor the disease at the population level has been restricted, especially among subsets of the vulnerable population groups at highest risk for periodontal disease, as well as specific geographic areas. Population-based surveillance of periodontal disease is very limited at the state and local levels, even though public health activities are designed to target state and local populations.[17,22,24] Existing state and local based oral health surveillance systems do not have the resources required to support clinically assessed periodontal data. The future of population-based periodontal disease surveillance at the national, state, and local levels relies on developing less resource-demanding measures that can be integrated into existing surveillance systems.[17,22,24]

In light of these considerations, the Division of Oral Health of the CDC collaborated with the American Academy of Periodontology (AAP) and convened a workgroup on Periodontal Disease Surveillance. The purpose of this workgroup was to respond to the need for surveillance measures to assess the prevalence of periodontal disease that can be used more broadly in a population.[17,24] The aim of the workgroup was to identify reliable and valid self-reported surveillance measures for periodontal infections, as well as possible sentinel sites, events, providers, and payers.[17,24]

Thus, in the past decade the CDC and AAP investigated the use of self-report measures for predicting prevalence of periodontitis in the US population. Findings from a number of analyses, including data from an Australian National Survey, identified six questions as possible predictors for periodontitis.[17] Results from several studies further suggest that measures obtained using self-report oral health questions, in combination with demographic information, are promising for predicting the prevalence of periodontitis in the adult US population.[17] The 2009–2010 NHANES uses clinically-based periodontal examination in which all teeth are included in the periodontal assessment.[17] Also, a series of questions is asked of survey participants 30 years and older about the condition of their teeth and factors related to periodontal health. **Box 4-5** outlines the questions used in NHANES to evaluate factors influencing periodontal status.

Measurement of Retention and Loss of Teeth

"No tooth loss" is equivalent to "tooth retention." "Complete tooth loss" reflects no remaining teeth regardless of the cause of the loss[16,18] Lack of any natural teeth is defined as edentulous or edentulism. An individual with at least one natural tooth is considered dentate. Tooth retention and tooth loss can be measured in oral health surveys.[16,18]

The ASTTD BSS methods specified for adult populations assesses edentulism on a per-person basis. A dichotomous measure is used during the screening of adults to record the absence of all natural teeth or the presence of all natural teeth.

In an epidemiologic examination, each tooth space can be assessed and scored to evaluate retention or loss of natural teeth.[16,18] Data collected about the presence or absence of each tooth are used as indicators of tooth retention and tooth loss at the tooth level, arch level, or individual level for population studies. The Tooth Count section of the clinical assessment evaluates the number and types of teeth retained by the individual.

Missing teeth can be assessed by tooth type and are scored by cause of loss (e.g., caries, periodontal disease, trauma, congenital absence, or orthodontia).[16-18] However, determining the exact cause of tooth loss is difficult and can be problematic for a dental examiner. Assessment of tooth retention and loss can be made in the primary or permanent dentition. The missing primary tooth score should be used only in an age group in which normal exfoliation would not sufficiently explain tooth absence.

Self-reported dentition status can be provided in a face-to-face interview or in a telephone interview.[25,26] Tooth loss was assessed in 2010 through the **Behavioral Risk Factor Surveillance System (BRFSS)** Core Question by asking survey participants the following question in a telephone interview[25]:

- How many of your permanent teeth have been removed because of tooth decay or gum disease? (Include teeth lost to infection but do not include teeth lost for other reasons such as injury or orthodontics. NOTE: If wisdom teeth are removed because of tooth decay or gum disease, they should be included in the count for lost teeth.)
  1. 1 to 5
  2. 6 or more but not all
  3. All
  4. None

BOX 4-5 Questions from NHANES to Assess Factors Related to Periodontal Health and Disease

Question	Responses
{Have you/Has survey participant} lost all of {your/his/her} upper and lower natural (permanent) teeth?	Yes (end of section) No Refused (end of section) Don't Know (end of section)
Gum disease is a common problem with the mouth. People with gum disease might have swollen gums, receding gums, sore or infected gums, or loose teeth. {Do you/Does survey participant} think {you/she/he} might have gum disease?	Yes No
Overall, how would {you/survey participant} rate the health of {your/his/her} teeth and gums?	Excellent Very Good Good Fair Poor
{Have you/Has survey participant} ever had treatment for gum disease, such as scaling and root planing, sometimes called *deep cleaning?*	Yes No
{Have you/Has survey participant} ever had any teeth become loose on their own, without an injury?	Yes No
{Have you/Has survey participant} ever been told by a dental professional that {you/she/he} have lost bone around {your/his/her} teeth?	Yes No
During the past 3 months, {have you/has survey participant} noticed a tooth that doesn't look right?	Yes No
Aside from brushing {your/his/her} teeth with a toothbrush, in the last 7 days, how many days did {you/survey participant} use dental floss or any other device to clean between {your/his/her} teeth?	Enter number of days
Aside from brushing {your/his/her} teeth with a toothbrush, in the last 7 days, how many days did {you/survey participant} use mouthwash or other dental rinse product that {you use/she/he uses} to treat dental disease or dental problems?	Enter number of days

From Centers for Disease Control and Prevention (CDC). National Health and Nutrition Examination Survey (NHANES) 2009–2010, Sample Person Questionnaire: Adult Supplement. Hyattsville, MD: National Center for Health Statistics, CDC; 2008.

    5. Don't know/Not sure

    6. Refused

    In addition, complete tooth loss can be tracked through personal interviews, and this method constitutes the basis of the measure used in the NHANES and **National Health Interview Survey (NHIS)**.[18,26] In addition to the clinical assessment NHANES has asked a single question in the interview component.[18] The question used in NHANES is: (have you/has survey participant) lost all of (your/his/her) upper and lower natural (permanent) teeth? Responses include yes, no, refused, or do not know. Two questions have been used in the NHIS to assess edentulous status of each arch, and responses of "yes" to both questions determined complete tooth loss.[26] The questions are (1) Have you lost all of your upper natural (permanent) teeth? Responses: Yes/ No, and (2) Have you lost all of your lower natural (permanent) teeth? Responses: Yes/No. The NHIS has changed and used a single question to assess edentulism: Have you lost all of your upper and lower natural permanent teeth? Responses: Yes/No.[26]

Appendix D summarizes the ways tooth loss has been monitored for *Healthy People 2010* and key data sources.

Measurement of Oral and Pharyngeal Cancer

Data to measure the number of deaths resulting from cancer of the oral cavity or pharynx are obtained from death certificates collected through the National Vital Statistics System, within the National Center for Health Statistics (NCHS) of the CDC; such data are available at the state and local levels.[13,17] This measure is based on the number of deaths resulting from oropharyngeal cancer per 100,000 people attributed to cancers classified in coded categories 140 to 149 of the tenth edition of the *International Classification of Diseases* (ICD-10). The original baseline statistic for *Healthy People 2010* was based on codes 140 to 149 of the ICD-9. Oral and pharyngeal cancers include cancers of the lip, tongue, buccal mucosa, floor of the mouth, and pharynx.

A second measure tracked is the proportion of oral and pharyngeal cancer lesions diagnosed at the earliest stage (e.g., stage 1, localized).[13,17] This measure is collected through state cancer registries and the surveillance, epidemiology, and end results (SEER) of the National Cancer Institute (NCI) of the NIH. Specific factors related to population groups (e.g., age, gender, race, or ethnicity) are often identified in assessments of oral and pharyngeal cancers in populations.

Another measure related to oral and pharyngeal cancer is the receipt of an examination to detect oral and pharyngeal cancer. The NHIS has assessed the receipt of an oral cancer examination through self-reports.[26,27] The face-to-face interview conducted for NHIS in 1998 included two questions to assess self-report of an oral cancer examination in 1998.[26] **Box 4-6** outlines a series of four questions used in a 2008 NHIS questionnaire for adults 18 years and older to evaluate examination for oral cancer.[27] Appendix D summarizes how oral and pharyngeal cancers have been monitored for *Healthy People 2010* and key data sources.

Measurement of Other Oral and Craniofacial Diseases, Conditions, and Injuries

Measurement of Malocclusion and Craniofacial Anomalies

Malocclusion through evaluation of occlusal characteristics can be assessed during a population-based oral health survey.[18] Some measurements focus on clinical measures of function, whereas other measurements are used to assess aesthetics. The evaluation of functional occlusal contacts was included in the epidemiologic examination protocol for persons 25 years and older for NHANES.[18] It included measurements using the functional occlusal contacts index (FOCI) that consisted of (1) an assessment of the posterior (premolar and molar) regions and then (2) a similar assessment for the sum of anterior tooth contacts.[18] The right and then left posterior regions were assessed for (1) the number of contacts between natural teeth, (2) natural teeth and pontics of fixed prostheses, (3) natural teeth and removable prostheses, and (4) the number of contacts between denture teeth.[18] Because there are few anterior teeth missing without prostheses in the US adult population, the anterior assessment is limited to a single assessment requiring at least one anterior mandibular tooth in contact with an opposing anterior tooth irrespective of the type of teeth involved in the dentition.

BOX 4-6 **Questions from National Health Interview Survey to Assess Receipt of Oral Cancer Examination**

Questions	Responses
Have you ever heard of an examination for oral or mouth cancer?	Yes No
Have you ever had an examination for oral cancer in which the doctor, dentist, or other health professional pulls on your tongue, sometimes with gauze wrapped around it, and feels under the tongue and inside the cheeks?	Yes No
Have you ever had an examination for oral cancer in which the doctor, dentist, or other health professional feels your neck?	Yes No
When did you have your most recent oral or mouth cancer examination? Was it within the past year, between 1 and 3 years ago, or over 3 years ago?	Within past year Between 1 and 3 years ago Over 3 years ago
Did you have your most recent oral cancer examination during a routine checkup or because you were having a specific problem?	Part of routine checkup For a specific problem
What type of health care professional performed your most recent oral cancer examination?	Doctor/Physician Nurse/nurse practitioner Dentists (include oral surgeons, orthodontists) Dental hygienist Other

From Centers for Disease Control and Prevention (CDC). National Health Interview Survey, 2008 questionnaire: Adult Supplement. Hyattsville, MD: National Center for Health Statistics, CDC; 2008.

WHO incorporates the Dental Aesthetics Index (DAI) in its epidemiologic examination protocol for a basic oral health survey.[16] The DAI considers an individual's social and psychologic well-being as the main benefit of orthodontic treatment. It includes objective measurements of aesthetic acceptability according to social norms.[28] Clinical assessments of missing incisors, canines, or premolars are recorded along with the following evaluations:
- Crowding and spacing in the incisal segments of both arches
- Diastema
- Largest anterior maxillary and mandibular irregularities (rotations or displacements from normal alignment)
- Anterior maxillary and mandibular overjet
- Vertical anterior open bite
- Anteroposterior molar relation

In the United States, craniofacial anomalies (including cleft lip and palate) are usually expressed as a proportion or rate based on recordings of congenital anomalies in birth certificates.[17,29] Recordings of craniofacial anomalies and oral clefts on birth certificates may not be universal.

Measurement of Orofacial Injuries

Tooth trauma can be assessed through oral epidemiologic examination procedures to evaluate clinical evidence of tooth injury and treatment received for the injury.[18] Incisor trauma has been assessed in NHANES because individuals aged 6 to 29 years received the Incisor Trauma Assessment for the maxillary and mandibular permanent incisors only.[18] A history of trauma is obtained by questioning individuals in the sample, and assessments are recorded for the eight permanent incisors in specific aged children and adults. The examiner proceeds to examine the eight permanent incisors carefully for evidence of traumatic injury. A positive history of trauma is determined for each permanent incisor tooth and an assignment of a specific code is given based on assessment of particular conditions and/or treatments. The assessment tracks the status of the tooth, from sound (no evidence of trauma) through a missing tooth caused by trauma, and reflects selected sequelae of trauma.[18] The classification scheme measures soundness or levels of tooth trauma and is applied to each of the incisor teeth or tooth spaces, as outlined in **Box 4-7**.

Measurement of Orofacial Pain and Temporomandibular Dysfunction

A temporomandibular joint (TMJ) assessment is included in the WHO basic oral health survey guide.[16] The guide suggests evaluation of signs such as the occurrence of clicking, tenderness on palpation, and reduced jaw mobility on opening greater than 30 mm during an epidemiologic examination. Brief interview questions are added to ascertain symptoms and include self-report of clicking, pain, or difficulties in opening or closing the jaw once or more within a week. An Orofacial Pain Assessment is included in NHANES with the use of the Orofacial Pain Questionnaire and Orofacial Pain Examination.[18] The Orofacial Pain Questionnaire assesses the frequency of experiences in the past 30 days with specific types of orofacial pain, including tooth-ache; sores or irritations; pain in the jaw joint; dull, aching pain across the face; and burning sensations in the mouth. Positive responses to questions about orofacial pain lead to quality-of-life questions assessing worry or concerns about the pain sensations and days lost to usual activities

BOX 4-7 Incisor Trauma Assessment

Score	Criteria
0	A permanent tooth has no evidence of traumatic injury.
1	An unrestored enamel fracture is present in a permanent tooth that does not involve the dentine.
2	An unrestored fracture in a permanent tooth that involves the dentine.
3	Untreated pulpal damage to a permanent tooth as evidenced by one of the following: (1) dark discoloration, as compared with other teeth—a discoloration of one tooth, or adjacent teeth, that are otherwise healthy is considered a sign of pulpal injury or, (2) swelling or a fistula in the labial or lingual vestibule adjacent to an otherwise healthy tooth
4	A fracture has been restored in a permanent tooth, either with a full crown or a less extensive restoration. It may be necessary to question the survey participant or responsible adult to ascertain the reason for the restoration.
5	The presence of a lingual restoration in a permanent tooth as a sign of endodontic therapy, and a positive history from the survey participant or responsible adult of root canal therapy following traumatic injury.
6	A permanent tooth is missing due to trauma.

From Centers for Disease Control and Prevention (CDC), National Center for Health Statistics. National Health and Nutrition Examination Survey (NHANES) Dental Examiners Procedures Manual (revised). Hyattsville, MD: CDC; 2004.

of daily life (e.g., work, school, self-care, and recreation) because of orofacial pain. In addition, an extraoral examination is conducted to assess orofacial pain by measuring the maximal incisal opening in millimeters and palpating the muscles of mastication and the TMJ region for tenderness.

Measurement of Dental Fluorosis

Dean's Fluorosis Index is the conventional index used to assess for dental fluorosis.[17,18] This index is one of the most universally accepted classifications for dental fluorosis. Each tooth present in an individual's mouth is rated according to these classifications: normal, questionable, very mild, mild, moderate, and severe. The classifications are based on specific criteria describing the enamel. The individual's fluorosis score is based on the severest form of fluorosis recorded for two or more teeth. Dean's Fluorosis Index is included in the WHO basic oral health survey methods.[16] Dental fluorosis has been classified in a number of other ways, including the Tooth Surface Index of Fluorosis, the Thylstrup-Fejerskov Index, and the Fluorosis Risk Index.[17]

The criteria for classifying and scoring dental fluorosis have been slightly modified from the system originally described by Dean in 1942 for the NHANES.[18] The assessment is conducted on survey participants 6 to 19 years of age, and only the maxillary anterior teeth (cuspids and incisors) are evaluated for fluorosis in NHANES. Each tooth is examined and assigned to one of six categories according to its degree of dental fluorosis. For analysis, classification of a person is based on the two teeth most affected by fluorosis. If the two teeth are not equally affected, the classification given to the person is the score for the less involved tooth. The modified criteria and the corresponding scores used in NHANES are provided **Box 4-8**.[18]

Measurement of Tooth Wear

The NHANES provided an opportunity to assess the prevalence of dental erosion and tooth wear across the lifespan among varied population groups to discern if health disparities existed nationally.[18] The survey permitted clinical assessments using the Tooth Wear Index in survey participants 13 years and older, as well as evaluation of dietary factors, medications, health conditions, and demographics on a nationally represented sample.[18] The Tooth Wear Index that Smith and Knight described in 1984, with modifications by Millward and colleagues from 1994, has been used in the assessment of dental erosion in epidemiologic surveys and studies.[18] The Tooth Wear Index

BOX 4-8 Modified Deans Index Used in National Health and Nutrition Examination Survey

Score	Criteria
0	Normal: No fluorosis detected
1	Very mild: Opaque, paper white areas involving less than one-quarter of the tooth surface
2	Mild: Opaque, paper white areas involving one-quarter to less than one-half of the tooth surface
3	Moderate: Opaque paper white areas involving one-half or more of the tooth surface
4	Severe: Discrete or confluent pitting in involved areas
5	Questionable: Slight aberration of normal enamel appearance, including white flecks

From Centers for Disease Control and Prevention (CDC), National Center for Health Statistics. National Health and Nutrition Examination Survey (NHANES) Dental Examiners Procedures Manual (revised). Hyattsville, MD: CDC; 2004.

used in the United Kingdom 1998 Adult Dental Health Survey was used in the NHANES.[18] Visual examination of the facial, lingual, and incisal surfaces of the teeth divided into four segments for the purpose of this assessment using a surface reflecting mirror, an examining light, and with each tooth surface being dried before inspection.[18] The Tooth Wear Scoring System specifies the criteria for assessment of tooth wear and is shown in **Box 4-9**.[18]

Measurement of Access to Oral Health Services

Measurement of Access to Community Prevention: Water Fluoridation

Community water fluoridation, a community preventive service, is measured by the percentage of persons served by public water systems containing optimally fluoridated water.[13] Optimal levels of fluoridation are achieved by adjusting fluoride to obtain a concentration between 0.7 and 1.2 parts per million (ppm).[30] The optimal fluoride concentration is determined by geographic areas based on mean daily temperature; thus states have different levels of optimal concentration of fluoride in water.[30]

To characterize a community as optimally fluoridated, it is necessary to compare tap water or water samples from water treatment plants with the level determined by the state to be optimal for that community. National information related to public water systems and community water fluoridation is obtained from the **Water Fluoridation Reporting System (WFRS),** an interactive

BOX 4-9 Tooth Wear Index

Score	Surface	Criteria
0	All	Sound natural tooth surface. Any wear is restricted to the enamel and does not extend into dentin.
1	All	Loss of enamel just exposing dentin.
2	B, L	Loss of enamel exposing dentin for more than an estimated one third of the individual surface area (B, L).
	O, I	Loss of enamel and extensive loss of dentin but not exposing secondary dentin or pulp. On occlusal/incisal surfaces exposed dentin facets with a buccolingual dimension of 2 mm or greater at the widest point will be seen.
3	B, L	Complete loss of enamel on a surface, pulp exposure or exposure of secondary dentin where the pulp used to be. Frank pulp exposure is most unlikely.
	O, I	Pulp exposure or exposure of secondary dentin.
8	All	Fractured tooth. Clear evidence of traumatic loss of tooth substance rather than wear.
9	All	Cannot assess. More than 75% of surface is obscured and no remaining incisal edge/tip that can be coded. Includes missing teeth, crowns, and abutments.

B, Buccal; *L,* lingual, *I,* incisal; *O,* occlusal.
From Centers for Disease Control and Prevention (CDC), National Center for Health Statistics. National Health and Nutrition Examination Survey (NHANES) Dental Examiners Procedures Manual (revised). Hyattsville, MD: CDC; 2004.

Internet-based monitoring and surveillance program available for use by state and tribal fluoridation managers.[30] WFRS is one of the first CDC surveillance systems to collect and edit data over
the Internet in "real time" (information entered instantaneously updates data records). The application was developed by the CDC in collaboration with the ASTDD to monitor fluoridation at
the local and state levels in the United States.

WFRS allows state and tribal fluoridation managers to update basic water system information
such as populations served, fluoridation status, communities and counties served, and contact
information for more than 52,000 community water systems directly over the Internet. WFRS
maintains the relationships among water systems that buy and sell water to each other, allowing
the fluoride content of a water system to be found, whether it produces its own water or purchases
water from another system.

Although knowing which systems are fluoridated is important, WFRS was also designed as a
tool to assist states and tribes in monitoring the quality of fluoridation. Users can enter monthly
data such as high, low, and average fluoride concentrations and split-sample analysis and can
indicate whether the water system met the daily testing requirements. Using criteria supplied by
the state or tribe, WFRS evaluates the data entered to determine whether the water system provided "optimally" (e.g., the fluoride concentration is within the desired range) fluoridated water
for the month. Numerous reports provide fluoridation managers with the tools they need to
improve the quality of fluoridation. This voluntary reporting system compiles information on the
number of people served by the fluoridated water system, the number of counties and cities served
by the fluoridated water system, and the quality of the fluoridated water system. These quality
measures will include the number of months the system is operating with optimal fluoride concentration. Data from WFRS are used to update the water fluoridation information and maps
on the NOHSS. CDC produces an annual report from the WFRS database.[30] Appendix D
includes a summary of ways community water fluoridation has been monitored for *Healthy People
2010* and key data sources.

Measurement of Access to the Oral Health Care System

Access to the oral health system consists of many facets, including availability, accessibility, accom-
modation, affordability, and acceptability.[31-35] Multiple factors have been assessed to explain the
use of clinical oral health services. These factors have been summarized as epidemiologic,
social, demographic, personal, and psychologic, as well as characteristic of the oral health care
system.[1,3,31-35]

A common measure of access to and use of the oral health care system is having an annual
dental visit.[13] This measure is assessed by determining the length of time since the last visit to a
dentist or dental clinic. Appendix D includes a summary of the ways to monitor the use of the
oral health care system for *Healthy People 2010* and key data sources.

Responses to interview questions have been used to measure the percentage of persons who
have had a dental visit in the past year.[13] The **Medical Expenditure Panel Survey (MEPS)**, which
uses a face-to-face interview to assess dental visits, is used to measure progress of the *Healthy
People 2010* objectives regarding dental attendance.[13] Other national surveys, such as NHANES
and NHIS, use face-to-face interviews with structured questionnaires to evaluate dental visits.[18,27]
Specific questions about dental visits are included in these questionnaires.[1,3,31-35]

The CDC, through its state-specific BRFSS, conducts telephone interviews to assess dental
attendance.[26] **Box 4-10** outlines the questions included in the 2010 BRFSS to evaluate access to
oral health care. In addition, self-administered questionnaires have been used by states and locali-

BOX 4-10 Questions Related to Access to Oral Health Care Included in the Behavioral Risk Factor Surveillance Survey (BRFSS)

Question	Responses
How long has it been since you last visited a dentist or a dental clinic for any reason? Include visits to dental specialists such as orthodontists.	1. Within the past year (anytime less than 12 months ago) 2. Within the past 2 years (1 year but less than 2 years ago) 3. Within the past 5 years (2 years but less than 5 years ago) 4. 5 or more years ago
How long has it been since you had your teeth cleaned by a dentist or dental hygienist?	1. Within the past year (anytime less than 12 months ago) 2. Within the past 2 years (1 year but less than 2 years ago) 3. Within the past 5 years (2 years but less than 5 years ago) 4. 5 or more years ago

From Centers for Disease Control and Prevention (CDC). 2010 Behavioral Risk Factor Surveillance System (BRFSS) Questionnaire. Atlanta: CDC; 2009.

ties to determine access to dental care.[9] The questionnaire may be completed by adult participants in surveys or by parents of children participating in school-based oral health surveys. The National Nursing Home Survey, conducted by the NCHS of the CDC in 1997 and 1999, measured the receipt of dental care services by nursing home residents in the past month.[13] For *Healthy People 2020*, the assessment of residents in long-term care facilities has been proposed to evaluate access to dental care in the past year.[6] Other important measures associated with access to oral care have been used in several national, state, and local surveys and include questions assessing the following[1,3,31-35]:

- Dental attendance for routine checkups or cleanings
- Assessment of dental insurance coverage
- Usual source of dental care
- Reason for not having a dental visit in the past year
- Difficulty in obtaining needed dental care
- Purpose of last dental visit

Box 4-11 outlines examples of questions about access to care that are included with the BSS methods developed by the ASTTD.[9] These questions can be included in a self-administered questionnaire or can be asked during a telephone or face-to-face interview.

Measurement of Oral Health, Well-Being, and Quality of Life

Quality of Life

Two major goals of *Healthy People 2010* were to (1) increase quality and years of healthy life and (2) eliminate health disparities.[5] **Quality of life** has been defined as individual's perceptions of their position in life in the context of the culture and value system in which they live and in relation to their goals, expectations, standards, and concerns.[4,5] It refers to a subjective evaluation, which induces both positive and negative dimensions and is embedded in a cultural, social, and environmental context.[1,4,5,17,36] Quality of life is a broad-ranging concept, incorporating in a complex way a person's physical health, psychologic state, level of independence, social relationships, personal beliefs, and relationship to salient features of the environment.[1,4,5,17,36] Six broad domains describe core aspects of quality of life cross-culturally,[37] as follows:

BOX 4-11 **Questions to Evaluate the Use of the Oral Health Care System***

1. During the past 6 months, did {you/your child} have a toothache more than once, when biting or chewing? [Source: *National Health Interview Survey,* 1989]
   1. Yes
   2. No
   3. Don't know/don't remember
2. About how long has it been since {you/your child} last visited a dentist? Include all types of dentists, such as orthodontists, oral surgeons, and all other dental specialists, as well as dental hygienists. [Source: *National Health Interview Survey,* 1997]
   1. 6 months or less
   2. More than 6 months but not more than 1 year ago
   3. More than 1 year ago but not more than 3 years ago
   4. More than 3 years ago
   5. Never have been
   6. Don't know/don't remember
3. What was the main reason that {you/your child} last visited a dentist? (Please check one.) [Source: *National Health Interview Survey,* 1986]
   1. Went in on own for checkup, examination, or cleaning
   2. Was called in by the dentist for checkup, examination, or cleaning
   3. Something was wrong, bothering, or hurting
   4. Went for treatment of a condition that dentist discovered at earlier checkup or examination
   5. Other
   6. Don't know/don't remember
4. During the past 12 months, was there a time when {you/your child} needed dental care but could not get it at that time? [Source: *National Health Interview Survey,* 1994]
   1. Yes
   2. No
   3. Don't know/don't remember
5. The last time {you/your child} could not get the dental care {you/he/she} needed, what was the main reason {you/he/she} couldn't get care? (Please check one.) [Source: *National Health Interview Survey,* 1994]
   1. Could not afford it
   2. No insurance
   3. Dentist did not accept Medicaid/insurance
   4. Not serious enough
   5. Wait too long in clinic/office
   6. Difficulty in getting appointment
   7. Don't like/trust/believe in dentists
   8. No dentist available
   9. Didn't know where to go
   10. No way to get there
   11. Hours not convenient
   12. Speak a different language
   13. Health of another family member

BOX 4-11 Questions to Evaluate the Use of the Oral Health Care System*—cont'd

14. Other reason
15. Don't know/don't remember
6. Do you have any kind of insurance that pays for some or all of {you/your child's} medical or surgical care? Include health insurance obtained through employment or purchased directly, as well as government programs like Medicaid.
   1. Yes
   2. No
   3. Don't know/don't remember
7. Do you have any kind of insurance that pays for some or all of {your/your child's} dental care? Include health insurance obtained through employment or purchased directly, as well as government programs like Medicaid.
   1. Yes
   2. No
   3. Don't know/don't remember
Additional questions for survey planners to consider:
8. During the past 12 months, was there a time when you felt that {you/your child} needed medical care or surgery but could not get it at that time? [Source: Modified from *National Health Interview Survey*, 1994]
   1. Yes
   2. No
   3. Don't know/don't remember
9. The last time {you/your child} could not get the medical care or surgery {you/he/she} needed, what was the main reason {you/he/she} couldn't get care? [Source: *National Health Interview Survey*, 1994]
   1. Could not afford it
   2. No insurance
   3. Doctor did not accept Medicaid/insurance
   4. Not serious enough
   5. Wait too long in clinic/office
   6. Difficulty in getting appointment
   7. Don't like/trust/believe in doctors
   8. No doctor available
   9. Didn't know where to go
   10. No way to get there
   11. Hours not convenient
   12. Speak a different language
   13. Health of another family member
   14. Other reason
   15. Don't know/don't remember

From Association of State & Territorial Dental Directors (ATSDD) Basic Screening Surveys. An Approach to Monitoring Community Oral Health—Preschool and School Children. Sparks, NV: ATSDD; 2008.
*For all questions, refused/no response is a coding option but is not listed as a choice on the questionnaire. For one-digit variables, 9 is coded. For two-digit variables, the refused/no response code is 99.

- Physical domain (e.g., energy, fatigue)
- Psychological domain (e.g., positive feelings)
- Level of independence (e.g., mobility)
- Social relationships (e.g., practical social support)
- Environment (e.g., accessibility of health care)
- Personal beliefs/spirituality (e.g., meaning in life)

In public health and in health care, the concept of **health–related quality of life (HRQOL)** refers to a person or group's perceived physical and mental health over time.[1,4,5,17,36] Health professionals have often used HRQOL to measure the effects of chronic illness in patients to better understand how an illness interferes with a person's daily life. Similarly, public health professionals use HRQOL to measure the effects of numerous disorders, short- and long-term disabilities, and diseases in different populations. Tracking HRQOL in different populations can identify subgroups with poor physical or mental health and can help guide policies or interventions to improve their health.

HRQOL reflects a personal sense of physical and mental health and the ability to react to factors in the physical and social environments. HRQOL is more subjective than life expectancy and can be more difficult to measure in surveys of populitions.[1,4,5,17,36] The following tools have been developed to measure HRQOL[1,17,36,37]:

- *Global assessments:* Person rates his or her health as "poor," "fair," "good," "very good," or "excellent"
- *Healthy days:* Estimate of the number of days of poor or impaired physical and mental health in the past 30 days
- *Years of healthy life:* A combined measure developed for the Healthy People initiative to assess national health goals in the United States by evaluating the difference between life expectancy and years of healthy life reflects the average amount of time spent in less than optimal health because of chronic or acute limitations

Oral Health–Related Quality of Life

A better understanding of cultural, social, behavioral, psychologic, and economic factors related to oral conditions and treatments can contribute to oral health efforts at the community level.[33,38-40] During an assessment, it is also important to consider the belief systems and cultural values, customs, traditions, and institutions related to the oral health of individuals and groups.[3] Measurements of knowledge, attitudes, beliefs, and behaviors traditionally have been used to evaluate personal oral health practices and use of the oral health care system.[1,3]

Data collection methods have been developed to assess oral health knowledge, attitudes, beliefs, and behaviors.[1,3] Multiple measurements have been designed to evaluate diverse factors as they relate to oral health care-seeking behaviors, oral hygiene and home care practices, dietary practices, use of tobacco and alcohol, age-appropriate safety measures, and use of protective gear.[1,38]

The development of sociodental indicators has been advocated to assess the nonclinical aspects of oral diseases.[3,17,36,39,40] Measures have been recommended to document the full impact of oral disorders and treatment within populations. Different measures have been used to evaluate economic impact and social and psychologic consequences of oral diseases, conditions, and injuries.[3,17,36,39,40] These measures have been developed to assess outcomes at the individual and societal levels. The term *oral health–related quality of life* **(OHRQOL)** has been adopted as a construct that considers multiple dimensions of oral health.[17,36,40]

OHRQOL is that part of a person's quality of life that is affected by his or her oral health.[17,36,40] It describes people's perspectives of the ways in which oral diseases, conditions, and treatments affect their symptoms, function, and well-being. OHRQOL is one aspect of an individuals' HRQOL, and a complete separation of OHRQOL and HRQOL is not possible because oral health is one aspect of overall health. Thus issues related to one's overall HRQOL are relevant to those related to OHRQOL and vice versa. This is a multidimensional construct that reflects (among other things) people's comfort when eating, sleeping, and engaging in social interaction; their self-esteem; and their satisfaction with respect to their oral health.[11,17,36,40] OHRQOL considers how oral health affects the person's quality of life based on the following dimensions[17,36,40]:

- Functional dimensions (being able to bite, chew, swallow, speak, and sleep)
- Sensations of pain and discomfort
- Psychological factors (concerning the person's appearance, self-esteem, and smile)
- Social well-being (eating or speaking in front of others, intimacy, personal contact/social integration, and social roles)

Perceived health status and general assessment of oral health are common measurements used in population-based oral health surveys. Global assessments use a ranking scale as a person rates his or her oral health. These questions have been included in many national health surveys and the International Collaborative Study of Oral Health Outcomes, sponsored by WHO.[41] The questions use a basic Likert measurement scale to assess self-perceived health status. The NHANES includes the following questions:[18]

- Would you say your health in general is excellent, very good, good, fair, or poor?
- How would you describe the condition of your teeth and gums? Is it excellent, very good, good, fair, poor, or very poor?

Satisfaction with oral health status is another measurement used in surveys. Satisfaction ratings to assess OHRQOL are measures used to ask individuals how satisfied (or dissatisfied) they are with their oral health status in relation to symptoms, physical function, appearance, social function, and psychologic status. Assessment instruments, such as the Geriatric Oral Health Assessment Instrument (GOHAI) and the Oral Health Impact Profile (OHIP), have been developed to evaluate OHRQOL.[1,17,36,40]

The psychosocial and functional dimensions of oral health have been used in studies of population groups.[1,34] These dimensions consider the crucial sensory, communicative, gustatory, and psychosocial functions of the structures related to the teeth, mouth, and face, such as social function, and the impact of oral disorders on intimacy, personal contact, social integration, and social roles.[1]

The functional dimensions of oral health have been assessed and include measurements of self-perceived oral functional status and well-being including self-reported evaluations of tooth loss, oral pain, eating ability, and ability to sleep. The impact of oral symptoms and pain can also be included in assessments.

Self-reported evaluations can assess presence or absence of pain in the teeth or soft tissues of the mouth from acute or chronic oral pain, dental pain, and facial pain. In addition, studies have considered social response to facial appearance by assessing social and psychologic outcomes of malocclusion, craniofacial anomalies, and oral cancer. Such assessments can include measurements of self-concept, psychosocial development, and social perceptions.

Social indicators are used to assess disability days, school loss days (children's restricted activity days because of dental problems or dental visits), work loss days caused by dental problems or dental visits, bed days, and restricted activity related to oral health considerations. Economic dimensions include indirect and direct economic impacts of oral health problems and their treatments.[1] A measurement of indirect economic impacts is self-reported reductions in normal activities related to dental conditions and dental attendance.[1] Answers to questions in a structured questionnaire can evaluate work-loss days, school-loss days, reduced activity days, and bed days resulting from acute dental conditions and dental visits. This measure has been included in the NHIS. Years of life lost can be calculated on the basis of premature deaths from oral and pharyngeal cancer.[1]

Direct economic impacts include direct costs related to dental and oral problems for society and individuals.[1] In addition, analyses of cost benefit and cost-effectiveness can be made for preventive and therapeutic treatments to evaluate direct economic impacts of oral health problems and their treatments.

Measures of oral health, well-being, and quality of life can be used to demonstrate the significance of oral health conditions for individuals and for society as a whole. It helps to ensure that treatments provided result in health gains that enhance not only the individual's clinical status but also his or her psychologic well-being. Assessing social, psychologic, and economic impacts can be used to identify population subgroups and oral diseases that need to be targeted for health promotion and disease prevention efforts.[1]

Future Directions for Assessing Oral Health–Related Quality of Life

In the United States, the impact of oral disease has been shown to disproportionately affect vulnerable groups, a finding that supports application of the *Healthy People 2010* major goals of improved quality of life and reduced health disparities.[1] With this situation under consideration the NHANES conducted in 2003–2004 evaluated OHRQOL for the first time using a subset of seven OHIP questions (i.e., the NHANES-OHIP).[42] In the cross-sectional survey of a nationally representative sample of US adults the prevalence was quantified as the proportion of adults who reported experiencing one or more impacts fairly often or very often within the past year. The questions used to assess OHRQOL in the NHANES conducted in 2005–2006 are outlined in **Box 4-12**.[43] The oral health questionnaire was provided before the physical examination, in the home, using the Computer-Assisted Personal Interviewing (CAPI; interviewer administered) system. The OHRQOL questions were asked of individuals 16 years of age and older, and the dental health perception was included for adults 18 years and older.

Measurement of Infrastructure, Capacity, and Resources

Infrastructure, capacity, and resources are key elements by which states and localities can effectively address oral health problems.[44-46] Infrastructure consists of systems, people, relationships, and resources that enable states and localities to perform public health functions and address oral health problems.[44-46] Within a public health agency, infrastructure includes assessment, surveillance, information systems, planning, policy development, applied research, training, standards development, quality management, coordination, and systems of care.[44-46]

Capacity enables the development of expertise and competence and the implementation of strategies.[44-46] Resources include personnel, financial capital, and available time.[44-46] The public health and personal health workforce must have the necessary capacity and expertise to effectively address oral health problems and issues in jurisdictions and states.[10]

BOX 4-12 **Oral Health–Related Quality of Life Questions**

Topic	Question and Responses
Condition of teeth	Now I have some questions about the condition of your teeth and gums. **Question:** How would you describe the condition of {your/survey participant's} teeth? Would you say … **Responses**: Excellent, Very good , Good, Fair, Poor
How often last year had aching in mouth?	**Question:** How often during the last year {have you/has survey participant} had painful aching anywhere in {your/his/her} mouth? Would you say … **Responses:** Very often, Fairly often, Occasionally, Hardly ever, Never
How often felt bad because of mouth?	**Question:** How often during the last year {have you/has survey participant} felt that life in general was less satisfying because of problems with {your/his/her} teeth, mouth or dentures? Would you say … **Responses:** Very often, Fairly often, Occasionally, Hardly ever, Never
Last year had difficulty with job because of mouth?	**Question:** How often during the last year {have you/has survey participant} had difficulty doing {your/his/her} usual jobs or attending school because of problems with {your/his/her} teeth, mouth or dentures? Would you say … **Responses:** Very often, Fairly often, Occasionally, Hardly ever, Never
Last year taste affected because of mouth?	**Question:** How often during the last year {have you/has survey participant's} sense of taste been affected by problems with {your/his/her} teeth, mouth or dentures? Would you say … **Responses:** Very often, Fairly often, Occasionally, Hardly ever, Never
Last year avoided some food because of mouth?	**Question:** How often during the last year {have you/has survey participant} avoided particular foods because of problems with {your/his/her} teeth, mouth or dentures? Would you say … **Responses:** Very often, Fairly often, Occasionally, Hardly ever, Never
Last year could not eat because of mouth?	**Question:** How often during the last year {have you/has survey participant} found it uncomfortable to eat food because of problems with {your/his/her} teeth, mouth or dentures? Would you say … **Responses:** Very often, Fairly often, Occasionally, Hardly ever, Never
Last year embarrassed because of mouth?	**Question:** How often during the last year {have you/has survey participant} been self-conscious or embarrassed because of {your/his/her} teeth, mouth or dentures? Would you say … **Responses:** Very often, Fairly often, Occasionally, Hardly ever, Never

From Centers for Disease Control and Prevention (CDC). National Health and Nutrition Examination Survey (NHANES) 2009–2010, Sample Person Questionnaire: Adult Supplement. Hyattsville, MD: National Center for Health Statistics, CDC; 2008.

Appendix D includes a summary of the ways to monitor the infrastructure and capacity of the public health system and oral health system for *Healthy People 2010* and key data sources.

To ensure achievement of the *Healthy People 2010* oral health objectives, it is necessary that instruments and methods be developed to assess the current status, best practices, and future development of infrastructure, capacity, and resources necessary to improve oral health at state and local levels.[44-46] States and localities that can evaluate and develop these key elements will be better prepared to maintain fully effective essential public health services for oral health and to achieve the oral health objectives.[44-46]

FUTURE CONSIDERATIONS FOR ORAL HEALTH SURVEILLANCE

A core foundation of successful planning in dental public health is information collected though oral health surveillance systems about the epidemiology of oral diseases and factors that could be targets for prevention. Assessment of key oral health indicators is crucial to effective public health planning that tailors oral health policies, programs, and practices based on oral health status and the progression of oral diseases among population groups. Oral health surveillance efforts are crucial to collect data on oral diseases, conditions and behaviors. These efforts have taken on a new focus because provisions for oral health promotion, disease prevention, and surveillance were included the Patient Protection and Affordable Care Act signed into law in 2010.

There is an impending need to develop new techniques to build oral health surveillance systems. Opportunity in the immediate future should enhance the monitoring of oral diseases, conditions as well as protective and risk factors. Also, testing the validity of self-reporting instruments, visual assessment, developing screening protocols for oral diseases, and implementing standardized assessments using electronic oral health records will be the focus of attention by federal agencies and national organizations collaborating to standardize methods and develop best practices for oral health surveillance. Surveillance activities for oral diseases will require developing a permanent process to share information and having the support of the research community for validation of new surveillance tools.

Future considerations should also address the challenges faced by federal, state, and local agencies to ensure that sufficient resources (e.g., staffing and funding) are available to develop and maintain oral health surveillance systems that will continue to mature and be linked at the national, state, and local levels. Data collection for surveillance requires ongoing funding. States and localities have reported cost-effective approaches such as linking to existing surveillance systems for oral health data (e.g., the CDC BRFSS) and adding new oral health questions to existing surveys or surveillance systems.

However, substantial resources are needed to collect primary oral health data through "open mouth" screenings. Although the unit cost of a survey screening using the BSS tool is more cost-efficient compared to an epidemiologic survey using the DMF Index for teeth, states and local agencies require ongoing resources to regularly and periodically collect oral health status data through screening surveys. These screening surveys will have to be repeated to monitor trends over time and to collect data for different population groups (e.g., preschool children, school-age children, adults, elders, and special needs individuals).

Oral health assessment methods should evolve as oral disease patterns and population demographics change. These changes demand new techniques and the development of skills by dental professionals working in public health. Future considerations need to seek cost-effective alternatives to assess the level of oral diseases, such as techniques to estimate the level of disease among populations, counties, or communities, without having to expand the survey sample for primary data collection.

SUMMARY

This chapter presents the goals and health objectives of *Healthy People 2020;* these benchmarks provide an important framework for the assessment of health in the United States in the coming decade. The chapter focuses on oral health surveillance as the ongoing and systematic collection, analysis, and interpretation of oral health indicators for use in planning, implementing, and evaluating dental public health practice. The chapter describes how assessments are important to monitor changes in the following:

- Oral health and disease patterns
- Use of services
- Social, demographic, and economic factors influencing oral health
- Workforce and service system capacity within the public, private, and nonprofit sectors

Specific measures used in assessing oral health in populations are discussed in the chapter. The chapter highlights examples of oral health surveys and discusses the importance of using standardized measurements to assess oral health trends.

Applying Your Knowledge

1. Apply your knowledge about community assessment and oral health surveys.
   a. Select three oral health objectives proposed for *Healthy People 2020.*
   b. For each objective, describe how you would assess it in the coming year in the following situations:
      i. *Objective 1*—in an urban inner-city community
      ii. *Objective 2*—in a suburban community
      iii. *Objective 3*—in a rural county
2. Read over the following situations and questions. Discuss your ideas and answers in small groups.
   a. The chair of the Healthy Communities Task Force contacts you at the State Health Department. The number one priority issue for the task force is fluoridation of the municipal water supply. The task force is interested in your technical assistance in developing this local initiative and would like your suggestions about assessments in the community that are necessary to get this initiative implemented in the coming year. What assessment issues might the task force need to address? Whom should task force members contact? What steps may it need to take? How could this community process instigate the development and implementation of a community oral health improvement plan?
   b. ARC, a community-based organization that provides vocational opportunities for disabled adults, has become concerned about its clients' dental status and lack of access to dental care. A legislator from this rural area takes up this issue and is interested in improving access to dental care for adults. She asks her legislative aide to evaluate the dental access problems and to study the options in the Medicaid program to provide dental coverage for low-income adults, especially adults with disabilities. Representatives from a State Disability Coalition meet with you at the State Health Department to discuss your insights. The next day, the Executive Director of the State Association of Community Health Centers calls you and asks you to describe some of the barriers to dental care that adults face in rural counties across the state. How would you capitalize on these unique circumstances

to develop a state oral health assessment? Whom would you contact? What steps would you take? How could these activities contribute to the development and implementation of a state oral health improvement plan?

Dental Hygiene Competencies

Reading the material in this chapter and participating in the activities of Applying Your Knowledge will contribute to the student's ability to demonstrate the following competencies:

Health promotion and disease prevention
HP.4 Identify individual and population risk factors and develop strategies that promote health-related quality of life.

Community involvement
CM.1 Assess the oral health needs of the community and the quality and availability of resources and services.

Patient/client care
PC.1 Systematically collect, analyze, and record data on the general, oral, and psychosocial health status of a variety of patients or clients using methods consistent with medicolegal principles.
PC.2 Use critical decision-making skills to reach conclusions about the patient's or client's dental hygiene needs based on all available assessment data.
PC.5A Determine the outcomes of dental hygiene interventions using indexes, instruments, examination techniques, and the patient's or client's self-report.

Community Case

In your position as the State Dental Director, you have received a request from the State Health Officer for the State Department of Public Health that the State Health Surveillance System be reorganized and changed based on the Healthy People 2020 Health Objectives. You are asked to develop a plan to integrate an updated oral health component for this State Health Surveillance System.

1. All of the following resources should be reviewed during the early planning of the oral health component for the State Health Surveillance System except:
   a. National Healthy People 2020 Oral Health Objectives
   b. National Oral Health Surveillance System (NOHSS)
   c. The Dental, Oral, and Craniofacial Data Resource Center (DRC)
   d. The Oral Health Impact Profile (OHIP)
2. What measure would be used to assess untreated tooth decay?
   a. Percentage of persons with ≥1 bleeding site
   b. Percentage of persons with ≥1 dft or DMFT
   c. Percentage of persons with ≥1 dt or DT
   d. Percentage of persons with all teeth extracted, edentulous
3. In conducting a survey to evaluate access to dental care, the following information is most often collected with the use of a questionnaire except?
   a. Oral cancer experience
   b. Usual source of dental care
   c. Annual dental visit
   d. Reason for not having a dental visit in the past year

4. Which survey method would you select to replicate in the state to assess the presence of dental sealants among third-grade students?
   a. National Health Interview Survey (NHIS)
   b. Association for State & Territorial Dental Directors (ASTDD) Basic Screening Survey (BSS)
   c. Behavioral Risk Factor Surveillance Survey (BRFSS)
   d. National Vital Statistics System
5. An important goal of an Oral Health Surveillance System is to assess disparities among different segments of a population. All of the following factors are important to include in a State Oral Health Surveillance System to track oral health disparities except?
   a. Geographic location
   b. Age
   c. Occupation
   d. Racial and ethnic background

References

1. Oral Health in America. A Report of the Surgeon General. Rockville, MD: US Department of Health and Human Services, National Institute of Dental and Craniofacial Research, National Institutes of Health; 2000.
2. US Department of Health and Human Services. A National Call to Action to Promote Oral Health. Rockville, MD: US Department of Health and Human Services, Public Health Service, Centers for Disease Control and Prevention, National Institutes of Health, National Institute of Dental and Craniofacial Research; May 2003.
3. Cohen LK, Gift HC, editors. Disease Prevention and Oral Health Promotion: Socio-dental Sciences in Action. Copenhagen: Munksgaard; 1995.
4. The Secretary's Advisory Committee on National Health Promotion and Disease Prevention Objectives for 2020. Phase I Report: Recommendations for the Framework and Format of Healthy People 2020. Washington, DC: The Secretary's Advisory Committee on National Health Promotion and Disease Prevention Objectives for 2020; October 28, 2008.
5. Healthy People 2010. Understanding and Improving Health. 2nd ed. Washington, DC: US Department of Health and Human Services; 2000.
6. US Department of Health and Human Services. Healthy People 2020 Public Meetings 2009 Draft Objectives. Washington, DC: US Department of Health and Human Services; 2009.
7. Beltran-Aquilar ED, Malvitz DM, Lockwood SA, et al. Oral health surveillance: Past, present, and future challenges. J Public Health Dent 2003;63:141.
8. Association of State & Territorial Dental Directors. Best Practice Approaches for State and Community Oral Health Programs: State-Based Oral Health Surveillance System. Association of State & Territorial Dental Directors; 2008.
9. Association of State & Territorial Dental Directors. Basic Screening Surveys: An Approach to Monitoring Community Oral Health—Preschool and School Children. Association of State & Territorial Dental Directors; 2008.
10. Association of State & Territorial Dental Directors. Guidelines for State and Territorial Oral Health Programs. Jefferson City, MO, 2007.
11. Kuthy RA, Siegal MA, Phipps K. Assessing Oral Health Needs: ASTDD Seven-Step Model. Jefferson City, MO: Association of State & Territorial Dental Directors; 2003.
12. Carnahan BW. Oral Health Examination Survey Manual (companion document to 1997 version of Assessing Oral Health Needs: ASTDD Seven-Step Model). Arlington, VA: National Center for Education in Maternal and Child Health; 1997.
13. US Department of Health and Human Services. Tracking Healthy People 2010. Washington, DC: US Government Printing Office; November 2000.
14. Giannobile WV, Burt BA, Genco RJ, editors. Clinical Research in Oral Health. Ames, IA: Wiley-Blackwell; 2010.
15. Drury TF, Winn DM, Snowden CB, et al. An overview of the oral health component of the 1988–1991 National Health and Nutrition Examination Survey (NHANES III, Phase 1) (special issue). J Dent Res 1996;75:620.
16. Oral Health Surveys. Basic Methods. 4th ed. Geneva: World Health Organization; 1997.
17. Chattopadhyay A. Oral Health Epidemiology: Principles and Practice. Sudbury, MA: Jones and Bartlett; 2011.

18. Centers for Disease Control and Prevention, National Center for Health Statistics. National Health and Nutrition Examination Survey: Dental Examiners Procedures Manual. Hyattsville, MD: National Center for Health Statistics, Centers for Disease Control and Prevention, US Department of Health and Human Services; Revised 2004.

19. Dye BA, Barker LK, Selwitz RH, et al. Overview and quality assurance for the National Health and Nutrition Examination Survey (NHANES) oral health component, 1999–2002. Community Dent Oral Epidemiol 2007;35:140.

20. Pitts N, editor. Detection, Assessment, Diagnosis and Monitoring of Caries: Monographs in Oral Science, Vol. 21. Basel, Switzerland: Karger; 2009.

21. Lewitt EM, Kerrebrock N. Child indicators: Dental health. Future Child 1998;8:133.

22. Dye BA, Thornton-Evans G. A brief history of national surveillance efforts for periodontal disease in the United States. J Periodontol 2007;78(7 Suppl.):1380.

23. American Academy of Periodontology. Position paper—epidemiology of periodontal diseases. J Periodontol 2005;76:1406.

24. Eke PI, Genco RJ. CDC periodontal disease surveillance project: background, objectives, and progress report. J Periodontol 2007;78(7 Suppl.):1366.

25. Centers for Disease Control and Prevention. 2010 Behavioral Risk Factor Surveillance System (BRFSS) Questionnaire. Atlanta: Centers for Disease Control and Prevention; 2009.

26. Dental, Oral and Craniofacial Data Resource Center. Questions Included in National Health Surveys. Rockville, MD: National Institute of Dental and Craniofacial Research, Centers for Disease Control and Prevention. Dental, Oral and Craniofacial Data Resource Center. Available at http://drc.hhs.gov. Accessed April 2010.

27. Centers for Disease Control and Prevention. National Health Interview Survey 2008 Questionnaire: Adult Supplement. Hyattsville, MD: National Center for Health Statistics, Centers for Disease Control and Prevention; 2008.

28. Cons NC, Jenny J, Kohout FJ. DAI: The Dental Aesthetic Index. Iowa City, IA: University of Iowa College of Dentistry; 1986.

29. Tolarova MM, Cervenka J. Classification and prevalence of orofacial clefts. Am J Med Genet 1998;75:126.

30. Bailey W, Duchon K, Barker L, et al. Populations receiving optimally fluoridated public drinking water—United States, 1992–2006. MMWR Morb Mortal Weekly Report 2008;57(27):737.

31. Vargas CM, Arevalo O. How dental care can preserve and improve oral health. Dent Clin North Am 2009;53:399.

32. Chattopadhyay A. Oral health disparities in the United States. Dent Clin North Am 2008;52:297, vi.

33. Glassman P, Subar P. Improving and maintaining oral health for people with special needs. Dent Clin North Am 2008;52:447, viii.

34. Chalmers JM, Ettinger RL. Public health issues in geriatric dentistry in the United States. Dent Clin North Am 2008;52:423, vii.

35. Davis MJ. Issues in access to oral health care for special care patients. Dent Clin North Am 2009;53:169, vii.

36. Rozier RG, Pahel BT. Patient-and population-reported outcomes in public health dentistry: Oral health-related quality of life. Dent Clin North Am 2008;52:345, vi.

37. World Health Organization, Quality of Life Group. What is quality of life? World Health Forum 1996;17;354.

38. Schou L, Blinkhorn AS. Oral Health Promotion. New York: Oxford University Press; 1993.

39. Weintraub JA. Uses of oral health–related quality of life measures in public health. Community Dent Health 1998;15:8.

40. Inglehart MR, Bagramian R. Oral Health-Related Quality of Life. Chicago: Quintessence Publishing; 2002.

41. Chen M, Andersen RM, Barmes DE, et al. Comparing Oral Health Care Systems: A Second International Collaborative Study. Geneva: World Health Organization; 1997.

42. Centers for Disease Control and Prevention. National Health and Nutrition Examination Survey (NHANES) 2003–2004, Sample Person Questionnaire: Adult Supplement. Hyattsville, MD: National Center for Health Statistics, Centers for Disease Control and Prevention; 2002.

43. Centers for Disease Control and Prevention. National Health and Nutrition Examination Survey (NHANES) 2005–2006, Sample Person Questionnaire: Adult Supplement. Hyattsville, MD: National Center for Health Statistics, Centers for Disease Control and Prevention; 2004.

44. Tomar SL. An assessment of the dental public health infrastructure in the United States. J Public Health Dent 2006;66:5.

45. Allukian M Jr, Adekugbe O. The practice and infrastructure of dental public health in the United States. Dent Clin North Am 2008;52:259, v.

46. Association of State & Territorial Dental Directors. Building Infrastructure and Capacity in State and Territorial Oral Health Programs. Sparks, NV: Association of State & Territorial Dental Directors; 2000.

Population Health

Jane E. M. Steffensen, RDH, BS, MPH, CHES

5

Objectives

Upon completion of this chapter, the student will be able to:
- Describe the current status of oral health in the United States.
- Discuss oral health trends in the United States.
- Compare the indicators for oral health included in the national oral health objectives for *Healthy People 2010* and *Healthy People 2020*.
- Identify oral health disparities and inequities among population groups.
- Discuss the factors that influence oral health in populations.

Key Terms

Healthy People 2010
Status
Trend
National Health and Nutrition
  Examination Survey
  (NHANES)
National Health Interview
  Survey (NHIS)

Medical Expenditure Panel
  Survey (MEPS)
National Oral Health
  Surveillance System
  (NOHSS)

Dental Health Professional
  Shortage Area (Dental
  HPSA)
Healthy People 2020

Opening Statement

The Burden of Oral Diseases in the United States[1-3]
- Of young children 2 to 4 years of age, 24% have already experienced dental caries and 19% have untreated tooth decay.
- Of children 6 to 8 years of age, 53% are affected by dental caries, and 56% of 15-year-old adolescents are affected by dental caries as well.
- Nearly one third (29%) of school children 6 to 8 years of age have untreated tooth decay.
- Only 32% of children 8 years of age and 21% of adolescents 14 years of age have received dental sealants.
- Nearly 70% of the population served by public water systems received optimally fluoridated water and the benefits for prevention of dental caries.
- Of adults 35 to 44 years of age, 16% have destructive periodontal disease.
- Oral diseases continue to burden older adults, and 24% of seniors (65 to 74 years of age) are edentulous and no longer have their natural teeth because of dental caries or periodontal disease.
- Approximately 36,540 Americans are found to have oral and pharyngeal cancer, and approximately 7880 people die of these cancers each year.

- More than two thirds (66%) of children and adults had dental insurance coverage; 35% had no dental insurance coverage.
- Nearly two thirds (55%) of children (>2 years of age) and adults have not had a dental visit in the past year.
- Only 25% of edentate adults 18 years and older had an annual dental visit in the preceding year.

PART ONE: ORAL HEALTH STATUS AND TRENDS

Global Burden of Oral Diseases

Oral health has a profound effect on general health and is an important indicator of quality of life. Oral health problems still persist in countries around the globe despite great improvements in the oral health among some populations.[4] Significant oral disease burdens exist among different age groups, especially for people with lower incomes and educational levels and for certain racial and ethnic groups in developing and developed countries.[5] Oral diseases, such as dental caries, periodontal diseases, tooth loss, oral mucosal lesions and oropharyngeal cancers, oral diseases associated with human immunodeficiency virus (HIV)/acquired immunodeficiency disease (AIDS), oral and craniofacial injuries, and noma (cancrum oris), are major public health problems worldwide.[4,5]

Communities throughout the world face dental public health problems as individuals experience preventable oral diseases, in particular, vulnerable and disadvantaged groups in developing countries.[4-9] Different oral disease patterns, as well as development trends between countries, reflect the impact of the application of effective evidence-based preventive oral health programs.[4-9] The important role of behavioral, social, cultural, and environmental factors in oral health and disease has been shown in epidemiologic surveys and data systems supported by the World Health Organization (WHO) Global Oral Health Program.[7-9]

In 1969, the WHO began building the Global Oral Data Bank.[9] Based on standard methods for data collection published in the *WHO Oral Health Surveys Basic Methods* manual, oral health indicators were surveyed and oral health data were submitted for comparisons between nations. In 1995, the WHO Oral Health Country/Area Profile Program (CAPP) was developed to organize and present data for various countries and regions so that oral health status and services could be described on the Internet. The CAPP was established in collaboration with the WHO Noncommunicable Diseases and Mental Health Cluster, several WHO Collaborating Centers, organizations, and individuals around the world. Today, 130 countries contribute oral health data to the Oral Health CAPP.[6,9]

These resources are now being integrated into the WHO Global Oral Health Databases and developed as part of the WHO Global InfoBase.[6,9] The expected results of the integrated data system will be oral health indicators mapped for target population groups at the global level to depict the oral disease burden. Also, a newly available resource, the Global Oral Health Atlas, has mapped oral health across the world. The publication describes oral health status, as well as key factors influencing trends in oral diseases, on a global level.[10]

National oral health indicators from the United States are included in the global and regional oral health surveillance systems. Selected oral health indicators are tracked by the 39 nations in the Americas, including those reported by the United States. The Pan American Health Organization (PAHO) serves as the WHO Regional Office for the Americas (AMRO) and leads this regional oral health surveillance effort on an international level.[6,9]

Oral Health in the United States

In the United States, progress has been made in reducing the extent and severity of common oral diseases.[1,11,12] Over the past half century, major strides in oral health have been seen nationally for many Americans, yet oral diseases remain common and widespread in the United States.[1,11-16] Oral diseases and conditions still afflict most people at some time throughout their lifespan.[1,13]

Factors that contribute to this burden of oral disease include poverty, literacy levels, limited oral health education and promotion efforts, and lack of access to timely and affordable clinical oral health services.* In addition to poor living conditions, major risk factors relate to unhealthy lifestyles (e.g., poor diet and nutrition, oral hygiene, use of tobacco and alcohol, etc.) and limited availability and accessibility of clinical oral health services. Several oral diseases are linked to noncommunicable chronic diseases primarily because of common risk factors. Moreover, general diseases often have oral manifestations (e.g., diabetes or HIV/AIDS). Furthermore, many communities lack dental public health programs, face limited capacity for oral health services, and have inadequate facilities and an inequitable distribution of dental professionals.†

Safe and effective disease prevention measures do exist to improve oral health and prevent oral disease.† These preventive measures include population-based measures (e.g., community water fluoridation, tobacco cessation programs, and school-based dental sealant and fluoride programs), self-care (e.g., daily oral hygiene, healthy diets), and personal oral health services (e.g., clinical dental visits, examination for oral cancer).[18-27] However, these measures are not consistently used by individuals or promoted by professionals and communities. In addition, several nations have not assured universal access to community preventive services such as community water fluoridation, salt fluoridation, school-based dental sealants, or oral health promotion in schools. For example, 31% of persons on public water supplies do not receive fluoridated water in the United States.[28] Furthermore, 68% of 8-year-old children and 86% of 14-year-old adolescents have not received any dental sealants on a permanent molar tooth in the United States, according to the 1999–2004 National Health and Nutrition Examination Survey (NHANES).[1,13] Preventive measures need to be adopted and applied by communities, individuals, and professionals to ensure marked improvements of the nation's oral health.†

Social Impact of Oral Diseases

Oral diseases are progressive and cumulative and become more complex over time.[11,12,23] These diseases can jeopardize physical growth, development, self-concept, and the capacity to learn. They influence eating and communicating.[29] Oral diseases affect economic productivity and compromise a person's ability to work at home or on the job or to concentrate in school.[30,31]

The social impact of oral disease is substantial.[30,31] More than 51 million school hours are lost each year as a result of dental problems.[11] Poor children experience nearly 12 times more restricted activity days than their counterparts from higher income families. Among those who lost school time, youngsters from low-income families, members of minority communities, and families without insurance missed more hours.[30] Children with early childhood caries—often a severe and painful form of dental caries—can demonstrate failure to thrive and be underweight.[32] Serious lifetime functional, aesthetic, and social consequences can be outcomes for children and adults

---

*References 4, 5, 8, 9, 11, and 17.
†References 4, 5, 8, 9, 11, and 12.

Table 5-1   Individual Items from Oral Health Impact Profile (OHIP) Questions Reported in the Dentate US Populations

Individual Items from OHIP Questions*	Never, Hardly Ever (%)	Occasionally (%)	Fairly Often, Very Often (%)	Rank†
Painful aching in mouth	80.4	12.7	6.8	1
Life less satisfying	89.7	5.7	4.6	5
Difficulty doing usual job	96.5	1.9	1.5	7
Taste affected	96.0	2.3	1.7	6
Avoided particular foods	84.1	9.8	6.1	3
Uncomfortable to eat	83.2	11.2	5.6	4
Self-conscious or embarrassed	87.1	6.5	6.4	2

*US National Health and Nutrition Examination Survey (NHANES) 2003–2004 evaluated oral health quality of life for the first time using a subset of seven OHIP questions (e.g., the NHANES-OHIP).
†Presented in rank order of prevalence scores (e.g., percentage of adults reporting one or more items fairly often or very often).

with severe developmental and acquired oral and facial conditions.[11] The Centers for Disease Control and Prevention (CDC) estimated that 16.2 years of life were lost per person who died prematurely of oral and pharyngeal cancer.[11] This figure exceeds the average 15.4 years lost for all cancer sites.

Dental diseases in adults affect their economic productivity and compromise their ability to get jobs. Employed American adults lose more than 164 million hours of work each year because of dental disease or dental visits.[11] Among those who miss work, women, African Americans, low-wage earners, employees with less education, and the uninsured miss the greatest number of hours. Employees of service industries lose from 2 to 3.5 times more hours of work than executives or professional workers.[31]

Oral diseases influence an individual's ability to eat, communicate, and interact in society.[29] The 2003–2004 NHANES evaluated oral health quality of life for the first time using a subset of seven Oral Health Impact Profile (OHIP) questions (e.g., the NHANES-OHIP among dentate adults aged 18 years and older as shown in **Table 5-1**).[29] The survey found that 6.8% of dentate individuals reported painful aching in mouth fairly often or very often, whereas 12.7% indicated this occurred occasionally.[29] Another 6.4% reported being self-conscious or embarrassed because of their teeth or mouth fairly often or very often, and 6.5% responded that this happened occasionally. Among adults, 5.6% reported that eating was uncomfortable fairly often or very often, and 11.2% stated occasional discomfort when eating foods because of problems with their teeth or mouth.

A study supported by the WHO found that among Navajo schoolchildren living in parts of the Navajo reservation in Arizona and New Mexico, 25% avoided laughing or smiling and 20% avoided meeting other people because of the way their teeth looked. Because of dental pain, almost 25% of Navajo adults were unable to chew hard foods, and nearly 20% reported difficulty sleeping.[33]

BURDEN OF ORAL DISEASES IN THE UNITED STATES

Despite improvements in oral health status, profound oral health disparities remain in specific population groups in the United States.[1,13,16] For some oral diseases and conditions, the magnitude

of the differences in oral health status among population groups is striking.[1,13] Oral health disparities are defined as differences in oral health status among population groups. Many different
demographic and social characteristics are associated with oral health disparities. These factors
include income, education, race/ethnicity, culture, geography (urban/rural), age, sex, disability
status, behavioral lifestyles, and other factors. These factors reflect the diversity of the US
population.

The burden of oral diseases is spread unevenly throughout the population.[11-13] People who
experience the worst oral health are found among the poor of all ages; poor children and poor
older Americans are particularly vulnerable. Members of racial and ethnic minorities experience
a disproportionate level of oral health problems. People who are medically compromised or who
have disabilities are at greater risk for oral disease; in turn, oral diseases further jeopardize their
overall health and well-being. This burden of oral disease restricts activities at school, work, and
home and often significantly diminishes quality of life.

ORAL HEALTH STATUS AND TRENDS

National benchmarks have been established to assess health in the United States through *Healthy
People*.[14,15] Tracking systems have been developed, and regular progress reports are used to monitor
the attainment of the national oral health objectives.[1,16] **Tables 5-2 and 5-3** summarize the
progress in reaching the ***Healthy People 2010*** oral health objectives.[1,14] The national trends reveal
progress for some oral health indicators. Other oral health indicators showed little or no improvement during the 2000s.

This chapter provides a broad overview of the status and trends associated with oral health.
Status is the current state or condition, whereas a **trend** is the direction of a condition on a
particular course over a period of time. The chapter concentrates on the national oral
health indicators for the United States and focuses on the indicators included in *Healthy
People*. Several surveys and data systems in the United States are used to track national oral
health indicators.[1,34,35] The following national surveys monitor key oral health indicators in the
United States:
- **National Health and Nutrition Examination Survey (NHANES)**
- **National Health Interview Survey (NHIS)**
- **Medical Expenditure Panel Survey (MEPS)**

The national oral health indicators used in *Healthy People* provide a framework for oral health
assessments at the state and local levels. Also, states and localities conduct and use several surveys
and data collection systems to monitor oral health including the Behavioral Risk Factor
Surveillance Survey (BRFSS). State oral health indicators are included in state-based oral health
surveillance systems and are integrated into the **National Oral Health Surveillance System
(NOHSS)**.[36] In addition, national surveys have been conducted to monitor health and wellness
indicators at the national and state level for children and children with special health care needs.
These resources include the National Survey of Children's Health and National Survey of Children
with Special Health Care Needs.[37] Progress in improving oral health will require diligent efforts
to assess oral health, mobilize resources, and ensure that necessary oral health policies, programs,
and services are in place and are received by individuals and communities across the United
States.[18-27,38,39]

Table 5-2   **Progress in Meeting** *Healthy People 2010* **Oral Health Objectives**

Number	Oral Health Objective	Age (year)	Baseline Data (%)	Trend Data (%) 2004*	Healthy People 2010 Goal (%)	Summary
21.1	Reduce dental caries experience in children					
	a. Young children (primary teeth)	2-4	18	24	11	Reversed
	b. Children (primary or permanent teeth)	6-8	52	53	42	Reversed
	c. Adolescents (permanent teeth)	15	61	56	51	Progress
21.2	Reduce untreated dental decay in children and adults					
	a. Young children (primary teeth)	2-4	16	19	9	Reversed
	b. Children (primary or permanent teeth)	6-8	28	29	21	Reversed
	c. Adolescents (permanent teeth)	15	20	18	15	Progress
	d. Adults (permanent teeth)	35-44	27	28	15	Progress
21.3	Increase adults with teeth who have never lost a tooth as a result of dental caries or periodontal disease	35-44	30	38	40	Progress
21.4	Reduce adults who have lost all their teeth	65-74	29	24	22	Progress
21.5	a. Reduce gingivitis in adults	35-44	48	Data not analyzed	41	No trend available
	b. Reduce destructive periodontal disease in adults	35-44	22	16	14	Progress
21.6	Increase detection of stage 1 oral cancer lesions	All	36	35	51	Reversed

Table 5-2   Progress in Meeting *Healthy People 2010* Oral Health Objectives—cont'd

Number	Oral Health Objective	Age (year)	Baseline Data (%)	Trend Data (%) 2004*	Healthy People 2010 Goal (%)	Summary
21.7	Increase number of oral cancer examinations	40+	13	Data not Available	20	No Trend Available
21.8	Increase dental sealants					
	a. Increase dental sealants for children	8 (first molars)	23	32	50	Progress
	b. Increase dental sealants for adolescents	14 (first and second molars)	15	21	50	Progress
21.9	Increase persons on public water receiving fluoridated water	All	62	69 (2006)	75	Progress
21.10	Increase use of the oral health care system	2+	44	45 (2004)	56	Progress
21.11	Increase use of dental services for those in long-term facilities (e.g., nursing homes)	All	19	Data not available	25	No trend available
21.12	Increase preventive dental services for low-income youth	<19	25	31	66	Progress
21.13	Increase number of school-based health centers with oral health component					
	a. School-based health centers with oral health component: dental sealants	K-12	12	24 (2008)	15	Progress
	b. School-based health centers with oral health component: dental care	K-12	9	10 (2008)	11	Progress
21.14	Increase number of community-based health centers with oral health components	All	52	70 (2006)	75	Progress

Continued

Table 5-2   Progress in Meeting *Healthy People 2010* Oral Health Objectives—cont'd

Number	Oral Health Objective	Age (year)	Baseline Data (%)	Trend Data (%) 2004*	Healthy People 2010 Goal (%)	Summary
21.15	Increase states with systems for recording and referring of children and youth with cleft lip and palate	All	16	32 (2006)	51 states	Progress
21.16	Increase number of states with state-based oral health surveillance systems	All	0	—	51 states	No trend available
21.17	Increase the number of tribal, state, and local dental programs with public health–trained directors					
	a. Increase the number of state and local dental programs with public health–trained directors		39	51 (2006)	41	Progress
	b. Increase the number of Indian Health Service and tribal dental programs with public health–trained directors		9	10 (2006)	9	Progress

From Centers for Disease Control and Prevention, National Center for Health Statistics, US Department of Health and Human Services. Data 2010: The Healthy People 2010 Database, January 2010 version. Available at http://wonder.cdc.gov/data2010/. Accessed May 2010.
*Trend data from 2004 except where noted.

Dental Caries

Children and Adolescents

Despite a tremendous decline in dental caries in children in the United States since the 1950s, tooth decay remains the single most common chronic disease of childhood.[11] It is five times more common than asthma and seven times more common than hay fever.[11]

Early childhood caries affects the primary teeth of infants and young children 1 to 5 years of age.[15] Sometimes referred to as baby bottle tooth decay or nursing caries, it can be a devastating condition, often requiring thousands of dollars and a hospital visit with general anesthesia during

Table 5-3   Progress in Meeting Selected *Healthy People 2010* Objectives Related to Oral Health

Number	Oral Health Objective	Age (year)	Baseline Data (%)	Trend Data* (%)	Healthy People 2010 Goal	Summary
01-8	Increase racial and ethnic representation in dental education programs					
	01-8m. American Indian or Alaska Native		0.5	0.3	1.0	Reversed
	01-8n. Asian or Pacific Islander		19.5	24.7	4.0	Progress
	01-8o. Black or African American		5.1	4.5	13.0	Reversed
	01-8p. Hispanic or Latino		5.3	6.3	12.0	Progress
03-6	Decrease oropharyngeal cancer deaths		2.7	2.7 (2006)	2.4	Progress
03-10	03-10c. Increase the number of dentists counseling about cancer prevention and tobacco cessation		59	No data available	85	No trend available
05-15	Increase annual dental examination for persons with diabetes	2 years and older	56	56 (2008)	71	No change
07-11	07-11t. Increase the number of local health departments that have established culturally appropriate and linguistically competent community oral health promotion and disease prevention programs		25	No data available	50	No trend available

From Centers for Disease Control and Prevention, National Center for Health Statistics, US Department of Health and Human Services. Data 2010: The Healthy People 2010 Database, January 2010 version. Available at http://wonder.cdc.gov/data2010/. Accessed May 2010.
*Trend data from 2004 except where noted.

treatment.[40] Substantial pain, psychologic stress, health risks, and expense are associated with restorative care for children affected by early childhood caries.[41] Infant feeding practices, in which children are put to bed with formula or other sweetened drinks and fall asleep while feeding, have been associated with this condition.[41]

The average number of decayed and filled teeth (DFT) among 2- to 4-year-olds remained unchanged over the 25 years leading to 2000.[15] According to the NHANES, 25% of young children 2 to 4 years of age experienced dental caries in their primary dentition during the years 1999–2004, which is an increase from 18% in 1988–1994.[1,13] Of these children, 19% had untreated caries in their primary teeth. Eighty-one percent of these children were free of dental caries.

The prevalence of dental caries among school-age children declined within the United States in the 1980s and 1990s. The decline is the result of various preventive measures such as community water fluoridation and increased use of fluoride toothpastes and mouthrinses, as well as the application of dental sealants.[11] But these improvements for children seemed to have stalled and for some indicators actually regressed in the 2000s.[13] More than half (53%) of children aged 6 to 8 years experienced dental caries in their primary or permanent teeth in 1999–2004, according to the NHANES.[1,13] This proportion has increased from 52% in the years 1988–1994.

The proportion of untreated dental caries in school-age children has plateaued overall.[13] Twenty-nine percent of 6- to 8-year-olds had untreated dental caries in 1999–2004, up from 28% in 1988–1994.[1,13] In the years 1988–1994, by the third grade, 60% of students had experienced tooth decay, and 33% of these third-graders had untreated dental caries.[1]

Caries experience is cumulative and thus is higher among adolescents than among young children.[13] By age 15 years, nearly two thirds (56%) of teenagers had experienced dental caries in their permanent dentition, according to a national survey in 1999–2004.[1,13] Forty-four percent of these teens were caries-free. In comparison, 61% of adolescents during the period 1988–1994 had experienced dental caries.[1,13] In the years 1999–2004, 18% of teens 15 years of age had untreated tooth decay and were in need of treatment.[1,13] This proportion has decreased slightly from 20% of teens with untreated dental caries in the period 1988–1994.[13]

As with general health, oral health status in the United States tends to vary based on social and demographic factors.[42,43] Dental caries, however, remains a significant problem in specific populations, particularly among poor children and adults from certain racial and ethnic groups.[1,11,13,44,45] Most tooth decay is experienced by only a few children.[46] National data indicate that for those aged 2 to 5 years, 75% of dental caries in the primary dentition was found in 8% of the population.[46] Also, for those 6 years and older, 75% of dental caries in the permanent dentition was found in 33% of the population.[45]

Children from minority racial and ethnic groups (e.g., American Indian, Alaska Native, Asian or Pacific Islander, Mexican American, and black or African American) whose parents have less than a high school education or who have a low income are often markedly at increased risk for dental caries.[42-44] Minority children 2 to 4 years of age in the United States are more likely to experience dental caries than white children.[1,13] Also, preschool-age African-American and Mexican-American children have more untreated tooth decay compared with their white peers.[1,13] America's youngest and poorest children, aged 2 to 4 years and living below the poverty level, have more than 2 times as much dental caries as children of higher-income families (>200% federal poverty level).[1,13]

Also, the level of untreated dental caries among African-American children aged 6 to 8 years (37%) and Mexican-American children (41%) was greater than for white children (25%) in the United States in 1999–2004.[1,13] A statewide oral health survey in California found 69% of Asian or Pacific Islander children 6 to 8 years of age had dental caries in 1993–1994.[15] In 1999, the oral health survey of Native Americans reported that 71% of American Indian or Alaska Native children 6 to 8 years of age had untreated dental caries.[15] Oral health disparities for dental caries are also found among adolescents in the United States. Oral health disparities for dental caries among children and adolescents are shown in **Figures 5-1 to 5-3.**

Young and Older Adults

In 1999–2004, 92% of dentate adults 20 to 64 years of age and 93% of dentate older adults 65 years of age and older had experienced dental caries.[1,13] According to NHANES 1999–2004, 32%

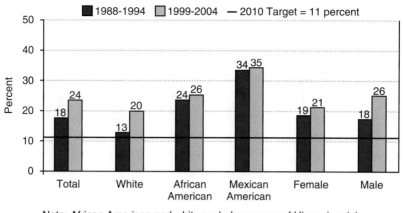

Figure 5-1 Percentage of children 2-4 years of age with dental caries experience in primary teeth, 1988–1994 and 1999–2004.

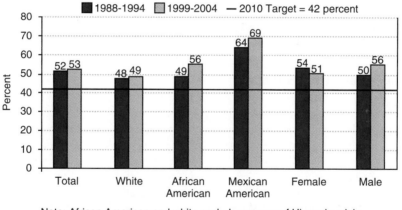

Figure 5-2 Percentage of children 6-8 years of age with dental caries experience in primary teeth or permanent teeth, 1988–1994 and 1999–2004.

of persons aged 65 to 75 years with teeth had experienced root caries (decayed or restored).[13] Also, 42% of people 75 years and older had root caries.[13] Approximately 28% of adults 35 to 44 years of age had untreated dental caries in 1999–2004.[1,13]

Findings from NHANES 1999–2004 showed disparities in dental caries among adults, with 40% of African-American and 40% of Mexican-American adults 35 to 44 years of age with untreated tooth decay compared with 23% of white adults.[1,13] In the same national survey, nearly three times as many young adults (35 to 44 years of age) with less than a high school education (50%) had untreated dental caries than did adults with some college education (16%).[1,13] Untreated

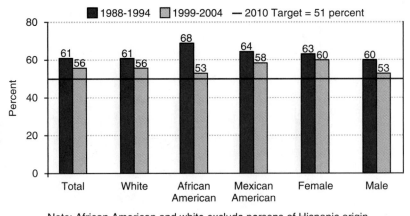

Note: African American and white exclude persons of Hispanic origin.
Persons of Mexican-American origin may be any race.
Source: National Health and Nutrition Examination Survey, National Center
for Health Statistics, Centers for Disease Control and Prevention.[1]

Figure 5-3 Percentage of adolescents 15 years of age with dental caries experience in permanent teeth, 1988–1994 and 1999–2004.

dental caries can lead to pain, abscesses, extensive dental treatment, extractions of teeth, and costly dental care. As the trends in aging continue, adults will lose fewer teeth as they age but will have more teeth that are at risk for dental caries throughout life.[11]

Community Preventive Services

Dental Sealants

Dental sealants can be very effective in preventing dental caries on the pit and fissure surfaces of teeth, but few children receive them.[1,13,20,24a] The percentage of school-age children with dental sealants has risen among specific groups in recent years as the public and private sectors increasingly provide this preventive measure, dental insurance pays for dental sealants, and parents request sealants for their children.[20,24a] Despite the effectiveness of dental sealants, only 32% of children 8 years of age and 21% of adolescents 14 years of age in the United States received dental sealants in 1999–2004.[1,13] Disparities in dental sealants have been shown among children based on race and ethnicity. In 1999–2004, 38% of white children 8 years of age had received sealants compared with 23% of their African-American and 19% of their Mexican-American peers had dental sealants.[1,13] This same survey found 23% of white adolescents 14 years of age had a dental sealant compared with 10% of their African-American and 18% of their Mexican-American counterparts.[1,13] Also, disparities for dental sealants have been shown for family income and parental education.[1,13] As few as 21% of poor 8-year-old children had dental sealants, in contrast to 42% of children from families with higher income levels, according to NHANES 1999–2004.[1,13]

In 1990, the NHIS found that 23% of adults in the United States reported that dental sealants prevented dental caries.[47] Hispanic adults (12%), African-American adults (12%), and adults with less than a high school education were less likely to know the purpose of dental sealants than white adults (25%).[47] **Figure 5-4** illustrates disparities for dental sealants among children 8 years of age and adolescents 14 years of age.

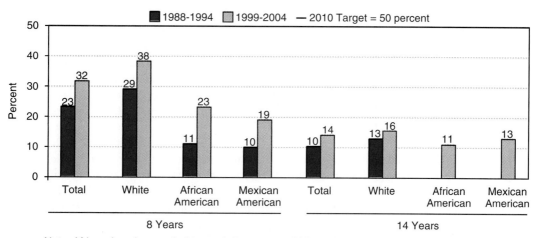

Note: African American and white exclude persons of Hispanic origin. Persons of Mexican-American origin may be any race.
Source: National Health and Nutrition Examination Survey, National Center for Health Statistics, Centers for Disease Control and Prevention.[1]

Figure 5-4 Percentage of children (8 years of age) and adolescents (14 years of age) with dental sealants, 1988–1994 and 1999–2004.

Community Water Fluoridation

Community water fluoridation is a cornerstone community preventive service in the United States.[18,38] During the second half of the twentieth century, a major decline in the prevalence and severity of dental caries resulted from the use of fluorides as an effective method of preventing caries.[11] Fluoridation of the public water supply is the most equitable, cost-effective, and cost-saving method of providing fluoride to the community.[48] Community water fluoridation is an effective, safe, and inexpensive way to prevent dental caries.[48] This method of fluoride provision benefits Americans of all ages and socioeconomic status. Fluoridation, which was started in Grand Rapids, Michigan, in 1945, has been used successfully for half a century in the United States as it benefits both children and adults. Communities with fluoridated drinking water in the United States, Australia, Britain, Canada, Ireland, and New Zealand show striking reductions in tooth decay—those with fluoridated drinking systems have 15% to 40% less tooth decay.[48] Because of these results, the CDC identified community water fluoridation as one of the 10 great public health achievements of the twentieth century and signifies it as a major contributor to the dramatic decline in dental caries over the past 55 years.[49]

A *Healthy People 2010* oral health objective is to increase to 75% the proportion of the US population served by community water systems who receive optimally fluoridated water.[15] The CDC analyzed fluoridation data for the period 1992 through 2006 from the 50 states and the District of Columbia to update reports on fluoridation in the United States and describe progress toward the *Healthy People 2010* oral health objective.[28] The results showed that the percentage of the US population served by community water systems who received optimally fluoridated water increased from 62% in 1992, to 65% in 2000, and 69% in 2006, and those percentages varied substantially by state.[28] Overall, approximately 184 million persons served by community water systems received fluoridated water; of that number, approximately 8 million persons received water with sufficient naturally occurring fluoride concentrations.[28] Approximately 88% of Americans receive their household water through a community system (the rest use well water), yet more than one quarter do not have access to optimally fluoridated water.

Public health officials and policymakers in states with lower percentages of residents receiving optimal water fluoridation should expand their efforts to promote fluoridation of community water systems to prevent dental caries.[2,18,28,38] State-specific percentages in 2006 ranged from 8% in Hawaii to 100% in the District of Columbia (median: 77%).[28] In 2006, the *Healthy People 2010* target of 75% had been met by 25 states and the District of Columbia.[28] During 1992–2006, 39 states reported increases in the percentage of their populations served by community water systems who received optimally fluoridated water; percentage-point increases ranged from 0.3 in Alabama to 69.9 in Nevada (median: 6.2).[28] Ten states had decreases as percentage-point decreases ranged from 0.2 in Kentucky and North Dakota to 17.0 in Idaho (median: 4.3).

In 2006, 25 states did not meet the national benchmark, based on *Healthy People 2010* objectives, of providing fluoridated water to 75 percent of their population on community water systems. In nine states—California, Hawaii, Idaho, Louisiana, Montana, New Hampshire, New Jersey, Oregon and Wyoming—the share of the population with fluoridated water had not reached even 50%.[28] The CDC updated its fluoridation statistics recently, and the new data were expected to be published in 2010.[50] The newer data should reflect additional progress in the past decade and gaining on the *Healthy People 2010* national oral health objective for community water fluoridation. These achievements are because of a state law in California that has produced expansions of community water fluoridation in cities including Los Angeles and San Diego.[50] Also, the updated data are expected to show that states, such as Delaware and Oklahoma, close to the national goal in 2006 now have met the 75% benchmark for *Healthy People 2010*. Of the 50 largest cities in the United States, 42 have community water fluoridation (and two cities have natural fluoride levels that are optimal).[48] The largest cities in the United States not benefiting from community water fluoridation include Long Island, NY; San Jose, CA; Honolulu; suburbs of Philadelphia; Bergen and Hudson Counties, NJ; Tucson, AZ; Portland, OR; and Fresno, CA.

The annual cost of fluoridation is approximately 50 cents per person in communities of 20,000 or more to approximately $3.00 per person in communities with 5,000 or less (in 1995 dollars) for all but the smallest water systems. Community water fluoridation saves money for families and the health care system.[51] A 2001 CDC study estimated that for every $1 invested in water fluoridation, communities save $38 in dental treatment costs.[52] It has been proposed that $1 billion could be saved every year if the remaining water supplies in the United States, serving 80 million persons, were fluoridated in the near future.

According to a national survey of adults in 1998, 70% of respondents indicated that water supplies should be fluoridated in communities.[53] In 1990, only 62% of adults had recognized that the primary purpose of water fluoridation is to prevent dental caries. Persons with lower levels of education, Hispanic adults, and African-American adults were less likely to know the purpose of water fluoridation.[54] When asked to identify the best method of preventing dental caries, only 7% of adults considered fluoride the correct answer, and 70% indicated toothbrushing and flossing to be the most effective.[47]

Periodontal Diseases

During the period 1988–1994, nearly half (48%) of adults 35 to 44 years of age had gingivitis (inflammation of the gums).[1] This figure represented an increase from the 41% of young adults with gingivitis in 1985–1986.[55] Periodontal diseases will probably remain a consideration in the future as tooth loss from dental caries declines and more adults retain their permanent dentition.[15]

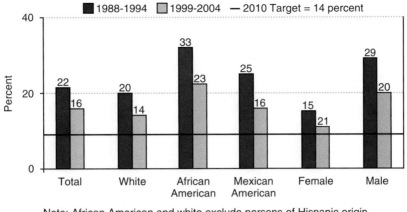

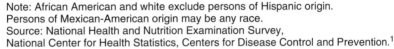

Note: African American and white exclude persons of Hispanic origin.
Persons of Mexican-American origin may be any race.
Source: National Health and Nutrition Examination Survey,
National Center for Health Statistics, Centers for Disease Control and Prevention.[1]

Figure 5-5 Percentage of adults with destructive periodontal disease, 1988–1994 and 1999–2004.

Destructive periodontal disease (defined as loss of attachment of 4 mm or greater) affected 16% of dentate adults 35 to 44 years of age in 1999–2004.[1,13] The incidence of this problem declined among young adults from 22% in 1988–1994.[1,13] Destructive periodontal disease seemed to increase with age, according to the most recent NHANES.[11]

Gingivitis occurred frequently among American Indians, Alaska Natives, Mexican Americans, adults with low incomes, and adults with less than a high school education.[1,11] Among certain population groups, the prevalence of destructive periodontal disease was higher. In 1999–2004, 23% of African-American, 16% of Mexican-American, 14% of white adults (35 to 44 years of age) had destructive periodontal disease.[1,13] In addition, gender differences were found in the same survey, with 12% of female adults and 20% of male adults (35 to 44 years of age) with destructive periodontal disease.[1,13] In addition, disparities for destructive periodontal disease have been shown among American Indian and Alaska Native adults, adults with low family incomes, adults with less than a high school education, and individuals smoking currently.[1,11] At all ages, more severe periodontal disease is seen among males and adults at the lowest income levels.[11] **Figure 5-5** describes the disparities for destructive periodontal disease.

Tooth Loss

Fewer adults are undergoing tooth extraction because of dental caries or periodontal disease. The percentage of people who have lost all of their natural teeth has been declining over the past half century.[11] Of adults 35 to 44 years of age, 38% had never lost a permanent tooth during the period 1999–2004.[1,13] Differences were found by gender, as males (42%) were more apt to have permanent tooth loss than females (34%).[1,13] White adults (41%) and Mexican-American adults (37%) were less likely to have any loss of permanent teeth compared with African-American (27%) adults (35 to 44 years of age) in 1999–2004.[1,13]

Approximately 24% of the American population aged 65 to 74 years was edentulous (i.e., have lost all of their natural teeth) in 1999–2004.[1,13] Among persons aged 65 to 74 years in 1999–2004,

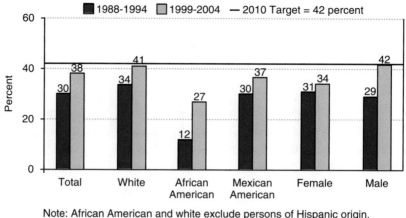

Figure 5-6 Percentage of adults 35-44 years of age without permanent tooth loss, 1988–1994 and 1999–2004.

43% of persons with less than a high school education were edentulous compared with 11% of persons with at least some college.[1,13] In this same age group, edentulousness was also higher among older African-American (26%) than among white (23%) and Mexican-American (18%) older adults.[5] Disparities related to tooth loss are shown in **Figure 5-6**.

Oral and Pharyngeal Cancer

Oral and pharyngeal cancers include different malignant tumors that affect the oral cavity and pharynx and are largely a preventable type of cancer.[56,57] Most of these tumors are squamous cell carcinomas.[56,57] These may include cancers of the lip, tongue, floor of the mouth, palate, gingival and alveolar mucosa, buccal mucosa, and oropharynx.[57] The American Cancer Society estimates that in 2010, 36,540 people will be found to have oral and pharyngeal cancers and 7880 persons will die of these cancers in the United States.[2] These cancers occur more frequently than Hodgkin lymphoma, and cancers of the brain, cervix, ovary, liver, bone, testis, and stomach.[2] Oral cancer accounts for 3% of all cancers diagnosed among males annually in the United States.[2]

Oral cancer rates have increased approximately 15% from the mid-1970s until 2004, according to the National Cancer Institute (NCI) survey.[58] There are significant disparities in some population groups, with higher rates of increase in minority men. Overall, 10.5 adults per 100,000 will develop oral cancer.[2] Oral cancer today occurs more often in males than in females with incidence rates more than twice as high in men as in women.[2,57,58] Oral cancer rates are significantly higher for males (15.5 per 100,000) than for females (6.1 per 100,000). Incidence has been declining in men since 1975 and in women since 1980, although recent studies have shown that incidence is increasing for those cancers related to human papillomavirus (HPV) infection.[2,57,58] Age is also a factor, as oral cancer rates tend to increase with age. The increase becomes more rapid after age 50 and peaks between 60 and 70 years of age.[2,57,58]

Disparities related to oral and pharyngeal cancers have been shown in national reports.[2,57,58] The occurrence of oral and pharyngeal cancers varies by race and ethnicity.[2,57,58] Oral cancer rates are higher for specific groups of males. African-American and white males have 17.2 and 15.7 new cases of oral and pharyngeal cancers per 100,000 per year, respectively, whereas Asians or Pacific Islanders, American Indian and Alaska Natives, and Hispanics have 10.9, 9.7, and 9.2 new cases per year, respectively, according to the Surveillance, Epidemiology, and End Results (SEER) Program, 2008.[58] In the United States, oral and pharyngeal cancers constituted the ninth most common cancer among all men and sixth most common cancer among African-American men.[36]

An estimated 7880 deaths from oral cavity and pharynx cancers are expected in 2010.[2] Death rates have decreased by more than 2% per year since 1980 in men and since 1990 in women.[2] In addition, oral and pharyngeal cancer deaths (per 100,000) differ among population groups.[1] In 2006, oropharyngeal cancer deaths for the overall population were 2.5 per 100,000, whereas they were 3.8 for males and 1.4 for females.[1] Differences among racial and ethnic groups were shown in 2006, with 3.2 oropharyngeal cancer deaths per 100,000 for African Americans, 2.4 for whites, 2.1 for American Indian and Alaska Natives, 2.0 for Asians and Pacific Islanders, and 1.5 for Hispanics.[1] Differences were shown by education level with 4.3 per oral and pharyngeal cancer deaths per 100,000 with less than a high school education compared with 2.5 for high school graduates and 1.0 for individuals with at least some college education.[1]

The NCI reported that oral cancer survival rates have increased approximately 15% from the mid-1960s until 2003.[58] In spite of this improvement, significant disparities remain in some population groups. Disparities in survival rates between white and black males have remained throughout this time period. For all stages combined, about 83% of persons with oral cavity and pharynx cancer survive 1 year after diagnosis.[2] Overall, 60% of persons with the diagnosis of oral cancer are alive 5 years after the diagnosis. Oral cancer survival rates are significantly lower for African Americans.[58] The 5-year survival rates for oral cancer are 61% for white males, 64% for white females compared with 35% for African-American males and 54% for African-American females.[58]

Diagnosing oral cancer at an early stage significantly increases 5-year survival rates. Only 35% of all individuals with oral and pharyngeal cancers were diagnosed at an early stage in 2000.[1] The rate is 40% for females and 33% for males.[1] Disparities by race and ethnicity have been reported, with only 21% of African Americans and 24% of American Indian and Alaska Natives having their oral cancer detected at the earliest stage compared with 29% of Asians and Pacific Islanders, 35% of Hispanics, and 37% of whites.[1] African-American males have experienced increases in both death rates and new case rates, and their 5-year survival rate is much poorer than that for whites (35% versus 61%).[58] African-American males have the highest incidence of and the lowest survival rates from oral and pharyngeal cancers. At every stage of diagnosis, the survival rate for African Americans is lower compared with other groups.[58]

Only 13% of adults (40 years of age and older) in the United States reported ever having an oral cancer examination, according to the most recent data reported from the NHIS in 1998.[1] Males (12%) were less likely to receive an annual oral cancer examination compared with females (14%).[1] Respondents who were more likely to have had an oral cancer examination included those with at least some college education (19%), whereas those with less than a high school education (5%) and high school graduates (10%) were less apt to report an examination for oral cancer.[1] Also, disparities for receipt of an annual oral cancer examination were noted for individuals based on race and ethnicity. Only 6% of Hispanic/Latinos and 7% of African Americans had an oral cancer examination, whereas 12% of Asians and Pacific Islanders and 14% of whites received an oral examination.[1]

Known risk factors for oral cancer include all forms of smoked and smokeless tobacco products and excessive consumption of alcohol. Combinations of tobacco and alcohol represent substantially greater risk factors than either substance consumed alone. Many studies have reported a synergism between smoking and alcohol use, resulting in a thirtyfold increased risk in individuals who both smoke and drink heavily.[51,59] The vast majority of oral cancers are attributed to the use of tobacco (smoked and smokeless tobacco) and alcohol use.[2,59] Those who chew tobacco are at high risk for oral lesions that can lead to oral cancer.[2,57] In 2005, 21% of adults smoked cigarettes, 2.3% used smokeless ("spit") tobacco, 2.2% smoked cigars, and 0.5% smoked pipes.[1] Twenty-six percent of high school students reported using tobacco in the past month; of these students, 20% smoked cigarettes, 14% smoked cigars, 8% used spit tobacco, and 2.9% smoked bidis in 2006.[1] Other factors that can place a person at risk for these cancers are viral infections, immunodeficiencies, poor nutrition, exposure to ultraviolet light (a major cause of cancer to the lips), and certain occupational exposures.[2,57] Human papillomavirus (HPV) infection is associated with certain types of oropharyngeal cancer.[51,57]

Overall, levels of knowledge about risk factors for oral cancer are low. In 2002, a statewide telephone study assessed awareness of oral cancer, knowledge of its major risk factors and clinical signs, and oral cancer examination experiences among Florida adults aged 40 years and older.[60] In Florida, 15% of adults 40 years of age and older had never heard of oral cancer and another 40% reportedly knew little or nothing about it.[60] About 50% of adults did not think oral white or red patches or bleeding could indicate oral cancer and 28% correctly identified three of the major risk factors for oral cancer.[60] After hearing an oral cancer examination described, only 19% of adults reported receiving one within the past year.[60] African-American and Hispanic individuals were significantly less likely than white respondents to have received a recent oral cancer examination.[60] Persons with low levels of education, those who lacked a regular dentist or source of preventive medical care, and adults who knew few or none of the clinical signs of oral cancer also were less likely to have received a recent oral cancer examination.[60]

There was extensive misinformation and a general lack of knowledge among adults about the signs, symptoms, and risk factors for oral and pharyngeal cancers in Florida. According to the NHIS in 1990, similar gaps in knowledge were reported among racial and ethnic groups, as well as disparities in frequency of recent visits for dental and medical care were identified nationally.[61] This lack of awareness and knowledge in adults regarding oral cancer and low levels of reported examination is a major concern and this is particularly crucial among groups experiencing disproportionately high incidence and late stage diagnosis for oral cancer. Increasing awareness of this disease and promoting primary and secondary prevention is essential to lessen the oral cancer burden and reduce disparities in its outcomes. Consideration needs to be given to income levels, education, availability of proper health care, and use of tobacco and alcohol by different population groups when examining disparities related to oropharyngeal cancers. **Figure 5-7** shows a comparison of the disparities related to early detection of oral and pharyngeal cancers based on race and ethnicity.

Other Oral Conditions

Cleft Lip and Cleft Palate

Cleft lip with or without cleft palate is one of the more common birth defects in the United States.[62] Cleft lip and/or palate can be isolated or one component of an inherited disease or syndrome.[62] Both genetic and environmental factors contribute to oral clefts. Although clefts can be repaired to varying degrees with surgery, researchers are working to understand the developmental processes that lead to clefting and how to prevent the condition or more effectively treat

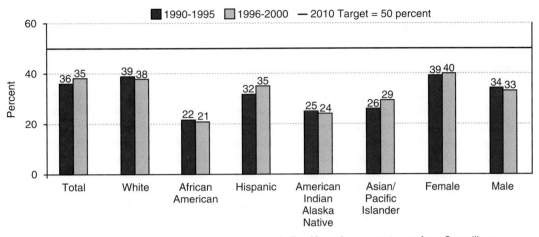

Note: Data are for stage 1 (localized) tumors, excluding Kaposi sarcoma tumor from Surveillance, Epidemiology, and End Results Program, National Institutes of Health, NCI. African American and white exclude persons of Hispanic origin. Persons of Hispanic origin may be any race.
Source: National Center for Health Statistics, Centers for Disease Control and Prevention.[1]

Figure 5-7 Percentage of individuals with early detection of oral and pharyngeal cancers, 1990–1995 and 1996–2000.

it. The lifetime cost of providing care to children born each year with cleft lip or cleft palate is estimated to be $697 million.[58]

Currently, there is a lack of national data for cleft lip or palate. The National Birth Defects Prevention Network (NBDPN) collects cleft lip and palate data annually from 11 states (Alabama, Arkansas, California, Georgia, Hawaii, Iowa, Massachusetts, North Carolina, Oklahoma, Texas, and Utah), which provides a means for estimating national data.[58] The average prevalence of cleft lip and palate was estimated as 6.39 per 10,000 live births for cleft palate and 10.48 per 10,000 live births for cleft lip with or with cleft palate.[58] The annual number of births affected each year in the United States was 2567 with cleft palate and 4209 with cleft lip with or without cleft palate, 1999 to 2001.[58]

States should have an efficient mechanism in place for identification, recording, referral, and follow-up of infants with oral clefts and craniofacial anomalies for treatment. Of 50 states plus the District of Columbia, 32 reported referral and reporting systems for children and youth with a cleft lip and/or palate in 2006.[1] Care by a multidisciplinary team has been shown to be an effective approach in providing services for people across the lifespan with craniofacial anomalies. Thus continued access to an integrated health care system is essential for children and adults to received necessary dental and health care services.

Malocclusion

It was found that 9% of persons 8 to 50 years of age had severe crowding of the anterior incisors and 25% had no crowding in a national survey with the latest published findings.[63] Approximately 9% of persons had a posterior crossbite, and this condition was most common in whites. Severe overbite was found in 8%, and a similar percentage had a severe overjet. Fewer than 5% of whites had an open bite. Findings from the NHANES were reported in the literature where children and adults were shown to have different rates and types of malocclusions that may benefit from orthodontic care.[64]

Craniofacial Injuries

Injuries to the head, face, and teeth are common. A national survey found that of all persons 6 to 50 years of age, 25% had sustained an injury that resulted in damage to one or more anterior teeth.[65] Incisal trauma data was collected in NHANES during 1999–2004. Incisal trauma is defined as a traumatic injury affecting either an upper or lower permanent incisor.

A recent report provided summary findings about incisal trauma among children 6 to 19 years of age from NHANES.[13] In 1988–1994, 9% of children 6 to 11 years of age had incisal trauma compared with 7% in 1999–2004.[13] For these children in 1999–2004, incisal trauma in the maxillary arch (6%) was more likely to occur than incisal trauma in the mandibular arch (1%). Groups indentified to have a greater rate of overall incisal trauma were males (8.62%), African Americans (10.13%), and older children 9 to 11 years of age (11%)[13]

For adolescents 12 to 19 years of age, 20% were observed to have experienced trauma of an anterior incisor tooth in 1999–2004.[13] The survey found that overall incisal trauma prevalence for adolescents remained basically unchanged between 1988–1994 and 1999–2004. The rates of incisal trauma increased with age among adolescents as 17.79% of those 12 to 15 years of age had incisal trauma and 22.51% of those 16 to 19 years of age were observed with this condition in 1999–2004.[13] In adolescence, higher rates were reported for 24.64% males compared with 15.53% females. Among adolescents 12 to 19 years of age, 13.29% were shown to have an unrestored fracture in enamel, the most common condition identified in the survey. Incisal trauma in the upper arch was most common for both age groups of adolescents as 16.08% of those 12 to 15 of age had this condition and 20.50% 16 to 19 years of age compared with 3.45% of the younger group and 4.63% of the older group having incisor trauma in the lower arch of their dentition.[13]

Different rates of emergency department visits for craniofacial injuries have been reported among demographic groups and for specific causes. In 1999, 11% of the emergency room visits were the result of craniofacial injuries.[66] Of these emergency department visits, 21% were by children younger than 15 years of age, 12% for those 15 to 24 years of age, and 10% were for adults 75 years and older.[66] The leading causes of injuries to the head, face, and teeth are falls, assaults, sports-related activities, and bicycle and automobile collisions.[13,66] Approximately one third of all dental injuries and 19% of head and face injuries are sports-related according to some epidemiologic surveys.[11,67,68] During 1997–1998, persons 5 to 24 years of age accounted for 2.6 million (70%) of the 3.7 million emergency department visits per year for sports-related injuries among persons of all ages. Approximately 22% of the average annual estimates of these visits were for craniofacial injuries to the brain and skull, face, scalp, and neck.[68]

More widespread use of effective population-based interventions could help reduce the morbidity, mortality, and economic burden associated with craniofacial injuries.[11,69] Community-based interventions, professional practices, and personal behaviors that increase the use of passenger restraints, air bags, helmets, protective gear, and mouth guards can prevent oral injuries in the future.[11,69]

Dental Fluorosis

In a 1999–2002 national survey, very mild or greater dental fluorosis was observed in 23% of persons 6 to 39 years of age examined with Dean's Fluorosis Index.[70] Thus 67% of survey participants were found not to have fluorosis.[70] Posterior teeth were more affected by fluorosis than were anterior teeth. An increase in the rate of very mild or greater fluorosis was observed among children and adolescents 6 to 19 years of age when findings from 1999–2002 were compared with those from the 1986–1987 survey of school children conducted by the National Institute of Dental Research (NIDR): from 23% in 1986–1987 to 32% in 1999–2002.[70] The results of this survey can serve as a benchmark for future national assessments of fluorosis in the United States.

PART TWO: ACCESS TO ORAL HEALTH CARE AND DENTAL PUBLIC HEALTH SYSTEMS

Access to the Oral Health Care System

With the recent crescendo of discussions about necessary changes to the US health care system that led to the historic health reform law, there also has been an increased concern for the inadequacies of the current oral health care system. Over the past decade, leaders from several sectors have called for greater prevention of oral diseases, elimination of oral health disparities, and changes that need to be instituted to ensure access to oral health services for children and adults.

Tomar and Cohen identified attributes of an ideal oral health care system that are important to assure consistency with the key principles recommended by leading public health authorities.[71] They proposed that an ideal oral health care system should include the following attributes: integration with the rest of the health care system, emphasis on health promotion and disease prevention, monitoring of population oral health status and needs, evidence-based, effective, cost-effective, sustainable, equitable, universal, comprehensive, ethical, linked with continuous quality assessment and assurance, culturally competent, and empowers communities and individuals to create conditions conducive to health.[71]

Moreover, several elements of an oral health care system have been specified as critical components for an integrated system in the provision of oral health care. Comparisons of the oral health care systems between nations have described these core elements that influence overall access to oral health care and ultimately have an impact on oral health outcomes.[72] Gift and Andersen described a conceptual framework of the essential components of an effective oral health care system.[72] They recommended that a comprehensive evaluation of a national oral health care system answer the following questions: (1) who provides? (2) what service? (3) for whom? (4) in what locations? (5) with what resources? (6) by what payment mechanism? and (7) with what effect?[72] **Figure 5-8** provides an overview of the components of an oral health care system. The next section discusses multiple factors and some selected indicators related to access to oral health services.

Barriers to Dental Care

Many children and adults in the United States do not receive clinical dental care that is essential for their healthy growth, development, and well-being. Americans of all ages can gain improved oral health with increased access to appropriate, timely, and quality dental care.[11,45] A host of barriers that prevent timely use of personal oral health services have been identified in several reports and include obstacles related to patients, professionals, the health care system, and society.[11,45,73-89] Some key barriers include the availability of providers, restrictive state dental practice acts, few school-based and community health centers that provide dental services, not

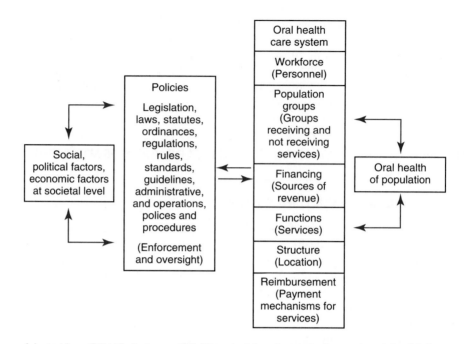

Adapted from Gift HC, Andersen RM. The principles of organisation and models of delivery of oral health care. In: Pine C, Harris R, editors. Community oral health (Chapter 17). Chicago, IL: Quintessence Publishing; 2007.

Figure 5-8 Key components of the oral health care system.

having a regular source of health or dental care, costs, not having health or dental insurance, lack of awareness of the importance of oral health and perceptions about need for regular dental care by both individuals and health professionals, cultural values and beliefs, and fear of dental visits.[11,17,73-89]

Access to oral health care has decreased for specific populations in recent years.[45] Vulnerable population groups, including low-income individuals, racial and ethnic minorities, pregnant women, prisoners, elderly individuals, recent immigrants, individuals with special health needs, homeless persons, homebound individuals, migrant and seasonal farm workers, persons with disabilities, individuals with HIV, individuals living in urban and rural areas, infants and young children face unique barriers, and often lack access to dental care.[1,45,73-89]

Regular Dental Visits and Use of Oral Health Services

The percentage of people in the United States who have had at least one dental visit annually and the average number of visits vary among population groups.[3,11] Regular dental attendance changes significantly according to social and demographic factors, including age, gender, race and ethnicity, level of education, family income, family structure, place of residence (urban, rural, etc.), geographic location in the United States, health insurance status, disability, dentition status, current health status, and institutionalization.*

According to the MEPS in 2004, 45% of the total US population older than 2 years of age had a dental visit in the past year.[1] Over half (52%) of children 2 to 17 years of age and 42% of

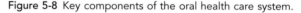

*References 1, 3, 11, 15, 78, and 88.

adults 18 years and older reported an annual dental visit in 2004.[1] This survey found that females (48%) were more likely than males (41%) to have had a dental visit during the past year.[1]

Disparities in regular dental attendance for children and adults over age 2 were reported in the MEPS among racial and ethnic groups, with 29% Hispanic, 30% African American, 33% American Indian and Alaska Native, 44% Asian and Pacific Islander, and 50% white survey participants indicating an annual dental visit in 2004.[1] For persons aged 25 and older, differences were shown based on educational attainment as the percentage of persons with a dental visit in the past year increased with each successive level of education.[1] The MEPS found that adults with at least some college education (59%) and high school graduates (41%) were more likely to have an annual dental visit than adults with less than a high school education (20%) in 2004.[1] A greater percentage of persons (2+ years of age) living at or above the federal poverty level had a dental visit during the past year compared with those living below the federal poverty level according to MEPS 2004.[1] Also, persons with disabilities (41%) were less likely to have regular dental visits than persons without disabilities (46%) in 2004, according to the MEPS.[1]

The percentage of people with an annual dental visit is lowest among children younger than 6 years of age.[3] Children 2 to 6 years of age are less likely to have had an annual dental visit, whereas a much larger proportion of these children have had well-child visits and have received immunizations, health care, or anticipatory guidance for their parents.[75] Between 1996 and 2004, the percentage of children younger than 21 years with an annual dental visit increased from 42% to 45%, with the highest utilization rates and greatest increases among children 6 to12 years of age.[3] Visits for children younger than age 6 increased from 21% to 25%, for 6 to 12 years of age from 54% to 59%, and for teens 13 to 20 years of age, visits remained stable at 48%.[75] According to the MEPS, 52% of children entering school (5 years) and 63% of third-grade children (8 to 9 years) had an annual dental visit in 2004.[1]

This same survey reported 31% of poor children, 34% of low-income children, 46% of middle income children, and 62% of high income children had an annual dental visit.[75] Only 31% of low-income youth received a preventive dental service in 2004 despite the dental coverage in Medicaid and the Children's Health Insurance Program (CHIP).[1]

Older people are less likely to schedule dental visits on a regular basis. Of people 65 years of age and older, 43% reported a dental visit in 2004.[1] Among dentate adults, 46% had a dental visit in the past year and the rate was 25% among edentulous adults 18 years of age and older.[1] In 1997, only 19% of residents in long-term care facilities received dental care during the last 30 days.[1] A greater percentage of younger residents in long-term care facilities received dental care compared with older residents. In addition, more males from long-term care facilities compared with females, and more African-American compared with white residents received dental care. According to MEPS 2004, disparities in dental utilization was found among adults. Less than a quarter (23%) of poor adults 21 to 64 years of age and 27% of those with low incomes had an annual dental visit, compared with 40% of middle income and 56% of high income peers.[3] For adults 65 years of age and older, only 28% of poor older adults and 30% of older adults with low incomes had a dental visit the previous year in comparison to 41% of their middle income and 60% of their high income counterparts.[3] Disparities related to annual dental visits are shown in **Figure 5-9**.

Unmet Dental Needs

Persons' perceptions of their unmet health care needs is an important indicator regarding access to health care. The national MEPS assesses the percentage of persons unable to get or delayed in getting needed medical care, dental care, or prescription medicines in the past 12 months.[76] In

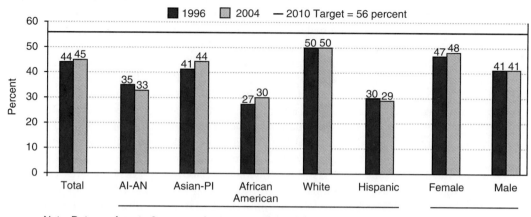

Figure 5-9 Percentage of population (2 years and older) with annual dental visit by selected factors, 1996 and 2004.

2007, approximately 10% of persons in the US civilian population not living in institutions (approximately 30 million persons) were unable to get or delayed getting needed medical care, dental care, or prescription medicines in the past year.[76] The survey found approximately 6% of the population unable to get or delayed getting needed dental care, which was higher than the 5% of persons who were unable to get or delayed getting needed medical care and the 3% of persons who were unable to get or delayed getting needed prescription medicines.[76]

Persons 25 to 64 years of age (7%) were more likely to be unable to get or delayed in getting needed dental care than persons 0 to 4 years of age (1%), 5 to 17 years of age (34%), 18 to 64 years of age (5%), and 65 years and older (4%).[76] For dental care, white (6%), African-American (6%), and Hispanic (5%) children and adults were more likely than their Asian (3%) peers to be unable to get or delayed getting needed dental care.[76] An estimated 10% of adults with at least a four-year college degree were unable to get or delayed getting needed dental care compared with 12% for adults with less than a high school degree, 13% with a high school degree, and 12% with a high school degree and some college.[76]

Persons with high family income were less likely (3%) than those who were poor (9%) or with low (8%) or middle (6%) family income to be unable to get or delayed in getting needed dental care in the last 12 months.[76] The largest difference was with persons in families who are poor who are about three times as likely as persons with high family income to be unable to get or delayed in getting needed dental care. Persons younger than age 65 and with any private health insurance (4%) were less likely than those with public only health insurance (7%) or uninsured persons (13%) to be unable to get or delayed getting needed dental care.[76] The greatest difference was with uninsured persons who are about three times as likely as persons with any private health insurance to be unable to get or delayed getting needed dental care.

Unmet dental needs were evaluated in the 2004 NHIS, and findings about children have been reported in the literature. In 2004, 7% of children 2 to 17 years of age had unmet dental needs, which meant they did not receive dental care in the past year because of financial reasons.[77] This proportion has wavered between 6% and 7% since 2000.[77] In 2004, children between the ages of

2 and 4 (3%) were much less likely than older children to have unmet dental needs compared with 6% of children 5 to 11 years of age and 9% of those 12 to 17 years of age.[77] According to the survey, African-American children were less likely than Hispanic children to have unmet dental needs (6% versus 10%, respectively)[77] The same survey found that 21% of uninsured children were much more likely than children enrolled in Medicaid with public insurance (8%) and children with private insurance (4%) to have unmet dental needs.[77] Ten percent of children in poor families and 11% of children from near poor families had unmet dental needs compared with 4% of children not from poor families.[77] When communities assess health care needs, dental care is frequently cited as a primary unmet need.

Dental Insurance Coverage

Expenditures

The societal costs of dental care are substantial in the United States. National dental care expenditures were $46.8 billion in 1996 and had increased to $95.2 billion in 2007. Expenditures for dental care among the US civilian population not in institutions were 7.4% of total health care expenditures in 2006.[97] Private insurance paid for 42.9% of dental expenditures in 2006 in the United States.[97] The percentage of dental expenditures paid out of pocket was 49.2% and public sources, such as federal, state, and local governments, paid 9.7% of dental expenditures in 2006.[97]

Dental insurance coverage is an important factor that influences access to oral health services. In the United States, dental care is financed primarily through out-of-pocket payments by individuals and dental insurance coverage.[89-91] Private dental insurance plans are received most often through employment but is occasionally purchased by individuals.[89-91] Public programs covering dental care include Medicaid and CHIP.[89,92-96] Medicare is a source of health insurance for the elderly in the United States but it is not a source of public dental insurance.[89,92] Medicare covers only extremely limited hospital-based oral surgery needed in conjunction with other treatment.[89,92] A few Medicare Advantage plans have included modest dental benefits recently.[85]

Private dental insurance differs from private health insurance in the amount of premiums, cost sharing by plan enrollees, and maximum annual benefits.[89-91] Although premiums for dental plans are much smaller than for health plans, enrollees of dental plans are required to pay out-of-pocket larger individual contributions for the cost of services compared with health plans. Additionally, many dental plans cap the amount paid out annually.[89,90] The differences between health and dental coverage are attributable to different assumptions about risk underlying each type of plan and how the risk is shared among plan enrollees.[89] The risk-sharing propositions of the different types of plans have been shown to have an impact on utilization and premiums rates with differentials in costs and cost sharing by beneficiaries.[89] Because of the low level of dental insurance coverage and the structure of dental benefits, out-of-pocket expenses account for a much larger percentage of total dental care spending for individuals in comparison to out-of-pocket costs for general health care paid by individuals. Dental care fees are usually charged by procedure and traditionally have been paid on a fee-for-service basis.[89]

While most large employers still offer private dental insurance, this rate has been decreasing. In the early 1970s, most dental care was paid for out-of-pocket. Employer-sponsored dental insurance grew in the 1970s through 1984 when it peaked as 77% of full-time private employees of medium and large firms had private dental coverage.[85] Dental benefits are vulnerable during economic downturns, and because of rising costs for health insurance and a difficult economic climate, private dental insurance rates had decreased to 57% for medium and large firms in 1997.[85]

A 2009 Bureau of Labor Statistics survey showed that overall, only 48% of full- and part-time workers have access to dental coverage through work and only 38% participate in the dental insurance plan.[98] The survey reported that employees least likely to participate in private dental insurance plans were part-time, non-union, and working in smaller businesses.[98] In 2009, 55% of employees working for employers with 500 or more employees participated in a private dental plan compared with a lower rate of 31% for those working in businesses with 1 to 99 employees, and 44% working in firms with 100 to 499 employees.[98] Geographic differences in the United States were also reported in the survey with participation among employees greatest in the Pacific region (49%) compared 27% the lowest level of participation in the West South Central region.[98] Another study using MEPS data assessed private dental insurance coverage among employers and also reported that well-established and larger employers with multiple worksites were more likely to offer private dental coverage.[91] This analysis found geographic differences among states depending on large employers within the states.[91]

Overall, dental insurance coverage is much less common than health insurance in the United States. More than 15% of persons 18 years of age and older have no form of health insurance, but more than two times as many are likely to not have any form of dental insurance.[3,99] In 2004, approximately 158 million people, or 54% of children and adults, had private dental coverage during the year.[3] Approximately 12% of this population had public dental coverage, and 35% had no dental coverage at all during the year.[3] Whereas 57% of children and adults with private dental coverage had a dental visit during 2004, 32% with public dental coverage and 27% with no dental coverage had a visit.[3] Disparities related to dental insurance coverage based on age are shown in **Figure 5-10**.

Dental Insurance Coverage: Children and Adolescents

According to MEPS for children from birth to 20 years of age, 46 million (54%) had private dental coverage during 2004.[3] Over a quarter (26%) of all children had public dental coverage, and slightly less than 20% of all children had no dental coverage. In 2004, 58% of children with

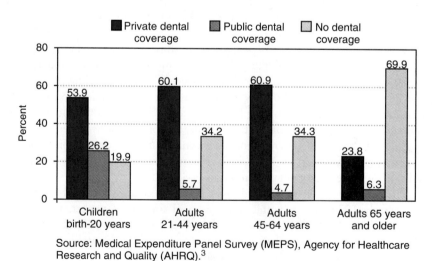

Source: Medical Expenditure Panel Survey (MEPS), Agency for Healthcare Research and Quality (AHRQ).[3]

Figure 5-10 Percentage of population with and without dental coverage by age, 2004.

private dental coverage had a dental visit, 34% of children with public dental coverage had a dental visit, and 28% of children without any dental coverage had a dental visit.[3] Overall, children with private dental coverage were twice as likely to have had a dental visit as children with no dental coverage.

Dental insurance coverage varied by age, family income, race and ethnicity, and family education among children. African-American and Hispanic children were more likely to have public dental coverage and less likely to have private dental coverage in 2004 than white children or children of other race and ethnic backgrounds.[3] Lack of dental insurance coverage can cause financial barriers that are a significant deterrent to receiving timely dental care, especially for children in families with low incomes. Children from a family with lower income were less likely to have private dental coverage and more likely to have public dental coverage in 2004 than children from a family with higher income.[3] Children from a family with low or middle income were more likely to have no dental coverage compared with poor children or children from a family with high income. Children with a caregiver with some or no school were more likely to have public dental coverage and less likely to have private dental coverage in 2004 than children with high school graduates or college graduates as caregivers.[3]

The percentage of children with public dental coverage increased from 1996 to 2004. In 2004, MEPS reported 26.2% of children with public dental coverage compared with 18.0% in 1996.[3] Children without dental coverage decreased from 28.8% in 1996 to 19.9% in 2004.[3] While no significant changes by age in the percentage of children with private dental coverage from 1996 to 2004 were noted, children of all ages were much more likely to have public dental coverage and less likely to have no dental coverage in 2004 than in 1996.[3] African-American, white, and Hispanic children were much more likely to have public dental coverage and less likely to have no dental coverage in 2004 than in 1996.[3] Children of other race and ethnicity backgrounds were less likely to have no dental coverage in 2004 than in 1996.[3]

Children from poor, low-income, and middle-income families were more likely to have public dental coverage and less likely to have no dental coverage in 2004 than in 1996.[3] Low-income and middle-income children were less likely to have private dental coverage in 2004 than in 1996. High-income children were more likely to have private dental coverage and less likely to have no dental coverage in 1996 compared with 2004. Children with a high school graduate caregiver had a statistically significant decrease in the likelihood of having private dental coverage from 1996 to 2004. Children of caregivers of all levels of education were much more likely to have public dental coverage and less likely to have no dental coverage in 2004 than in 1996.[3]

Dental Coverage: Younger and Older Adults

About 60% of adults (103 million adults 21-64 years of age) had private dental coverage, and 34% of adults had no dental coverage during 2004.[3] For older adults 65 years and older approximately 9 million older adults (24%) had private dental coverage in 2004.[3] Approximately 70% of all older adults did not have any dental coverage.[3]

More than half (56%) of adults with private dental coverage had a dental visit in 2004 compared with 28% of adults with public dental coverage and 22% of adults without any dental coverage.[3] In 2004, 65% of the older adults with private dental coverage had a dental visit, 26% of older adults with public dental coverage had a dental visit, and 37% of older adults without any dental coverage had a dental visit.[3] Adults without dental coverage had a statistically significant decrease in the likelihood of having a dental visit from 1996 to 2004. Older adults with public dental coverage were more likely to have a dental visit in 2004 than 1996.[3]

Dental coverage varied by age, family income, race and ethnicity, and education among younger and older adults in 2004 according to MEPS.[3] Adults from a family with lower income were less likely to have private dental coverage and more likely to have public coverage. Adults from a poor family were almost three times more likely to have no dental coverage as those from a high-income family (59% and 21%, respectively).[3] Poor adults and adults from a family with low income were more likely to have no dental coverage in 2004 than adults from a family with middle or high income.[3] Older adults who were poor, as well as those from a family with low or middle income were less likely to have private dental coverage and more likely to have no dental coverage compared with their counterparts with higher income.[3]

African-American and Hispanic adults were more likely to have no dental coverage in 2004 than their white peers or adults from other race or ethnicity backgrounds.[3] Hispanic older adults were less likely to have private dental coverage in 2004 than African-American older adults or white older adults.[3] Adults with less than a high school education were more likely to have no dental coverage in 2004 than high school or college graduates. Older adults with less than a high school education were less likely to have private dental coverage in 2004 than college graduates.[3]

The percentage of adults with private dental coverage increased from 58% in 1996 to 60% in 2004.[3] For this age group, there was a decrease in the percentage of adults with no dental coverage from 1996 to 2004. Overall there were no significant changes in the percentage of older adults with private, public only, or no dental coverage from 1996 to 2004. Older adults from a middle-income family were less likely to have private dental coverage and more likely to have no dental coverage than older adults from a family with either lower or higher income in 2004 than in 1996.[3]

Publicly Funded Health Insurance Programs

The costs for dental care can be a significant burden on low-income Americans. Often, dental care in the private sector is not accessible for many Americans, especially those from vulnerable groups.[45,91] Medicaid is the nation's principal safety-net health insurance program as it covered health and long-term care services for 59 million low-income Americans, including children and parents, people with disabilities, and seniors in 2005.[99,100] Most children and parents covered by Medicaid are in working families, and without Medicaid the vast majority of its enrollees would be uninsured.

Since its enactment in 1965, Medicaid has increased access to care for low-income people, functioned as the main payer of nursing home and other long-term care, and supported the safety net of providers that serve low-income and uninsured people.[99-101] In 2005, Medicaid provided coverage to 29.4 million children; 15.2 million adults (primarily poor working parents); 6.1 million elders; and 8.3 million individuals with disabilities. More than one in four children, including over 60% of poor children and 40% of those near poverty, rely on the Medicaid program for coverage.[99] Largely because of Medicaid and the smaller CHIP, the rate of children without health insurance fell by more than one third between 1997 and 2005, from 23% to 14%, despite declining employer-based health coverage.[99] Over the same period, the uninsured rate rose among adults, for whom Medicaid eligibility is much more restrictive.[99] During economic downturns, rising unemployment and declines in income cause more workers and their families to lose their health coverage, and by design the Medicaid program expands at such times, mitigating increases in the number of uninsured.[99-101]

To qualify for Medicaid, a person must meet financial criteria and also belong to one of the categorically eligible groups: children, parents with dependent children, pregnant women, people with severe disabilities, and the elderly.[99-101] Federal law has required that states offer Medicaid to all people in these groups up to specified income thresholds. Also, states have broad authority to expand Medicaid beyond these federal minimum standards, and they have done so to varying degrees.[99,100]

The federal government and the states jointly finance Medicaid, and the states administer the program within broad federal guidelines.[100] The federal share of Medicaid spending is at least 50% in every state.[99] It varies based on state per capita income relative to the national average and ranges as high as 76% in the poorest state. Overall, the federal government finances approximately 57% of Medicaid spending.[99] Medicaid purchases health care services primarily in the private sector, contracting with managed care plans or paying for care on a fee-for-service basis.[99] Medicaid covers a wide range of benefits to meet the complex needs of the diverse populations it serves. State Medicaid programs are generally required to cover: inpatient and outpatient hospital services; physician, midwife, and certified nurse practitioner services; laboratory and radiography services; nursing home and home health care for individuals age 21 and older; Early and Periodic Screening, Diagnosis, and Treatment (EPSDT) for children younger than age 21; family planning services and supplies; and rural health clinic and federally qualified health center services.[99-101] States can also receive federal matching funds for many optional services, including prescription drugs, prosthetic devices, hearing aids, and dental care for adults.[99-101]

Quality dental coverage is essential to ensure access to dental services and improvement of oral health. All states provide dental benefits for children under the mandatory Medicaid benefit EPSDT, since federal law requires states to cover comprehensive preventive care, diagnostic services, and dental treatment for children up to age 21, according to the Centers for Medicare & Medicaid Services (CMS).[85,102] The EPSDT requirements encompass both coverage and arranging for care. The benefits required under EPSDT include preventive dental care, as well as all dental care that is medically necessary to restore teeth and maintain dental health (including orthodontics), as well as assistance in arranging for covered services such as scheduling and transportation.[95,96,102] A distinctive focus of EPSDT is an orientation to prevention that maximizes health and development of children and that diverts the health implications and financial expenses of long-term treatment and disability.

Also, the CHIP program has provided important opportunities for improving access to dental care for children from low-income and modest-income families since its inception in 1997 (then named the State Children's Health Insurance Program, or SCHIP).[85,95,96,103] In CHIP programs that are Medicaid expansions, the EPSDT mandate applies for oral health services.[95,96] However, in separate (non-Medicaid) CHIP programs, dental benefits are optional and there is no requirement that states cover all medically necessary health care. Consequently, dental benefits in states with separate CHIP programs have varied by state and may change over time. Because dental benefits in CHIP have been optional, state governments have had the prerogative to include benefits in CHIP programs and a few states did not include dental benefits over the years.[95,96] In 2008, fourteen states with separate CHIP programs offered children the same benefit package provided to children in Medicaid; other states provided more limited benefits similar to private dental insurance as seven states capped annual dental expenditures or limited the number of dental services allowed annually. By 2008, all states had chosen to cover some oral health services under CHIP.[85,95,96]

Provisions in the Children's Health Insurance Program Reauthorization Act of 2009 (CHIPRA) guaranteed dental benefits under CHIP.[103] Beginning October 1, 2009, all CHIP programs were required to cover dental services for children necessary to prevent disease and promote oral health, restore oral structures to health and function, and treat emergency conditions based on a benchmark standard and the states were required to report annually on utilization of dental services.[103] CHIPRA also gave states a new option to offer a dental-only supplement or cost-sharing protection for dental services to children who would qualify for CHIP except that they have other health coverage.[103] In addition, the law included new measures to improve the oral health of children in both Medicaid and CHIP. These provisions include (1) parents of newborns enrolled in Medicaid or CHIP are to receive education about their child's oral health, (2) states allow community health centers to contract with private dentists for dental care, (3) states produce a list dental providers participating in Medicaid and CHIP that is accessible through the federal Insure Kids Now website, and (4) a Government Accountability Office (GAO) study on children's access to care and the feasibility of using new types of dental providers to meet children's needs.[103]

Medicaid and CHIP, the nation's safety-net health insurance programs, are a major source of coverage for children in the United States.[85,95,96] In 2007, the two programs covered more than 25% of all children and about 50% of children from families with low incomes, Medicaid covered about 29 million poor and near-poor children, and CHIP built on this foundation of coverage, providing health insurance for an additional 7 million low-income children.[85,95,96] In 2006, 69% of children from families with low incomes in the United States received dental coverage through Medicaid and CHIP during at least part of the previous year. This was a substantial increase compared with 1999, when the rate was just about 50%. In the absence of Medicaid and CHIP, most children covered by these programs would be uninsured. Reflecting on this reality and the impact of broader public coverage among children, the share of children from families with low incomes with no dental coverage fell by 10 percentage points between 1999 and 2006, from 25% to 15%.[85,95,96]

Children from families with low incomes enrolled in Medicaid or CHIP fared at least as well as their low-income peers with private insurance in having a dental visit.[85,95,96] In 2006, 43% of low-income children enrolled for a full year in Medicaid or CHIP had a dental visit in the past year, similar to 40% of children from low-income families enrolled with private dental insurance for a full year. Uninsured children were less likely to have a dental visit (34%). Relative to uninsured children, children with public dental insurance coverage are also more likely to have a usual source of dental care and to receive preventive dental care, and they are less likely to have unmet dental needs.[85,95,96] In focus groups and other studies, dental care for children emerges as one of the benefits of Medicaid and CHIP that are valued most by families. Children with Medicaid and CHIP coverage fare much better than their low-income uninsured counterparts, but their access to oral health care falls short of meeting oral health care needs.[85,95,96]

Reports have described the successes and shortcomings of Medicaid and CHIP as well as the interlinked deficits of the other components of the oral health care system that influence overall access issues.[78-89] Although surveys report that more children have dental coverage because of dental programs in Medicaid and CHIP compared with the 1990s, much more needs to be done to assure that all children enrolled receive needed dental care. It is essential that there are improvements in government performance because reports indicate as many as 62% of children 1 to 18 years of age enrolled in Medicaid had not received dental care in 2007.[111] CHIP is much smaller than Medicaid; 4.8 million children were enrolled in CHIP, compared with 22.7 million children enrolled Medicaid in 2008. Little is known about dental access for children covered by CHIP. There has been a lack of data because CHIP programs were not required to report utilization data comparable to annual Medicaid reporting requirements until a change in the law that was enacted in 2009.[103] While some of the access problems observed in Medicaid are often found in CHIP as well, dentists appear more willing to serve children covered by CHIP in states that have set higher dental payment rates in their CHIP programs than in Medicaid.

Several reports have proposed explicit recommendations to improve the oral health components of Medicaid and CHIP that would assure accountability so that more children enrolled in the programs receive comprehensive dental care.[81,83,85-88,96] Early primary prevention and greater continuity of dental care for young children at highest risk for dental caries have been emphasized in recent reports. This early intervention (EI) for early childhood caries holds promise for improving health and lowering public expenditures. States have instituted several strategies to improve access for low-income children.[81,83,85-88,96] Many have worked to raise Medicaid and CHIP payment rates, simplify reporting requirements, and expedite payment. Other states have been focused on workforce issues. States have used loan repayment and other financial incentives to encourage dentists to serve the uninsured and participate in Medicaid and CHIP, examined the scope of practice laws in the state that govern the work dental hygienists can do under different levels of supervision, and expanded the supply of providers capable of providing care to children by educating and reimbursing physicians and nurses to provide oral health guidance to parents and children and to apply fluoride varnishes to young children. It has been recognized that long-standing, complex barriers limit the potential of Medicaid and CHIP to provide necessary oral health services for children across the nation, but states have shown successful ways to make improvements to the Medicaid and CHIP programs.[81,83,85-88,96]

Medicaid is the primary mechanisms for dental coverage among adults with low incomes.[92-94] While state Medicaid programs are required by federal rules to cover comprehensive oral health services for children, coverage for adult dental services is considered optional.[92-94] States often choose to offer adults a more limited set of covered services than children or offer no coverage at all.[91,92] Because of this optional status, adult dental coverage is often one of the first areas states turn to when making reductions in Medicaid. Among elderly Americans, traditional Medicare is not a source of dental insurance as it does not pay for any general oral health care. Medicare pays for dental care in only extremely limited hospital-based dental care required in conjunction with other treatments, such as organ transplantation. Therefore approximately 70% of Americans aged 65 and older do not have any form of dental coverage.[3]

A report on Medicaid coverage of adult oral health services found as of early 2008, before the recession, that 45 states, including Washington, DC, provided some type of coverage of dental benefits to at least some adults enrolled in Medicaid. However, this coverage ranged from comprehensive dental care to coverage limited to emergencies, or coverage for only specific groups of enrollees.[93] A wide variation in dental coverage for adults on Medicaid was reported among states as the types of dental services and degree of coverage differed between states. Also, dental benefits varied in total amount, duration, and scope of coverage. For example, dental coverage described in this report indicated adult Medicaid programs in some states provided selected dental benefits for specific groups, such as low income individuals with disabilities living in institutions, but did not provide coverage to the general adult population with low incomes. The study found sixteen states offering more comprehensive dental coverage (coverage in all categories, with no annual maximum) to adults, and twenty-two offered emergency services or no coverage at all.[93] In 2005, a survey using different methods for assessing the extent of adult benefits found that only seven states had coverage of every service category without any annual caps on costs for all adult beneficiaries in Medicaid, down from twelve states in 2002.[93] Twenty-six states were reported to offer emergency services only or no dental coverage at all.[93] Recent fiscal constrains in states have led states to reduce or eliminate dental benefits for adults and the elderly, including Medicaid beneficiaries with disabilities as cost-saving measures. These cuts leave millions of adults unable to access dental care in the face of pain and infection.

The improvements made by CHIP Reauthorization Act have the promise to strengthen the ability of Medicaid and CHIP to expand access to oral health care for children.[103] Advocates worked with partners to promote the inclusion of oral health provisions in the Patient Protection and Affordable Care Act enacted in 2010. This legislation will bring health care to millions of Americans because key provisions related to oral health in Medicaid and CHIP were included in the landmark legislation.[104,105] These provisions include the following:

- Expansion of Medicaid coverage: States are required to set Medicaid income eligibility cap no lower than 133% of the federal poverty level (FPL), resulting in Medicaid being provided to approximately 16 million additional children and adults.
- Extension of CHIP through fiscal year 2015.
- Requirement for pediatric dental benefits under new state insurance exchanges.
- Provision of funding for Medicaid and CHIP Payment and Access Commission (MACPAC).

Oral health coverage for adults and elders was not included in the provisions for health reform enacted in 2010.[104,105] A great opportunity to assure universal access to dental coverage for all, including adults and the elderly, was lost. This dark shadow will continue to be a major challenge to expanding access to necessary oral health care for the increasing number of adults and elders retaining their teeth throughout their retirement years. Dental public health professionals will be called on to foster linkages for adults to access dental care in communities across the country. Also, programs will need to be developed to provide direct oral health services to individuals lacking dental care and not covered by the provisions in the health reform law. Addressing the oral health care needs of adults especially among vulnerable populations will be an ongoing struggle for communities in the coming decade unless significant policy changes are made.

ORAL HEALTH WORKFORCE

Population Trends and Future Dental Workforce

The oral health care system depends on the size, composition, characteristics, and distribution of the oral health workforce.[79] Factors such as scope of practice, productivity, practice settings, and participation of providers, have an impact on the capacity of the workforce to serve vulnerable populations.[79,106-111] Concerns have been raised about the adequacy of the number of oral health professionals available to provide needed oral health services in the United States. Several factors have been implicated including the marked decline in the number of dentists, the growth in number of dental hygienists, the number and demographic shifts among students graduating from academic dental institutions; the number and location of dental professionals retiring; population and demographic trends; changing oral disease patterns; and barriers to care faced by children and adults.[79,106-111] These factors are likely to influence the dynamics of the oral health care system as changes in the organization and financing of health service occur in the coming decades. Dental public health professionals can serve in leadership roles to facilitate progress and positively affect access to oral health services for underserved population groups.[110]

Changing demographics within the United States will have a long-term impact on the oral health care system in the future. By 2030, minorities are expected to increase to one half of the US population (235.7 million), including half of all children.[112] The number of elderly Americans will double from 35 million to more than 88.5 million by 2050.[112] Also, those in the baby boomer generation, as well as elders, are retaining more teeth and there is a growing focus on increasing access to health care and preventive dental care.[1,11,13] There were approximately 54.4 million individuals (18.7% of the population) with a disability living in communities across the country and 35.0 million (12%) severely disabled in 2005.[113] Today, only 5% of the population older than age 65 (1.8 million) live in nursing homes where dental care is problematic, but the number of individuals using long-term care services (e.g., whether at home or in residential care such as assisted living or skilled nursing facilities) is expected to grow to 27 million by 2050.[114]

These population trends and other demographic shifts will have far-reaching effects not only for the oral health care service system but also for patients and oral health care providers in the coming decades. Moreover, public health professionals can provide leadership locally, at the state and national levels to assure universal access to effective oral health services. These professionals will have opportunities to contribute to improvements in oral health outcomes of individuals and communities by shaping policies, programs, and practices that will influence the future development of an integrated system of quality health services including oral health care.

Supply of Dental Professionals

The US Bureau of Labor Statistics (BLS), which placed the number of practicing dentists at 141,900 in 2008, projects a 16% growth in the number of dentists through 2018.[115] At the same time, large numbers of dentists are expected to retire over the next few decades at a 2:1 ratio to new graduating dentists.[116] The estimated number of dentists who will retire between 2002 and 2022 is estimated to be between 63,440 to 83,430.[117] Four new accredited dental schools have opened, and as many as ten new schools may be graduating students by 2020. It is estimated that this will increase the number of dental school graduates by approximately 5300 per year by 2020.[117] Dental schools graduated an estimated 4700 graduates in 2008.[118] Favorable economic conditions will encourage retirements, and poor economic conditions will be a disincentive to retire as the stock market returns are lower during such a time period. The likely result is that the number of dental school graduates will not keep pace with the increasing demand for oral health care resulting from growth in the US population. A projected decline in the dentist workforce and the population's growth, as well as demand for oral health services, are likely to accelerate access problems for historically underserved and disadvantaged segments of the US population.[79,106,107]

Currently, about 79% of dentists are practitioners in general dentistry and the remaining 21% of dentists practice in one of nine recognized specialty areas: (1) endodontics, (2) oral and maxillofacial surgery, (3) oral pathology, (4) oral and maxillofacial radiology, (5) orthodontics, (6) pediatric dentistry, (7) periodontics, (8) prosthodontics, and (9) public health dentistry.[79,106,118] Of the nation's dentists, 91% professionally active dentists provide dental care in the private sector of the oral health care system.[106,118] Most of these practitioners are in privately owned solo or two-person group practices.[106,118] The employment status for dentists in 2007 shows that 67% are sole proprietors, 24% are independent non-solo practitioners, 6% are employees and 3% are independent contractors.[106,118]

The number of general dentists in the United States started declining around the turn of the twentieth century,[79,106] and this decline likely will continue throughout the next decade.[79,106,118] There are potential consequences of this trend, particularly in the supply of dentists in nonurban areas.[74,88,106,119] The overwhelming majority of specialists work in urban areas. As the number of general dentists decreases, it is predicted to have negative impact on the supply of dentists in rural areas.

The allied oral health workforce is central to meeting increasing needs and demands for dental care. Historically in the United States, the allied dental workforce has been comprised of dental hygienists, dental assistants, and dental laboratory technologists. During the past decade, new types of oral health professionals have been included in the dental workforce as education programs have started and individuals have become educated to provide oral health services. A number of states have passed or considered legislation that would create new providers. Multiple new oral health professionals are proposed, enrolled in education programs, or now working in communities. These include the Alaska Dental Health Aide Therapists, Minnesota Dental Therapists, Community Dental Health Coordinators, and Advanced Dental Hygiene Practitioners. Also, oral health education has been integrated into formal and continuing education programs for health professionals such as nurses, physicians, physician assistants, and nurse practitioners, and other health professionals.[106,109,111]

About 174,100 dental hygienists, 295,300 dental assistants, and 53,000 dental laboratory technologists were in the US workforce in 2008.[115] Both dental hygiene and dental assisting have an expected growth of 36% through 2018 and are among the fastest growing occupations in the country.[115] More than two thirds (67%) of all dentists employ at least one dental hygienist, and 93% of dentists work with dental assistants and 88% work with receptionists.[107,118] The current dental workforce is thought to have a reserve capacity largely through allied dental personnel.

Academic Dental Institutions: Educating Future Dental Professionals

Each year academic dental institutions (ADIs), including dental schools, allied dental programs, and postdoctoral and advanced dental education programs, graduate new practitioners to join the dental workforce. These academic dental institutions are private and public educational institutions across the United States, including 60 dental schools, 600 allied dental education programs, and 700 advanced dental education programs with more than 12,000 faculty members who educate nearly 50,000 students and residents attending these institutions.[115,118] It is at these ADIs that future practitioners and researchers gain their knowledge, the majority of dental research is conducted, and significant dental care is provided in clinical dental settings.

Approximately, 4714 predoctoral dental students graduated in 2007.[118] About half of these new graduates begin to practice as general dentists and others join the military, the US Public Health Service, or advance their education in a dental specialty. Approximately 2800 graduates along with hundreds of practicing dentists apply to residency training programs.[107,118] Unlike education programs for physicians, there is no universal requirement for education in dental residencies. However, about 65% of dental school graduates, a substantial proportion of dentists, now enroll in dental specialty or general dentistry residency programs.[107,118] Nearly 23,000 allied dental health professionals graduate from academic dental institutions each year and join the dental workforce.[107,118] Approximately 14,000 dental hygiene students, 8000 dental assistants, and 800 dental laboratory technologists graduate annually.[107,118] In the United States, there were 301 dental hygiene programs (2008), 281 dental assisting programs (2009), and 20 dental laboratory technology programs (2008) accredited by the Commission on Dental Accreditation.[115] Allied dental education has experienced a major expansion in capacity in the past twenty years, reflected in a nearly 25% increase in first-year dental hygiene enrollment and a 46% increase in first-year dental assisting enrollment over the last 10 years.[107,118]

The greatest gains in dental school enrollment have been an expansion in the representation of females. Female enrollees in dental schools in the United States increased from 2% in 1970 to 43% in 2007.[107,118] Approximately, 64% of graduates from dental schools were female during the years 1997–2006.[107,118] It has been projected that women will comprise 30% of professionally active dentists by 2020.[107,118]

Several national reports have focused attention on the growing diversity within the US population and the lack of diversity among many health professions.[120-122] Representation by underrepresented minorities has been low among predoctoral dental students enrolled in dental schools. During the 2008–2009 academic year, 0.7% of dental students were Native American or Alaska Native, 5.8% were African American, 6.2% were Hispanic or Latino, 23.4% were Asian American or Pacific Islander, 59.9% were white, and 4.0% were other.[107,118] Based on current dental school enrollment trends and growth in the diversity of the population by race and ethnicity, the future dental workforce will remain unrepresentative of the population to be served in the United States. This imbalance will become more exacerbated with the significant changes in racial and ethnic composition of the United States over the coming years.

African-American dentists report that nearly 62% of their patients are African Americans, and approximately 45% of the patients of Hispanic dentists are Hispanic.[123] Minority dentists are more likely to provide care to minority populations, but minority dentists are a small portion of the dental workforce. The number of minorities in the dental professions is inadequate and underrepresented compared with the overall population. In 2006, 89% of dentists were white, 5% were Asian and Pacific Islander, 4% were Hispanic, 2% were African American, and 0.1% were Native American and Alaska Native compared with the overall population of 86% white, 12% African American, 11% Hispanic, 4% Asian and Pacific Islander, and 0.9% Native American and Alaska Native.[118] African Americans, Hispanics, and Native Americans are severely underrepresented in the health professions. Expanding diversity is justified based on the grounds of civil rights, public health and educational benefits, and business gains. Improving the diversity of the health professions requires multiprong strategies addressing the educational pipeline, admissions policies and the institutional culture at health professions schools, and the broader policy environment. Several reports have recommended strategies that academic dental institutions can implement to enhance diversity, as well as address oral health care issues in their communities.[124-130]

Distribution of Dental Professionals

Recent national reports have highlighted a dental shortage and discussed the maldistribution of dentists to meet the nation's oral health needs.[79,105-111] No matter how the situation is described, there definitely is a significant problem accessing oral health care for millions of children and adults across the United States. The current dental workforce is unable to meet present day demand and need for dental care. If every individual were to have a dental home, then the nation would clearly have an insufficient number of dentists to care for the population. The nation needs the political will to assure that everyone who needs and wants dental care is able to receive oral health care. The need and demand for dental services continues to increase; in large measure this is due to the changing population trends. Even when the numbers of dentists may be adequate, the distribution of dentists remains a major challenge.

The distribution of dentists in relation to the population (dentists per 100,000 people) is dramatically different from the distribution of dentists. However, the ratio of dentists to population is decreasing. By 2010, that ratio is predicted to be at its lowest level in nearly 100 years. The dentist-to-population ratio peaked twice during the twentieth century: once prior to the Great Depression and again in the late 1980s.[107] According to the US Surgeon General, the ratio of dentists to the total population has steadily declined and it is projected that there will not be enough active dentists to care for the population.[11]

The dentist-to-population ratio has declined since the 1980's peak. In 1980, there were an estimated 53.6 dentists per 100,000 persons.[1] This ratio peaked at 59.1 per 100,000 people in the late 1980s and decreased to 58.3 in 2000. By the year 2010, the ratio of dentists to population is expected to decrease to 57.2.[107,108] It is projected to decline even further, to 53.7 in 2020 and only 50 dentists per 100,000 people in 2050. By 2010, that ratio will be at its lowest level in nearly 100 years. By 2020, the dentist-to-population ratio is projected to be comparable to the ratio experienced during World War II.[107]

Availability of dentists differs markedly among states—the dentist-to-population ratio ranges from 31.3 per 100,000 to 69 per 100,000, with Washington, DC, at 94.9 per 100,000.[66] The four states with the highest dentist to population ratio were New York, New Jersey, Connecticut, and Hawaii. The four states with the lowest dentist to population ratio were Mississippi, New Mexico, Nevada, and North Carolina.[66] Dentists in the United States are distributed unevenly and are underrepresented in areas of high need. Privately owned dental practices tend to be disproportionately concentrated in suburban areas, with dentists less available in inner cities or rural areas.[11] In 2008, there were 22 general practice, pediatric, or public health dentists per 100,000 persons in rural areas compared with 30 in urban areas, nationally.[119] Also, rural areas on a national level had a higher percentage of generalist dentists aged 56 or older than urban areas (42% versus 38%). This percentage was 44% in remote rural locations.[119]

The distribution of dentists varies across regions in the United States and within each state. A **Dental Health Professional Shortage Area (Dental HPSA)** is one of the three types of health professional shortage areas defined by the federal government.[131] Factors for identifying health professional shortage areas include primary care provider-to-population ratios, access to primary health care according to distance and time, incomes at poverty levels, and infant mortality and low-birth-weight incidences. In addition to communities, special populations and institutions may be designated as shortage areas.[131]

At the present time, the HPSA criteria require three basic determinations for a geographic area request: (1) the geographic area involved must be rational for the delivery of health services, (2) a specified population-to-practitioner ratio representing shortage must be exceeded within the area, and (3) resources in contiguous areas must be shown to be over utilized, excessively distant, or otherwise inaccessible.[131] Dental HPSAs have limited access to primary oral health care services because of financial, geographic, cultural, and language barriers.[131] The federal government designates areas as having practitioner shortages if a minimum number of specified criteria are met and the designation is made in collaboration with local communities and state health departments.

HPSA designation is used for a variety of purposes by federal programs. Dental HPSA is used to evaluate the eligibility of a given area or population for a number of federal and state programs to expand the oral health workforce.[131] These programs include the National Health Service Corps (NHSC), federal and state loan repayment programs, Community Health Center programs, and several Title VII Health Professions Programs.

The number of Dental HPSAs designated by the US Health Resources and Services Administration (HRSA) has grown from 792 in 1993 to 3527 in 2006.[118,131] In 2009, there were 4230 Dental HPSAs with 49 million people living in communities that lack a sufficient number of dental providers to ensure comprehensive dental care.[131] In 1993, HRSA estimated 1400 dentists were needed in the dental HPSA areas. By 2009, the number grew as it was predicted that 9642 practitioners were needed to meet oral health needs in these communities at a population-to-practitioner ratio of 3000 to 1.[131]

The dental safety net includes the facilities, providers, and payment programs that support dental care for underserved populations, including those individuals from various disadvantaged social, economic, and health conditions. Its components are made up by health centers, dental schools, clinics, Medicaid-oriented dental practices, free-care programs, hospital emergency rooms, and other places that tend to vary in availability, comprehensiveness, continuity, and quality.[132] Safety-net facilities located in dental academic institutions, community health centers, city and county health departments, migrant and rural health clinics, school-based programs, and mobile van programs target the underserved populations in primarily inner city and rural areas are few in number.[126,132,133]

For more than 40 years, HRSA-supported health centers have provided comprehensive, culturally competent, and quality primary health care services to underserved communities and vulnerable populations.[133] Health centers are community-based and patient-directed organizations that serve populations with limited access to health care. These include low-income populations, the uninsured, those with limited English proficiency, migrant and seasonal farm workers, homeless individuals and families, and those living in public housing.

More than 1000 Community health centers operate 6000 service sites. In 2008, more than 80% (850) of health centers across the country offered on-site dental services and 3.1 million patients were provided oral health care during 7.3 million visits. During that same year, health centers provided medical care to 14.9 million patients.[132] The proportion of community health centers with an oral health component increased from 52% in 1997 to 70% in 2006.[1] Between 1998 and 2008, the number of dental patients at health centers increased by 158% (from more than 1.2 million in 1998 to 3.1 million in 2008). The National Network for Oral Health Access (NNOHA) estimated that more than 12 million health center patients do not have access to dental services.[132] Nationwide in 2008, health centers employed 2300 full-time equivalent (FTE) employees as dentists and 900 as dental hygienists.[132]

Geographic maldistribution of dental professionals contributes to poor access to dental care in many communities, especially in rural and urban areas as local programs struggle to meet the oral health needs within their communities.[134-136] The safety-net dental delivery system is under pressure and in short supply.[132,133] The nation's oral health safety-net programs are meeting a small part of the great need for dental care.[132] The distribution of the dental workforce is placing stress on the public, nonprofit, and private sectors that provide services in the oral health care system and is causing reductions in access to oral health services.[134-139]

Reports have examined a number of components, including stresses on state health departments, community health centers, and the US Public Health Services Commissioned Corps.[81,140-142] Other reports have emphasized the need for adequate reimbursement levels, less complex administrative requirements, effective provider and patient outreach, and care coordination.[81,83,85-88,96] Model public health interventions and promising practices for safety net delivery systems to improve access to dental care for vulnerable population groups have been described in the literature.[137-142] Reviews of education assessed the needs of schools of dentistry, programs in dental hygiene, schools of public health, advanced education including dental public health residencies, and preventive research centers.[140] Several publications have noted inadequacies of the workforce that contributed to problems with dental public health capacity. This included lack of board-certified public health dentists and lack of diversity among the dental workforce and students.[140] Also, regulatory issues related to state licensure boards and state practice acts regarding dental hygiene practice were evaluated in the reports.[81,83,86,106-109]

Innovative strategies are needed to recruit and retain dental professionals who will seek careers in oral health and public health, today and in the future.[140-142] Strategies must be implemented to ensure that the dental workforce is culturally competent to provide oral health services to increasingly diverse individuals and communities.[125] As demands for oral health services increase both nationally and through programs for specific, vulnerable populations, groups, or communities, collaboration among state and local oral health programs and key stakeholders is essential to enhance development of the dental workforce.[134,137] Partnerships are necessary among state dental and dental hygienists' associations, dental and dental hygiene schools, state dental licensing boards, state primary care associations, community health centers, hospitals, and safety net oral health programs to increase the dental workforce, expand access to oral health services, and improve oral health outcomes.[137]

With the enactment of the Patient Protection and Affordable Care Act in 2010, the nation has an opportunity to expand quality dental care for children and adults who are not receiving needed services currently.[104,105] The provisions when implemented will expand the number of dental care professionals in high-need areas who can provide dental care to underserved and vulnerable populations.[104,105] These provisions include the following:

- **Funds for Community Health Centers** (CHCs): CHC funds to construct, expand, and sustain community health centers.
- **Support for school-based health centers:** A grant program with preference for centers that serve large numbers of children enrolled Medicaid or similar programs. Oral health assessments and referrals are part of the core services that the school-based health centers must include in the grant program.
- **Authorization of a demonstration grant program for new workforce models:** A 5-year program used for education or employment of new types of dental providers to increase access to oral health services in rural and other underserved communities. The term used in the law is *alternative dental health care providers,* and the law specifies the inclusion of community dental health coordinators, advance practice dental hygienists, independent dental hygienists, supervised dental hygienists, primary care physicians, dental therapists, and dental health aides (or other models the Secretary of the Department of Health and Human Services [DHHS] approves). Only pilot programs authorized by state law can be funded beginning no later than March 23, 2012. The program is authorized but has not yet been funded through appropriations. There is also a required contract with the Institute of Medicine (IOM) to study the demonstration programs to assess their impact on expanding access.
- **Expansion of the dental health aide therapist model for tribal lands:** The Indian Health Service can help expand the dental health aide therapist (DHAT) model into states where the use of DHATs or other midlevel dental providers is authorized under state law. A tribe must elect to participate, but this provision gives tribes the opportunity to work within the states to develop strategies for improving access to dental care, with a focus on increasing the number of oral health care providers and this provision is effective immediately.
- **Funds for provider education:** Awards education grants or contracts to academic institutions, including dental and dental hygiene schools, residency and advanced education programs in general, pediatric, and public health dentistry to support and develop education programs and faculty loan repayment.
- **Primary care residency funding:** Authorizes 3-year grants to be awarded to create new accredited or expanded primary-care residency programs, including dental programs. Also, provides funding for new and expanding graduate medical education, including dental education.

Organizations and agencies at the national, state, and local levels have begun to discuss and implement innovative ways to address dental care access problems for children and adults.[81,138,139,143] Recently, published policy briefs and reports have described effective innovations that can be implemented to increase access to oral health services for children and adults.[81,138,139,143] It is essential that discussions that have often focused on children be expanded to ensure access to dental services for all children and adolescents, as well as assure access to dental care for all adults and elders in communities across the United States. With the current oral health disparities and expected population growth, creative measures are crucial to improve oral health, including developments in education, research, and health promotion and expansions of clinical care within the private, public, and nonprofit sectors.

DENTAL PUBLIC HEALTH PROGRAMS

Status and Trends

The burden of oral diseases and needs of populations are in transition, and oral health systems and scientific knowledge are changing rapidly. The challenges of improving oral health are great in many countries and communities. The downturn in the global economy has contributed to major budget constraints for federal, state, and local government agencies in recent years. This comes at a time when the incomes of many families are stressed, and an increase has occurred in the oral health needs of many children and adults, as well as those in vulnerable population groups. The infrastructure and capacity of many dental public health programs at the national, state, and local levels are limited and stretched compared with the oral health needs in states and communities.[140-142] Published reports in the United States have reviewed the challenges faced in ensuring a viable dental public health infrastructure, as well as state- and community-based programs to ensure access to dental care for the underserved population in the United States.[140-142]

Public Health Infrastructure and Capacity

The structures of public health agencies are undergoing significant changes. These public health agencies and the related oral health programs at the federal, state, and local levels vary greatly in size, structure, staffing and funding.[73] The Association of State & Territorial Dental Directors (ASTDD) report, Building Infrastructure and Capacity in State and Oral Health Programs highlighted resources and funding ranges needed to maintain fully effective dental public health programs at the state and territorial levels.[144] The ASTDD identified essential elements under the core functions of assessment, policy development and assurance to build infrastructure and capacity for state oral health programs. Oral health infrastructure consists of systems, people, relationships, and the resources that would enable federal, state, and local oral health programs to perform public health functions.[144] Oral health capacity enables the development of oral health expertise and competence and the implementation of oral health strategies.[144] The ASTDD infrastructure project found that state oral health programs that have (1) competence in surveillance, (2) a full-time dental director and skilled staff, (3) a state oral health plan, (4) the support of policymakers, (5) strong public/private partnerships and community coalitions, and (6) an ability to obtain funds for services will be better prepared to achieve *Healthy People 2020* Oral Health Objectives for their state and for the nation.[144] Oral health programs in some localities have shown significant progress in collaboration with partnering organizations and agencies to address infrastructure and build capacity.

The HRSA's Maternal and Child Health Bureau (MCHB) uses a pyramid to describe the four levels of core public health services for the population served by programs in the bureau.[145] **Figure 5-11** illustrates the MCHB pyramid of public health services. Starting at the base, these are (1)

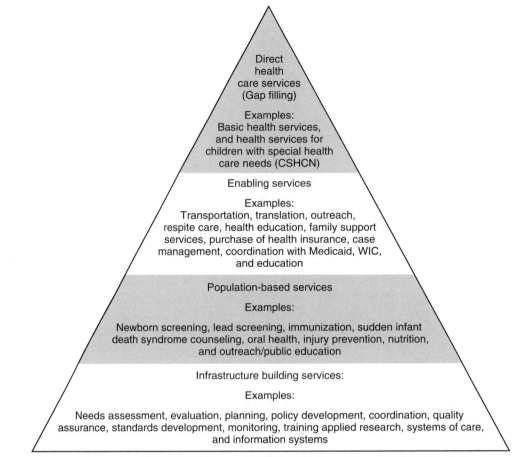

Source: Maternal and Child Health Bureau. Strategic Plan: Fiscal Year 2003-2007. Rockville, MD: Maternal and Child Health Bureau; 2003.

Figure 5-11 Key public health services provided by Maternal and Child Health (MCH) Agencies.

infrastructure building services, (2) population-based services, (3) enabling services, and (4) direct health care (gap-filling) services.[145] Infrastructure building and population-based services provide the broad foundation on which enabling and direct care services rest. The pyramid provides a useful framework for understanding programmatic directions of the MCHB for linking oral health and public health programs that can contribute to collaborative partnerships in meeting the mission and accomplishing the goals of the MCHB.

The MCHB and the Division of Oral Health of the CDC have adapted the essential elements and the MCH pyramid to support the development of oral health programs at the state and local levels.[146] Also, these frameworks have been used for evaluation of state and local oral health programs as well as the formation of a basis for performance measures.[146] The ASTDD has specified that a key infrastructure element is having leadership to address oral health problems, with a full-time state dental director and an adequately staffed oral health unit with competence to perform core public health functions.[144] Surveys conducted by ASTDD demonstrated that substantially more oral health–related assessment, policy development, and assurance activities occur in states with a direct commitment of human resources.[144] Lack of continuity in dental public health leadership is a serious problem and can interfere with long-term strategic planning and evaluation.[140-142] The presence of more activities related to the essential public health functions was found in states with full-time dental directors compared with those states with part-time directors, no directors, or no oral health program in the state health agency.[144]

Current Status: Structure and Funding

Most state oral health programs are located within a health department or a broader department of human services.[73] Where the oral health program is placed in the organizational structure has been shown to affect the oral health program director's level of authority, reporting relationship, hiring process, funding, and the program's focus.[144] Whatever the designation, most states place oral health programs or functions under a broader organizational umbrella such as maternal and child health, family health, rural health, primary care, chronic disease or disease prevention, or health promotion.[73] In 2003, 23 states reported having a statutory basis for their program, meaning a state law requiring an oral health program or the requirement for a state dental director.[147] In a 2007 ASTDD survey, 47% of 42 responding states had a statutory basis for their program and 47% had a statutory requirement for the director position.[73] These are not necessarily the same states because the survey found that four do not have a statutory basis for their program but do for the director position, whereas four have a statutory basis for the program but not for the director.

For fiscal year 2007–2008, 47 of the 50 states and Washington, DC, reported having a full-time dental director.[148] Although the majority of dental director positions are full-time, many have other responsibilities in addition to administering the state oral health program. The same report indicated that 17 directors devoted at least 20% of their time to Medicaid dental issues.[148] Many serve in an advisory capacity to other programs or state agencies. While the majority reported were state employees, 10 were appointed by the state health officer, governor, or other official, three were contractual and three others had some other arrangement. The position status of a dental director can greatly influence the selection process and requirements as well as the continuity of a program if the director changes with a change in administration.[73,144] Professionals in state dental director positions need public health experience and skills to function effectively in the public health environment found today.[144] Of 42 states responding to the 2007 ASTDD survey, 30 required public health experience; an earlier survey that year reported 22 of 47 states required a master's degree, but not necessarily in public health.[73] About 60% of the directors held a master's in Public Health (MPH); three others held a doctor of laws (JD), master of arts (MA), or a doctor of philosophy (PhD) degree.[73] Eleven states did not require a state dental or dental hygiene license for professionals serving as dental director.[73]

Staffing patterns for oral health programs vary substantially in terms of numbers of personnel, job categories, responsibilities, level and type of education, lines of supervision, employee or contractor status, and job location.[144,149] Most staff who have positions in the state office function in non-clinical roles such as managers, coordinators, regional consultants, public health educators, program planners or evaluators.[144] In fiscal year 2007–2008, 18% of responding state programs had two or fewer FTE employees and contractors, 49% had 3 to 9, 12% had 10 to 19, 19% had more than 20, and one state did not respond.[148] Some programs may also hire, contract with, or share with other state programs an epidemiologist, statistician, evaluator, fluoridation engineer, or other specialized staff.[73,144] Higher numbers of employees are likely to reflect states that administer programs that provide services directly. These programs often employ clinicians, clerical, and administrative personnel in prevention programs (e.g., school-based dental sealant programs), community clinics, and mobile clinics.[73,144] In other states the oral health programs provide grants to local programs that hire employees who are not considered state employees.[73,144]

Historically, most state dental public health activities were funded with federal MCHB support through mechanisms like the MCH Block Grant. Also, the CDC Preventive Health Services Block Grant has funded community preventive services such as community water fluoridation in some states.[144] Since 2003, grants for oral health programs through CDC and HRSA have focused on building the infrastructure and capacity of state oral health programs. MCHB provided State Oral Health Collaborative Systems grants to most states from 2003 to 2007. A new cycle of Targeted State Oral Health Service System cooperative agreements provided funds to 19 states and one territory in 2007–2011. The CDC's Division of Oral Health provided funding to 12 states and one territory for cooperative agreements to increase their oral health infrastructure in 2003–2008. Another round of funding by the CDC for State-Based Oral Disease Prevention Programs provided funding for 16 states in 2008–2013. In addition, a third round of states and territories will be supported by the CDC in 2010–2013. Also, the HRSA Health Professions has provided funding to state health agencies through four rounds of state Oral Health Workforce grants since fiscal year 2006.

The state synopsis shows that many states have more diversified support from multiple funding streams such the HRSA's MCHB and Health Professions, the CDC's Division of Oral Health, state general revenues, and foundations.[148] Of the 42 states that provided information on source of funding for fiscal year 2006–2007, 22 (50%) reported receiving 75% to 100% of their funding from just one source.[148] For seven states (17%), this sole source is their state general revenue funds; for 10 states (23%), their main source is HRSA; and for four states (9%), the primary source is the CDC.[148] In the same survey, 23% of states reported decreases in their budget, whereas 37% reported increases.[148] At least 50% of states still receive 75% to 100% of their funding from just one source.[148] Reliance on one funding source can affect program sustainability over time.

State programs funded consistently and continuously have shown evidence of building and maintaining state oral health program infrastructure and capacity. These resources help states prevent oral diseases and promote oral health by establishing systems that foster oral disease surveillance, coalition-building, and partnerships. States are then able to leverage support for increased promotion and coordination of effective public health preventive interventions such as school-based dental sealant programs and community water fluoridation.[149,150]

Current Status: Oral Health Program Performance

State, territorial, tribal, and local governments are uniquely situated within government structures to develop partnerships and resources that provide leadership for oral health initiatives. There is consensus that well-established oral health programs are critical to the oral health of the United States. Strengthening dental public health programs through systematic oral health surveillance linked with planning, implementation, and evaluation of effective measures to prevent oral diseases and promote oral health is essential.[151,152] A recent report graded the performance of states in relation to their oral health programs.[83] The Pew Children's Dental Campaign assessed and graded all 50 states and Washington, DC, on whether and how well they were implementing cost-effective preventive strategies and promising policy approaches.[83] The report evaluated key performance indicators related to approaches with the potential to improve oral health of children and their access to care including: (1) school-based dental sealant programs; (2) community water fluoridation; (3) improvements to state Medicaid programs to increase the number of children receiving oral health services; (4) innovative workforce models that expand the number of qualified dental providers, including medical personnel, dental hygienists, and new primary care dental professionals; and (5) collecting oral health data to track changes and drive progress for improving oral health program performance.[83]

Several states have demonstrated progress by implementing some of these approaches, but many states have limitations so the approaches are not yet initiated or widespread. The analysis shows that about 60% of states do not have key policies in place.[83] Only six states merited the highest grade by meeting at least six of the eight policy benchmarks (i.e., they had particular policies in place that met or exceeded the national performance thresholds).[83] Although these states were doing well on the benchmarks, all states needed improvement because no state met all targets. Even those with good policy frameworks can do far more to provide additional children with access to prevention and dental care based on current benchmarks. According to this national report card, six states merited an A grade, two earned B grades, three states and Washington, DC, were awarded a grade of C or below, and nine of those states that received an F met only one or two policy benchmarks. This report serves as a warning sign and a wake-up call for policymakers to take serious action to make greater progress in the future.[83] To meet these challenges effectively, public health administrators and decision-makers need to assure sufficient levels of funding for tools, capacity, and application of evidence-based practices to assess and monitor health needs, implement intervention strategies, and design policy options appropriate for their unique circumstances to improve the performance of the public health system, as well as the oral health system.[18,146] Although there have been some gains in the size and strength of the dental public health programs in the United States, these programs generally remain small, understaffed, and underfunded with great variation in capacity to meet oral health needs.[142] Limited resources ensure that the public health missions of these programs will fall short because they are unable to protect and enhance the oral health of communities in their jurisdictions.[142] Sources of funding for oral health programs from local, state, and federal revenue streams need to be sustained and increased in the future.

The Patient Protection and Affordable Care Act enacted in 2010 includes provisions for prevention and wellness.[104,105] Advocates are working to ensure that appropriations are included in federal budgets to implement provisions for oral health promotion and oral disease prevention.[104,105] These provisions are as follows:

- **Increasing funds for CDC grants:** Establishes cooperative agreements to improve oral health infrastructure in all 50 states, territories, and Indian tribes. Government agencies would receive funding, dependent on the availability of funding, through fiscal year 2014.
- **Expanding school-based sealant programs:** With the appropriation of funding, the provision allows the CDC and HRSA to provide grants to the 50 states, territories, Indian tribes, and organizations for the development of school-based dental sealant programs to improve the access of children to primary prevention.
- **Expanding access to optimally fluoridated water:** Increase community understanding of water fluoridation and other preventive activities. The Secretary of DHHS, acting through the director of the CDC, will work with each of the 50 states, territories, and tribal organizations to implement a national, science-based public education campaign focused on oral health. A 5-year campaign is to include oral disease prevention messages about water fluori-

dation, early childhood caries, periodontal disease, and oral cancer beginning no later than 2012, with funding authorized from fiscal years 2010–2014. Using effective methods to educate the public about community water fluoridation should increase understanding and support for fluoridation in communities.

- **Monitoring oral health trends:** Comprehensive and accurate data are critical for states to track oral health status and develop effective strategies. This provision supports the continuation of NOHSS by increasing participation of all 50 states, territories, and the District of Columbia. Also, this provision expands the collection of oral health data in other national health surveys but is subject to available funding.

Oral health programs need to maximize opportunities for securing funding from all available sources to implement evidence-based oral health measures. Sustained resources are crucial for oral health programs to build capacity and infrastructure for program planning and management, implementation, building of partnerships, and evaluation. A range of complementary strategies can be implemented in partnership with local, state, national and international agencies. At the crux of a public health approach is the need to empower local communities to become actively involved in dental public health efforts.

FUTURE DIRECTIONS

Oral Health in America: A Report of the Surgeon General described the oral health successes of the twentieth century and also discussed the oral health challenges confronting the nation. A National Call to Action to Promote Oral Health proposed opportunities to reduce oral health disparities in the twenty-first century. *Healthy People 2010* outlined oral health benchmarks for the United States, and some oral health indicators showed promise of improvements in the 2000s. The National Oral Health Objectives in ***Healthy People 2020*** now provide the road map for the next decade. These reports provide the framework that, when combined with political will, can produce oral health improvements for all in the United States. Political will is critical at the national, state, and local levels for improved oral health outcomes to come to fruition in 2020 and beyond. The Patient Protection and Affordable Care Act enacted in 2010 offers opportunities to expand oral health promotion, strengthen disease prevention, increase access to dental care, enhance professional education, and build public health programs to improve oral health outcomes in the nation.[104,105] Also, the 2010 National Oral Health Initiative released by the DHHS provides greater focus and direction for oral health actions at the national level.[153] The forthcoming two national reports from the IOM based on the deliberations of the consensus study committees and commissioned background papers can generate momentum to drive oral health action in the coming decade.[154,155] Oral health programs at the national, state, and local levels need the following key elements to be better prepared to achieve the *Healthy People 2020* Oral Health Objectives:

- A workforce educated and competent in dental public health representing the diversity of the United States.
- Adequate workforce and sufficient administrative presence with skilled staff and leadership from full-time oral health program directors at the international, national, state, and local levels.
- Collaborative oral health planning and implementation that integrates evidence-based public health principles and practices.
- Support of informed policymakers to develop and promote oral health policies.
- Strong and vibrant public-private partnerships.

- Ability to obtain and leverage sufficient financial resources.
- Legal authority to use personnel in an effective and cost-efficient manner.
- Infrastructure and capacity to plan, implement, and evaluate oral health policies, practices, and programs that are sustainable in the future.
- Evidence-based population-based interventions to prevent oral diseases in communities.
- Health systems interventions to ensure access to oral health care for children and adults.

Specific focus areas should include surveillance of oral disease, reporting the burden of disease, facilitating the development and implementation of oral health coalitions, oral health plans, dental sealant programs, community water fluoridation coordination, and management of program capacity and infrastructure to sustain an oral health program.

SUMMARY

This chapter presents the oral health indicators used for tracking and monitoring national oral health objectives. These benchmarks provide an important framework for the assessment of oral health in the United States in the past and in the coming decade. The current status and trends of oral health and access to oral health services used as key indicators in the United States are also described. Finally, important oral health disparities among population groups based on race and ethnicity, family income, education level, gender, geographic location, and disability are highlighted in the chapter.

Applying Your Knowledge

1. Select an oral health indicator such as dental caries or periodontal disease. For each oral health indicator discuss current status, past trends, and disparities among population groups. Use information presented in the chapter, websites listed in the appendixes, library resources, and the Internet for updated information now available to describe the oral health status of the selected indicator.
2. Describe how you would use the information found on the selected oral health indicator to plan, implement, and evaluate dental public health programs in your role as the following:
   a. State Dental Director
   b. County Oral Health Director
   c. Dental Director in a Community Health Center

Dental Hygiene Competencies

Reading the material in this chapter and participating in the activities of Applying Your Knowledge will contribute to the student's ability to demonstrate the following competencies:

Health promotion and disease prevention
HP.4 Identify individual and population risk factors and develop strategies that promote health-related quality of life.

Community involvement
CM.1 Assess the oral health needs of the community and the quality and availability of resources and services.

Patient/client care

PC.1 Systematically collect, analyze, and record data on the general, oral, and psychosocial health status of a variety of patients or clients using methods consistent with medicolegal principles.

PC.2 Use critical decision-making skills to reach conclusions about the patient's or client's dental hygiene needs based on all available assessment data.

PC.5A Determine the outcomes of dental hygiene interventions using indexes, instruments, examination techniques, and the patient's or client's self-report.

Community Case

As the State Dental Director, you are working with a state oral health coalition to plan a statewide oral health survey. You decide to review the current status of key oral health indicators from information you have for the nation and various states. This information is presented in **Table A** and the graph in **Figure B**.

1. Based on the information in **Table A**, which state has the highest rate of untreated tooth decay?
   a. Oklahoma
   b. Nevada
   c. Illinois
   d. Oregon
2. Based on the information in **Table A**, which state has the lowest rate of untreated tooth decay?
   a. Colorado
   b. Alaska
   c. Louisiana
   d. Massachusetts
3. Based on the information in **Table A**, which state does not meet the national oral health objective of 33% of third-grade children with untreated tooth decay by 2010?
   a. Wisconsin
   b. Idaho
   c. Texas
   d. California

Table A   Percentage of Third-Grade Students with Untreated Tooth Decay

State	School Year	Percent (%) with Untreated Tooth Decay
Alaska	2007–2008	26.2
California	2004–2005	28.7
Colorado	2006–2007	24.5
Idaho	2008–2009	22.5
Illinois	2008–2009	29.1
Louisiana	2007–2009	41.9
Massachusetts	2006–2007	17.3
Nevada	2005–2006	44.0
Oklahoma	2007–2008	32.3
Oregon	2006–2007	35.4
Texas	2007–2008	42.7
Wisconsin	2007–2008	20.1

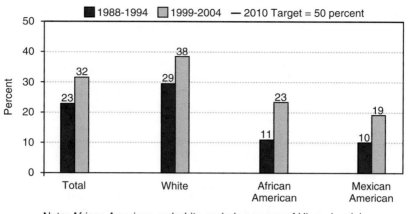

Note: African American and white exclude persons of Hispanic origin.
Persons of Mexican-American origin may be of any race.
Source: National Health and Nutrition Examination Survey, National Center
for Health Statistics, Centers for Disease Control and Prevention.[1]

Figure B Percentage of children (8 years of age) with dental sealants, 1988–1994 and 1999–2004.

4. Based on the information in the bar graph in **Figure B**:
   Statement 1: White children 6 to 11 years of age in 1999–2004 had two times the rate of dental sealants than their Mexican-American counterparts.
   Statement 2: African-American children 6 to 11 years of age in 1999–2004 had the highest rate of dental sealants.
   a. The first statement is true and the second statement is false.
   b. The first statement is false and the second statement is true.
   c. Both statements are true.
   d. Both statements are false.
5. Based on the information in the bar graph in **Figure B**, which group of 6- to 11-year-old children had the greatest need for dental sealants in 1999–2004?
   a. Mexican-American and African-American children have the same need.
   b. Mexican-American children.
   c. African-American children.
   d. All of the groups had the greatest need for dental sealants.

References

1. Centers for Disease Control and Prevention, National Center for Health Statistics, US Department of Health and Human Services: Data 2010: Healthy People 2010 Database. Atlanta: Centers for Disease Control and Prevention; January 2010.
2. American Cancer Society. Cancer Facts and Figures 2010. Atlanta: American Cancer Society; 2010.
3. Manski RJ, Brown E. Dental use, Expenses, Dental Coverage, and Changes, 1996 and 2004, MEPS Chartbook No.17. Rockville MD: Agency for Healthcare Research and Quality; 2007.
4. Petersen PE. The world oral health report 2003: Continuous improvement of oral health in the 21st century—the approach of the WHO Global Oral Health Programme. Community Dent Oral Epidemiol 2003;31:3.
5. Petersen PE, Bourgeois D, Ogawa H, et al. The global burden of oral diseases and risks to oral health. Bull World Health Organ 2005;83:661.
6. World Health Organization. Oral Health. Geneva: World Health Organization. Available at www.who.int/oral_health/en/. Accessed May 2010.
7. Petersen PE, Bourgeois D, Bratthall D, et al. Oral health information systems–towards measuring progress in oral health promotion and disease prevention. Bull World Health 2005;83:686.

8. Petersen PE. Global policy for improvement of oral health in the 21st century–implications to oral health research of World Health Assembly 2007, World Health Organization. Community Dent Oral Epidemiol 2009;37:1.

9. Kwan S, Petersen PE. Oral health: equity and social determinants. In: Blas E, Kurup AS, editors. Equity, Social Determinants and Public Health Programmes. Geneva: World Health Organization; 2010.

10. Beaglehole R, Benzian H, Crail J, et al. The Oral Health Atlas: Mapping a Neglected Global Health Issue. Brighton, UK: Myriad Editions for FDI World Dental Federation; 2009.

11. US Department of Health and Human Services. Oral Health in America: A Report of the Surgeon General. Rockville, MD: US Department of Health and Human Services, National Institute of Dental and Craniofacial Research, National Institutes of Health; 2000.

12. US Department of Health and Human Services. A National Call to Action to Promote Oral Health. Rockville, MD: US Department of Health and Human Services, Public Health Service, Centers for Disease Control and Prevention, National Institutes of Health, National Institute of Dental and Craniofacial Research; May 2003.

13. Dye BA, Tan S, Smith V, et al. Trends in Oral Health Status, United States, 1988–1994 and 1999–2004. National Center for Health Statistics; Vital Health Stat Series 11 Number 248, 2007.

14. US Department of Health and Human Services. Healthy People 2000: National Health Promotion and Disease Prevention Objectives. Washington, DC: U.S. Department of Health and Human Services; 1990.

15. US Department of Health and Human Services. Healthy People 2010: Understanding and Improving Health, 2nd ed. Washington, DC: US Department of Health and Human Services; 2000.

16. National Centers for Health Statistics, Centers for Disease Control and Prevention. Healthy People 2010 Progress Review Focus Area 21—Oral Health: Briefing Book Materials–Objective Charts and Disparity Charts for Focus Area 13—Oral Health, February 7, 2008.

17. Cohen LK, Gift HC, editors. Disease Prevention and Oral Health Promotion: Socio-dental Sciences in Action. Copenhagen: Munksgaard; 1995.

18. Task Force on Community Preventive Services. Promoting oral health: Interventions to prevent dental caries, oral and pharyngeal cancers, and sports-related craniofacial injuries: A report on the recommendations of the Task Force on Community Preventive Services. MMWR Morb Mortal Wkly Rep 2001;50(RR-21):1.

19. Gooch BF, Griffin SO, Malvitz DM. The role of evidence in formulating public health programs to prevent oral disease and promote oral health in the United States. J Evid Based Dent Pract 2006;6:85.

20. Gooch BF, Griffin SO, Gray SK, et al. Preventing dental caries through school-based sealant programs: Updated recommendations and reviews of evidence. J Am Dent Assoc 2009;140:1356.

21. Centers for Disease Control and Prevention. Recommendation for using fluoride to prevent and control dental caries in the United States. MMWR Morb Mortal Wkly Rep 2001;50(RR-14):1.

22. American Dental Association Council on Scientific Affairs. Professionally applied topical fluoride: Evidence-based clinical recommendations. J Am Dent Assoc 2006;137:1151.

23. Centers for Disease Control and Prevention. Preventing Dental Caries with Community Programs. Atlanta: Centers for Disease Control and Prevention; April 2010.

24a. Beauchamp J, Caufield PW, Crall JJ, et al. Evidence-based clinical recommendations for the use of pit-and-fissure sealants: a report of the American Dental Association Council on Scientific Affairs. J Am Dent Assoc 2008;139:257.

24b. Rethman MP, Carpenter W, Cohen EE, et al. Evidence-based clinical recommendations regarding screening for oral squamous cell carcinomas. J Am Dent Assoc 2010;141:509.

25. Fiore MC, Jaen CR, Baker TB, et al. Treating Tobacco Use and Dependence: 2008 Update. Clinical Practice Guideline. Rockville, MD: US Department of Health and Human Services. Public Health Service; May 2008.

26. Task Force on Community Preventive Services. Strategies for reducing exposure to environmental tobacco smoke, increasing tobacco-use cessation, and reducing initiation in communities and health-care systems: A report on recommendations of the Task Force on Community Preventive Services. MMWR Morb Mortal Wkly Rep 2000;49(RR12):1.

27. US Preventive Services Task Force. Guide to Clinical Preventive Services. 2nd ed. Baltimore, MD; 1996.

28. Bailey W, Duchon K, Barker L, et al. Populations receiving optimally fluoridated public drinking water—United States, 1992–2006. MMWR Morb Mortal Wkly Rep 2008;57:737.

29. Sanders AE, Slade GD, Lim S, et al. Impact of oral disease on quality of life in the US and Australian populations. Community Dent Oral Epidemiol 2009;37:171.

30. Blumenshine SL, Vann WF Jr, Gizlice Z, et al. Children's school performance: Impact of general and oral health. J Public Health Dent 2008;68:82.

31. Gift HC, Reisine ST, Larch DC. The social impact of dental problems and visits. Am J Public Health 1993;82:1663.

32. Acs G, Lodolinni G, Kaminski S, et al. Effect of nursing caries on body weight in a pediatric population. J Pediatr Dent 1992;14:302.

33. Chen M, Andersen RM, Barmes DE, et al. Comparing Oral Health Care Systems: A Second International Collaborative Study. Geneva: World Health Organization; 1997.

34. National Institute of Dental and Craniofacial Research, Centers of Disease Control and Prevention. Dental, Oral and Craniofacial Data Resource Center. Rockville, MD: Dental, Oral and Craniofacial Data Resource Center; 2010.

35. US Department of Health and Human Services. Tracking Healthy People 2010. Washington, DC: US Government Printing Office; November 2000.

36. Centers of Disease Control and Prevention, Oral Health Program. National Oral Health Surveillance System. Atlanta: Centers for Disease Control and Prevention; 2010.

37. Child and Adolescent Health Measurement Initiative. Data Resource Centers for Child and Adolescent Health. Portland, OR: Child and Adolescent Health Measurement Initiative; 2010.

38. Truman BI, Gooch BF, Evans CA Jr, editors. The guide to community preventive services: Interventions to prevent dental caries, oral and pharyngeal cancers, and sports-related craniofacial injuries. Am J Prev Med 2002;23(1 Suppl):21.

39. Task Force on Community Preventive Services. The guide to community preventive services: Tobacco use prevention and control. Am J Prev Med 2001;20(2 Suppl):1.

40. Bertness J, Holt K. Promoting Awareness, Preventing Pain. Facts on Early Childhood Caries (ECC), 2nd ed. Washington, DC: National Maternal and Child Oral Health Resource Center; 2004.

41. Reisine S, Douglas JM. Psychological and behavioral issues in early childhood caries. Community Dent Oral Epidemiol 1998;26:32.

42. Patrick DL, Lee RS, Nucci M, et al. Reducing oral health disparities: a focus on social and cultural determinants. BMC Oral Health 2006;15:S4.

43. Fisher-Owens SA, Gansky SA, Platt LJ, et al. Influences on children's oral health: A conceptual model. Pediatrics 2007;120:e510.

44. Chattopadhyay A. Oral health disparities in the United States. Dent Clin North Am 2008;52:297.

45. Vargas CM, Arevalo O. How dental care can preserve and improve oral health. Dent Clin North Am 2009;53:399.

46. Macek MD, Heller KE, Selwitz RH, et al. Is 75 percent of dental caries really found in 25% of the population? J Public Health Dent 2004;64:20.

47. Gift HC, Corbin SB, Nowjack-Raymer RE. Public knowledge of prevention of dental disease. Public Health Rep 1994;109:397.

48. Centers for Disease Control and Prevention. The Benefits of Fluoride. Atlanta: Centers for Disease Control and Prevention; August 2009.

49. Centers for Disease Control and Prevention. Achievements in public health, 1900–1999: fluoridation of drinking water to prevent dental caries. MMWR Morb Mortal Wkly Rep 1999;48:933.

50. Bailey W, Duchon K. Water Fluoridation Prevalence and Occurrence. In: Water, Public Health, and Health Promotion, Plenary Session 3152.0 Philadelphia, PA. American Public Health Association 137th Annual Meeting Water and Public Health: The 21st Century Challenge; Abstract 206556, November 9, 2009.

51. Centers for Disease Control and Prevention. Cost Savings of Community Water Fluoridation. Atlanta: Centers for Disease Control and Prevention; September 2009.

52. Griffin SO, Jones K, Tomar SL. An economic evaluation of community water fluoridation. J Publ Health Dent 2001;61:78.

53. American Dental Association. 1998 Consumers' Opinions Regarding Community Water Fluoridation. Chicago: American Dental Association; 1998.

54. Centers for Disease Control and Prevention. Knowledge of the purpose of community water fluoridation: United States, 1990. MMWR Morb Mortal Wkly Rep 1992;41:919.

55. Centers for Disease Control and Prevention, National Center for Health Statistics. Healthy People 2000 Review, 1999–2000. Hyattsville, MD: Public Health Service; 1999.

56. Centers for Disease Control and Prevention. Preventing and controlling oral and pharyngeal cancer: Recommendations from a national strategic planning conference. MMWR Morb Mortal Wkly Rep 1998;47(RR14):1.

57. American Cancer Society. Detailed Guide: Oral Cavity and Oropharyngeal Cancer. Atlanta: American Cancer Society; 2009.

58. National Institute of Dental and Craniofacial Research. Data and statistics. Bethesda, MD: National Institute of Dental and Craniofacial Research; March 2010.

59. Pelucchi C, Gallus S, Garavello W, et al. Cancer risk associated with alcohol and tobacco use: Focus on upper aerodigestive tract and liver. Alcohol Res Health 2006;29:193-8.

60. Tomar SL, Logan HL. Florida adults' oral cancer knowledge and examination experiences. J Publ Health Dent 2005;20:221.

61. Horowitz AM, Nourjah PA, Gift HC. U.S. adult knowledge of risk factors and signs of oral cancers: 1990. J Am Dent Assoc 1995;126:39.

62. Chattopadhyay A. Oral Health Epidemiology: Principles and Practice. Sudbury, MA: Jones & Bartlett; 2009.

63. Brunelle JA, Bhat M, Lipton JA. Prevalence and distribution of selected occlusal characteristics in the U.S. population, 1988–1991 (special issue). J Dent Res 1996;75:706.

64. Proffit WR, Fields HW Jr, Moray LJ. Malocclusion prevalence and orthodontic treatment need in the United States: Estimates from the NHANES III survey. Int J Adult Orthodon Orthognath Surg 1998;13:97.

65. Kaste LM, Gift HC, Bhat M, et al. Prevalence of incisor trauma in persons 6 to 50 years of age: United States, 1988–1991 (special issue). J Dent Res 1996;75:696.

66. National Institute of Dental and Craniofacial Research, Centers for Disease Control and Prevention. Dental, Oral and Craniofacial Data Resource Center: Oral health US, 2002. Rockville, MD: Dental, Oral and Craniofacial Data Resource Center; 2002.

67. Burt CW, Overpeck MD. Emergency visits for sports-related injuries. Ann Emerg Med 2001;37:301.

68. Bourguignon C, Sigurdsson A. Preventive strategies for traumatic dental injuries. Dent Clin North Am 2009;53:729.

69. Andreasen JO, Andreasen FM, Anderson L. Textbook and Color Atlas of Traumatic Injuries to the Teeth. 4th ed. Oxford, UK: Blackwell Munksgaard; 2007.

70. Beltrán-Aguilar ED, Barker LK, Canto MT, et al. Surveillance for dental caries, dental sealants, tooth retention, edentulism, and enamel fluorosis. Morb Mortal Wkly Rep Surveill Summ 2005;54:1.

71. Tomar S, Cohen L. Developing a new paradigm for the dental delivery system. J Public Health Dent 2010;70(special issue):S6.

72. Gift HC, Andersen RM. The principles of organisation and models of delivery of oral health care. In: Pine C, Harris R, editors. Community Oral Health (Chapter 17). Chicago, IL: Quintessence Publishing; 2007.

73. Association of State & Territorial Dental Directors. Guidelines for State and Territorial Oral Health Programs. Sparks, NV: Association of State & Territorial Dental Directors; 2010.

74. Rural Health and Human Service Issues, National Advisory Committee. The 2004 Report to the Secretary: Rural Health and Human Service Issues. Rockville, MD: National Advisory Committee on Rural Health and Human Services; April 2004.

75. Edelstein BL, Chinn CH. Update on disparities in oral health and access to dental care for America's children. Acad Pediatr 2009;9:415.

76. Chevarley FM. Percentage of Persons Unable to Get or Delayed in Getting Needed Medical Care, Dental Care, or Prescription Medicines: United States, 2007, Statistical Brief 282. Rockville MD: Agency for Healthcare Research and Quality; 2007.

77. Child Trends Databank. Unmet Dental Needs. Washington, DC: Child Trends; 2010.

78. Glassman P, Subar P. Creating and maintaining oral health for dependent people in institutional settings. J Public Health Dent 2010;70(special issue):S40.

79. Institute of Medicine. The U.S. Oral Health Workforce in the Coming Decade. Workshop summary. Washington, DC: National Academies Press; 2009.

80. Haley J, Kenney G, Pelletier J. Access to Affordable Dental Care: Gaps for Low-income Adults. Menlo Park, CA: Kaiser Commission on Medicaid and the Uninsured, Henry J. Kaiser Family Foundation; July 2008.

81. Shirk C. Oral Health Checkup, Progress in Tough Times? Washington, DC: National Health Policy Forum, George Washington University; Issue Brief Number 836, March 29, 2010.

82. Center for the Health Professions. Improving Oral Health Care Delivery Systems in California. California Dental Access Project, an Initiative to Improve the Oral Health of California's Underserved. San Francisco, CA: Center for the Health Professions, University of California, San Francisco; December 2000.

83. Pew Center on the State, Pew Children's Dental Campaign. The Cost of Delay: State Dental Policies Fail One in Five Children. Philadelphia, PA: Pew Charitable Trusts; 2010.

84. Lewis CW. Dental care and children with special health care needs: A population-based perspective. Acad Pediatr 2009;9:420.
85. Snyder A, Gehshan S. State Health Reform: How do Dental Benefits Fit In? Options for Policy Makers. Washington, DC: National Academy for State Health Policy; 2008.
86. Mertz E, O'Neil E. The growing challenge of providing oral health care services to all Americans. Health Aff (Millwood) 2002;21:65.
87. Fisher-Owens SA, Barker JC, Adams S, et al. Giving policy some teeth: Routes to reducing disparities in oral health. Health Aff (Millwood) 2008;27:404.
88. Skillman S, Doescher M, Mouradian WE, et al. The challenge to delivering oral health services in rural America. J Public Health Dent 2010;70(special issue):S49.
89. Bailit H, Beazoglou T. Financing dental care: Trends in public and private expenditures for dental services. Dent Clin North Am 2008;53:281.
90. Chapin R. Dental benefits improve access to oral care. Dent Clin North Am 2008;53:505.
91. Manski RJ, Cooper PF. Characteristics of employers offering dental coverage in the United States. J Am Dent Assoc 2010;141:700.
92. Manski RJ. Public programs, insurance, and dental access. Dent Clin North Am 2009;53:485.
93. McGuinn-Shapiro M. Medicaid coverage of adult dental services. State Health Policy Monitor 2008;2:1.
94. Maas WR. Access to care—what can the United States learn from other countries? Community Dent Oral Epidemiol 2006;34:232.
95. Henry J. Kaiser Family Foundation. Oral Health Coverage and Care for Low-Income Children: The Role of Medicaid and CHIP. Menlo Park, CA: The Kaiser Commission on Medicaid and the Uninsured, Henry J. Kaiser Family Foundation; April 2009.
96. Gehshan S, Snyder A, Paradise J. Filling an Urgent Need: Improving Children's Access to Dental Care in Medicaid and SCHIP. Menlo Park, CA: The Kaiser Commission on Medicaid and the Uninsured, Henry J. Kaiser Family Foundation; July 2008.
97. Rohde F. Dental Expenditures in the 10 Largest States, 2006. Rockville, MD: Agency for Healthcare Research and Quality; Statistical Brief 263, September 2009.
98. Department of Labor. National Compensation Survey: Employee Benefits in the United States, March 2009. Washington, DC: Department of Labor; Bulletin 2731, September 2009.
99. Henry J. Kaiser Family Foundation: The Uninsured and the Difference Health Insurance Makes. Menlo Park, CA: The Kaiser Commission on Medicaid and the Uninsured, Henry J. Kaiser Family Foundation; September 2009.
100. Henry J. Kaiser Family Foundation: Medicaid, a Primer. Menlo Park, CA: The Kaiser Commission on Medicaid and the Uninsured, Henry J. Kaiser Family Foundation; January 2009.
101. Institute of Medicine. America's Uninsured Crisis: Consequences for Health and Health Care. Washington, DC: National Academies Press; 2009.
102. Centers for Medicare & Medicaid Services. Guide to Children's Dental Care in Medicaid. Baltimore, MD: Centers for Medicare & Medicaid Services, US Department of Health and Human Services; October 2004.
103. Georgetown University's Center for Children and Families, Children's Dental Health Project. CHIP Tips, Children's Oral Health Benefits. Menlo Park, CA: The Kaiser Commission on Medicaid and the Uninsured, Henry J. Kaiser Family Foundation; March 2010.
104. Children's Dental Health Project. Summary of Oral Health Provisions in Health Care Reform. Washington, DC: Children's Dental Health Project; April 2010.
105. Gehshan S. A New Law, A New Opportunity: How the Health Care Reform Law can Help Provide the Dental Care that Underserved Children Need. Philadelphia, PA: Pew Charitable Trusts; 2010.
106. Mertz E, Mouradian WE. Addressing children's oral health in the new millennium: Trends in the dental workforce. Acad Pediatr 2009;9:433.
107. Solomon ES. Dental workforce. Dent Clin North Am 2009;53:435.
108. Health Policy Institute of Ohio. The Report of the Ohio Dental Workforce Roundtable. Columbus, OH: Health Policy Institute of Ohio; 2005.
109. Edestein BL. Training New Dental Health Providers in the US. Battle Creek, MI: The W.K. Kellogg Foundation; 2009.
110. Association of State & Territorial Dental Directors. Best Practices Approaches for State and Community Oral Health Programs: Access to Oral Health Care, Workforce Development. Jefferson City, MO: Association of State & Territorial Dental Directors; 2003.

111. Pew Center on the States, National Academy for State Health Policy. Help Wanted: A Policy Maker's Guide to New Dental Providers. Philadelphia, PA: The Pew Charitable Trusts; 2009.

112. US Census. An Older and More Diverse Nation by Midcentury. Washington, DC: US Census; August 2008.

113. Brault MW. Americans with Disabilities: 2005. Washington, DC: US Census; Household Economic Studies Current Population Reports P70-117, December 2008.

114. US Department of Health and Human Services, US Department of Labor. The Future Supply of Long-term Care Workers in Relation to the Aging Baby Boom Generation: Report to Congress. Washington, DC: Office of the Assistant Secretary for Planning and Evaluation; 2003.

115. Bureau of Labor Statistics, US Department of Labor. Occupational Outlook Handbook, 2010–2011 edition. Washington, DC: Superintendent of Documents, US Government Printing Office; Bulletin 2800, 2006.

116. Beazoglou T, Bailit H, Brown LJ. Selling your practice at retirement: Are there problems ahead? J Am Dent Assoc 2000;131:1693.

117. Guthrie D, Valachovic R, Brown LJ. The impact of new dental schools on the dental workforce through 2022. J Dent Ed 2009;73:1353.

118. American Dental Education Association. Trends in Dental Education. Washington, DC: American Dental Education Association; 2010.

119. Doescher MP, Keppel GA, Skillman SM, et al. The Crisis in Rural Dentistry: Policy Brief. Seattle: WWAMI Rural Health Research Center, Department of Family Medicine, University of Washington; April 2009.

120. Smedley BD, Stith AY, Nelson AR, editors. Committee on Understanding and Eliminating Racial and Ethnic Disparities in Health Care, Unequal treatment: Confronting Racial and Ethnic Disparities in Health Care. Washington, DC: Institute of Medicine, National Academies Press; 2005.

121. Smedley BD, Stith AY, Bristow lR, editors. In the Nation's Compelling Interest: Ensuring Diversity in the Health Care Workforce. Washington, DC: Institute of Medicine, National Academies Press; 2004.

122. Sullivan Commission on Diversity in the Health Care Workforce. Missing Persons: Minorities in the Health Profession. Battle Creek, MI: W.K. Kellogg Foundation; 2004.

123. Brown LJ, Lazar V. Minority Dentists: Why do we Need Them? Washington, DC: Closing the Gap, Office of Minority Health; July 1999.

124. Andersen RM, Davidson PL. Evaluating the Dental Pipeline Program: Recruiting Minorities and Promoting Community-based Dental Education. Washington, DC: American Dental Education Association; Special Supplement Journal Dental Education Volume 73, Number 2, February 2009.

125. Garcia RI, Cadoret CA, Henshaw M. Multicultural issues in oral health. Dent Clin North Am 2008;52:319.

126. Haden NK, Catalanotto FA, Alexander CJ, et al. Improving the oral health status of all Americans: Roles and responsibilities of academic dental institutions: The report of the ADEA President's Commission. J Dent Educ 2003;67:563.

127. Atchison KA, Thind A, Nakazono TT. Community-based clinical dental education: Effects of the Pipeline Program. J Dent Educ 2009;73(2 Suppl.):S269.

128. Hood JG. Service-learning in dental education: meeting needs and challenges. J Dent Educ 2009;7:454.

129. McKinnon M, Luke G, Bresch J, et al. Emerging allied dental workforce models: Considerations for academic dental institutions. J Dent Educ 2007;71:1476.

130. Bresch JE, Luke GG, McKinnon MD, et al. Today's threat is tomorrow's crisis: Advocating for dental education, dental and biomedical research, and oral health. J Dent Educ 2006;70:601.

131. Bureau of Health Professions. Shortage Designation: HPSAs, MUAs & MUPs, HPSA Designation Criteria, Guidelines and Process. Rockville, MD: Bureau of Health Professions, Health Resources and Services Administration; May 28, 2010.

132. Edelstein B. The dental safety net, its workforce, and policy recommendations for its enhancement. J Public Health Dent 2010;70(special issue):S32.

133. National Network for Oral Health Access. Health Center Fundamentals in Health Center Oral Health Program. Operations Manual. Denver, CO: National Network for Oral Health Access; 2010.

134. Mertz EA, Finocchio L. Improving oral healthcare delivery systems. J Public Health Dent 2010;70(special issue):S1.

135. Hilton I, Lester A. Oral health disparities: A framework for workforce innovation and solutions. J Public Health Dent 2010;70(special issue):S15.

136. Wendling W. Private sector approaches to workforce enhancement. J Public Health Dent 2010;70(special issue):S24.

137. Garcia RI, Inge RE, Niessen L, et al. Envisioning success: The future of the oral health care delivery system in the United States. J Public Health Dent 2010;70(special issue):S58.

138. Helgeson MJ. The Minnesota Oral Health Care Solutions Project: Implications for People with Special Needs. J California Dent Assoc 2005;33:641.
139. Ballard C, Highsmith N. Catalyzing Improvements in Oral Health: Best practices from the State Action for Oral Health Initiative. Hamilton, NJ: Center for Health Care Strategies; 2006.
140. Tomar SL. Assessment of the Dental Public Health Infrastructure in the United States. Gainesville, FL: University of Florida College of Dentistry; Contract number 263-MD-012931, National Institute of Dental and Craniofacial Research, National Institutes of Health, July 2004.
141. Allukian M Jr, Adekugbe O. The practice and infrastructure of dental public health in the United States. Dent Clin North Am 2008;52:259.
142. Tomar SL, Reeves AF. Changes in the oral health of US children and adolescents and dental public health infrastructure since the release of the Healthy People 2010 Objectives. Acad Pediatr 2009;9:388.
143. Silow-Carroll S, Alteras T. Economic & Social Research Institute. Community-based Oral Health Programs: Lessons Learned from Three Innovative Models, Case Studies on ABCD/E Kids Get Care–WA; Apple Tree Dental–MN; Community DentCare–NY. Battle Creek, MI: WK Kellogg Foundation; October 2004.
144. Association of State & Territorial Dental Directors. Building Infrastructure and Capacity in State and Territorial Oral Health Programs. Jefferson City, MO: Association of State & Territorial Dental Directors; 2000.
145. Maternal and Child Health Bureau, Health Resources Services Administration. Strategic Plan: Fiscal Year 2003–2007. Rockville, MD: Maternal and Child Health Bureau, Health Resources Services Administration; 2003.
146. Gooch BF, Malvitz DM, Griffin SO, et al. Promoting the oral health of older adults through the chronic disease model: CDC's perspective on what we still need to know. J Dental Educ 2005;69:1058.
147. Association of State & Territorial Dental Directors. Best Practice Approach Report: Statutory Mandate for a State Oral Health Program. Jefferson City, MO: Association of State & Territorial Dental Directors; 2003.
148. Association of State & Territorial Dental Directors. Summary Report: Synopses of State Dental Public Health Programs, Data for Fiscal Year 2006–2007. Jefferson City, MO: Association of State & Territorial Dental Directors; 2008.
149. Association of State & Territorial Dental Directors. Synopses of State and Territorial Dental Public Health Programs, 2005–2009. Association of State & Territorial Dental Directors; 2010.
150. Centers for Disease Control and Prevention. State-based Oral Disease Prevention Program: Full Program Announcement. Washington, DC: US Department of Health and Human Services; 2010.
151. Tomar SL. Planning and evaluating community oral health programs. Dent Clin North Am 2008;52:403.
152. Tomar SL, Garcia AI. Dental public health, the big picture specialty. J Am Coll Dent 2009;76:31.
153. US Department of Health and Human Services. Oral Health Initiative 2010. Washington, DC: US Department of Health and Human Services; 2010.
154. Institute of Medicine. Oral Health Access to Services Consensus Study. Washington, DC: Institute of Medicine; 2010.
155. Institute of Medicine. An Oral Health Initiative Consensus Study. Washington, DC: Institute of Medicine; 2010.

6

Oral Health Programs in the Community

Sherry R. Jenkins, RDH, BS
Kathy Voigt Geurink, RDH, MA
Linda M. Altenhoff, DDS

Objectives

Upon completion of this chapter, the student will be able to:
- Identify oral health programs at the national, state, and local level.
- Discuss the essential public health services for oral health.
- Describe the four phases of organizing an effective community oral health program.
- Define goals and objectives.
- Explain how program goals and objectives are used in program planning, implementation, and evaluation.
- Discuss the benefits of primary prevention programs, including fluoride, sealants, and oral health education.
- Describe the importance of community water fluoridation as a public health measure.
- Identify the different funding streams and structures for obtaining dental services through public health systems.

Key Terms

Access to dental care	Planning	Fluoride varnishes
Evidenced-based practices	Implementation	Sealants
Essential public health services for oral health	Evaluation	Oral health education
	Goals	Dental home
Oral health coalition	Objectives	
Assessment	Community water fluoridation	

Opening Statements

- Dental caries is a transmissible, chronic disease that can be prevented.
- School-based pit and fissure sealant programs reduce dental caries as much as 60%.
- Community water fluoridation decreases tooth decay by 29% to 51% in children and adolescents.
- Fluoride varnish applied every 6 months is effective in preventing caries in the primary and permanent teeth of children and adolescents.
- Integration of oral health into coordinated school health programs becomes a reality.
- Association of State & Territorial Dental Directors (ASTDD) develops a Basic Screening Survey (BSS) to assess the oral health of older adults.

GENERAL HEALTH AND ORAL HEALTH

The mission of public health is to "fulfill society's interest in assuring conditions in which people can be healthy."[1] Without public health, including community oral health, society as a whole suffers because of lost productivity, decreased learning among school-age children as a result of health-related absences, and increased health care costs. Surgeon General David Thatcher, in the May 2000 Surgeon General's Report,[2] refers to dental disease as a "silent epidemic that restricts activities in school, work, and home, and often significantly diminishes the quality of life." He further states:

> To improve the quality of life and eliminate health disparities demands the understanding, compassion, and will of the American people. There are opportunities for all health professionals and communities to work together to improve health.[2]

This chapter discusses community oral health programs as opportunities to address the **access to dental care** problems for children and adults. **Evidenced-based practices,** those that have been scientifically proven to be effective, are offered in these programs as a means to achieve improved oral health and consequently, overall health for all populations.

NATIONAL, STATE, AND LOCAL PROGRAMS: ROLE OF THE HEALTH DEPARTMENT

National Level

National, state, and local dental public health programs have similar roles but widely varying organizational schemes. Nationally, several governmental programs are involved in oral health promotion.

Among these programs are the US Department of Health and Human Services (DHHS), which is the federal government's principal agency for protecting the health of all Americans and providing essential services, especially for people who are least able to help themselves. DHHS is the largest grant-making agency in the federal government ($\approx$60,000 grants per year). DHHS works with state and local governments and funds services at the local level through state or county agencies or through private sector grantees. DHHS also provides regulatory oversight and monitoring of the expenditures made by grantees. DHHS has multiple public health service operating divisions, including the following:
- National Institutes of Health (NIH)
- Food and Drug Administration (FDA)
- Centers for Disease Control and Prevention (CDC)
- Indian Health Service (IHS)
- Health Resources and Services Administration (HRSA)

State Level

Approximately two thirds of the states have full-time state dental directors who provide leadership and guidance in the planning, funding, and implementation of oral health promotion programs for the residents of the states that they serve. These programs vary in their scope of services and organization across the United States.

A state's program may include, in addition to the state dental director, regional dental directors, public health educators, clinical dentists, dental hygienists, and dental assistants who provide oral health services to underserved populations. These public professionals also promote oral health through educational programs in public and private schools and through collaborative efforts with dental and dental hygiene schools; Head Start centers; Women, Infant, and Children (WIC) programs; county and city health departments; community-based organizations; faith-based organizations; civic groups; and local dental providers and dental hygienists.

Local Level

Individual county and city health departments across the nation have recognized the need within their communities for the provision of oral health services to various members of their populations. Many of these clinics are federally funded, offering services on a sliding scale fee schedule and accepting clients who receive public assistance through Medicaid. These clinics employ both public health dentists and dental hygienists and sometimes have supplemental clinical coverage provided by local dental professionals.

Hours of operation are tailored to best meet the needs of the population they serve. The clinics provide diagnostic, preventive, and restorative oral health services to older adults and to the indigent population and the working poor.

Essential Public Health Services for Oral Health

The core public health functions of assessment, policy development, and assurance shape the basic practice of public health at state and local levels. These core public health functions and the essential public health services (see Chapter 1) provided input into the **Essential Public Health Services for Oral Health** developed by the Association of State & Territorial Dental Directors (ASTDD) (**Box 6-1**).[3] These guidelines describe the roles of state oral health programs and have been used in the development and evaluation of public health activities at the state level.

Many states have developed programs that include the essential services for oral health. For example, in the state of Washington, the "Smile Survey" was initiated to provide statewide screenings for children to assess the status of their oral health and to identify gaps in access to care. Preventive programs, such as sealants and oral health education, have followed as an answer to the problem of tooth decay. In addition, the Washington State Oral Health Coalition was formed in 1993 to further support improvements in oral health. A coalition is a diverse group of individuals, organizations, and agencies that unite to reach a common goal. An **oral health coalition** is therefore a cooperative effort on the part of many individuals and organizations to build systems and develop programs that improve community oral health.

The Washington State Oral Health Coalition has proved to be an excellent means of bringing dedicated professionals together to resolve oral health issues through policy development. This coalition is also involved in continual assessment of oral health and in the assurance of oral health solutions. More than 20 different locations in Washington have established oral health coalitions, with representation from consumers, schools, community clinics, health care and dental providers, health departments, and agencies that come in contact with low-income and minority populations. Anyone interested in achieving the goal of optimal oral health for Washington residents is invited to join. The strength and unity of a coalition make this goal attainable. The Washington Department of Health and the DHHS have developed a document, *Community Roots for Oral*

BOX 6-1 Essential Public Health Services for Oral Health

Assessment
- Assess oral health status and needs so that problems can be identified and addressed.
- Analyze determinants of identified oral health needs, including resources.
- Assess the fluoridation status of water systems and other sources of fluoride.
- Implement an oral health surveillance system to identify, investigate, and monitor oral health problems and health hazards.

Policy Development
- Develop plans and policies through a collaborative process that supports individual and community oral health efforts to address oral health needs.
- Provide leadership to address oral health problems by maintaining a strong oral health unit within the health agency.
- Mobilize community partnerships between and among policymakers, professionals, organizations, groups, the public, and others to identify and implement solutions to oral health problems.

Assurance
- Inform, educate, and empower the public regarding oral health problems and solutions.
- Promote and enforce laws and regulations that protect and improve oral health, ensure safety, and ensure accountability for the public's well-being.
- Link people to needed population-based oral health services, personal oral health services, and support services, and assure the availability, access, and acceptability of these services by enhancing system capacity, including directly supporting or providing services when necessary.
- Support services and implementation of programs that focus on primary and secondary prevention.
- Assure that the public health and personal health workforce has the capacity and expertise to effectively address oral health needs.
- Evaluate effectiveness, accessibility, and quality of population-based and personal oral health services.
- Conduct research and support demonstration projects to gain new insights and applications of innovative solutions to oral health problems.

Adapted from Association of State & Territorial Dental Directors (ASTDD). Guidelines for State and Territorial Oral Health programs. Sparks, NV: ASTDD, 1997.

Health: Guidelines for Successful Coalitions, that is available to people interested in forming an oral health coalition to improve the oral health of residents in their community (**Box 6-2**).[4]

ASSESSMENT, PLANNING, IMPLEMENTATION, AND EVALUATION

Four components necessary in initiating an oral health program are **assessment, planning, implementation,** and **evaluation.** Dental hygienists in private practice and in the community use these components to deliver oral health care. Community health extends the role of the dental hygienist from the traditional private practice to the community as a whole.

BOX 6-2 Oral Health Coalitions

- Provide public recognition and visibility.
- Leverage resources; expand the scope and range of services.
- Provide a comprehensive approach to programming.
- Enhance clout in advocacy and resource development.
- Enhance competence.
- Avoid duplication of services, and fill gaps in service delivery.
- Accomplish what single members cannot.

Adapted from Children's Alliance: Washington State Oral Health Coalition. Available at www.doh.wa.gov/.

BOX 6-3 Components Necessary for Initiating an Oral Health Program

Community				Private Practice
Community survey	→	ASSESSMENT	←	Patient examination
Plan the program	→	PLANNING	←	Plan patient treatment
Conduct the program	→	IMPLEMENTATION	←	Treat the patient
Review program/evaluate	→	EVALUATION	←	Evaluate patient treatment

In this setting, the community is viewed as the patient. The community survey is comparable to the patient's examination for assessment. The program plan and implementation are similar to the treatment plan and treatment of the patient. Evaluation and review of the program can be compared to the evaluation of the patient's treatment (**Box 6-3**).

With increased emphasis on improving public access to oral health care, the responsibilities of the dental hygienist to promote oral health in the community take on renewed importance. Therefore it is important that the dental hygienist understand the basic concepts of assessment, planning, implementation, and evaluation as they apply to oral health programs.

Definitions of the components of initiating an oral health program are as follows[5]:

1. *Assessment* is an organized and systematic approach to identify a target group and to define the extent and severity of oral health needs present.
2. *Planning* is an organized response to reduce or eliminate one or more problems.
3. *Implementation* includes the process of putting the plan into action and monitoring the plan's activities, personnel, equipment, resources, and supplies. This step should include feedback from personnel and participants as well as ongoing evaluation mechanisms.
4. *Evaluation* is the method of measuring results of the program against objectives developed during the early planning stages. This process is ongoing and should identify problems and solutions to assist in revising the program as needed.
   a. Formative evaluation, or the internal evaluation of a program, is an examination of the processes or activities of a program as they are taking place.
   b. Summative evaluation involves judging the merit or worth of a program after it has been in operation. This step is an attempt to determine whether a fully operational program is meeting the goals for which it was developed.

These components are portrayed in the planning cycle model in **Figure 3-4**. The model provides a continuous cycle of steps to assess, plan, implement, and evaluate.[6]

Assessment

Assessing the relative importance of needs can be a complex process. It depends on human values, some of which are universally agreed on and others are more controversial. For example, a need that involves life or death generally receives higher priority; however, a choice between a health need that might affect the lives of a few people and one that affects the lives of large numbers of people is less clear-cut. Although many would argue that the needs of larger numbers must take priority, others want to consider factors such as age and the future impact on society. For example, a community may need to decide about initiating a free influenza vaccine program for its older population, enhancing the immunization program for children, or adding a clinic offering reduced dental care for indigent families (see Guiding Principles).

GUIDING PRINCIPLES

Establishing Health Priorities
- What is the magnitude of the problem? (Does it cause death or disability?)
- How many people are affected (one person, small community, or entire country)?
- What types of resources are available (personnel, money, facilities, and technology)?
- What has already been done in the community?
- What are the prevailing attitudes toward the problem?
- Which groups are expressing the most interest in the problem?
- What are the legal constraints?

Compounding the problem of establishing the priorities of health needs is the fact that each community is unique, with its own values and ideas. If a community's basic need for food and security are not being met, dental needs assume a low priority. An issue that often arises is the idea that if a community's perception of needs is adhered to exclusively, actual clinical health problems may go untreated because the people are not knowledgeable about many areas of health care. The solution to this dilemma involves striking a delicate balance between negligence and overzealousness. Although it is unethical to impose one's own perceptions on a community, it is the professional's responsibility to inform people of existing problems and their consequences.[7]

A needs assessment can identify health care problems within the community. The assessment provides information not only about the problem but also about the community itself. The data collected can be used to develop a community profile that will assist in finding the appropriate solution. Conducting a needs assessment for a community can be expensive with regard to labor and time. If funds are not available, coordination with other agencies interested in obtaining similar health information on the given population may be the solution.

Another possibility is to investigate dental surveys that have been done by other organizations. Dental surveys are conducted by professionals at dental schools, local and state health departments, and community health centers. Coordination with other agencies and organizations to know what has been done and what needs to be accomplished can prevent duplication of services.[8] Data can be obtained and analyzed by various methods (see Chapter 3). After the needs assessment is performed, developing the appropriate goals and objectives is the next step.

Planning

Developing goals, objectives, and program activities is part of the planning process. During this stage, it is essential to have community involvement and participation. The formulation of program goals and objectives is an active process, offering specific proposals for changes to be made in the community. These changes address the specific problems identified in the needs assessment.

Goals

Goals provide a broadly based statement of what changes will take place, from which specific objectives are developed. For example, the school-based fluoride mouth rinse program will improve the oral health of school-age children.

Objectives

Objectives are more specific than goals; they describe in a measurable way the desired end result of program activities. They should tell the learner what he or she needs to do to be successful.

The performance verb is the key to a measurable objective (**Box 6-4**); it is an action word, such as "write," "demonstrate," or "recite." Other elements of the objective are the condition, which tells under what circumstance the activity occurs, and the criterion, which tells how well the activity must be performed. The performance verb is essential in writing a measurable objective. The inclusion of a condition and a criterion makes the objective more specific and useful to the learner. In summary, the objectives should include the following:

1. A performance verb tells the activity and outcome.
2. A condition tells under what circumstance the outcome will occur.
3. A criterion tells how well the action and outcome must be accomplished to be effective.

BOX 6-4 Performance Verbs for Writing Behavioral Objectives

Adjust	Estimate	Map	Sort
Analyze	Examine	Measure	Spell
Apply	Explain	Observe	State
Attempt	Express	Organize	Test
Brush	Find	Perform	Try
Calculate	Form	Plan	Unite
Categorize	Gather	Practice	Weigh
Choose	Group	Predict	Write
Classify	Hypothesize	Produce	
Complete	Identify	Prove	
Copy	Invent	Recognize	
Create	Join	Record	
Define	Keep	Repeat	
Demonstrate	Label	Select	
Describe	List	Show	
Design			

An example of an objective for the aforementioned goal would be as follows: On completion of today's six-step demonstration of how to rinse, the children will demonstrate the six steps without error.

Performance verb: demonstrate

Condition: on completion of today's six-step demonstration

Criterion: without error

Another example of a measurable objective: On completion of the calibration exercise, the three examiners will record their findings with 85% accuracy.

Performance verb: record

Condition: on completion of the calibration exercise

Criterion: 85% accuracy

Once the problem has been identified and program goals and objectives have been established with a description of a solution, the next step is to state how to bring about the desired results. This area of program planning, referred to as program activities, describes how the objectives will be accomplished.

In planning these program activities, one must carefully consider the type of resources available, as well as program constraints. For example, in planning a school fluoride mouthrinse program in which the chosen activity would be weekly rinsing, resources might include selecting (1) the site at which the rinsing is conducted, (2) personnel, (3) supplies, and (4) the financial means to pay for the supplies. Constraints might include (1) availability of dental personnel to conduct screenings, (2) negative attitudes from some parents, (3) the amount of time it takes to rinse, or (4) lack of funding.

Planning is a crucial element to a successful program. A community oral health program that is well planned, with specific activities and consideration given to resources and constraints, is usually successful in terms of implementation.

Implementation

The process of putting the plan into action, the implementation phase, is ongoing and should be supervised and evaluated to ensure program effectiveness. Implementation, like planning, involves individuals, agencies, and the community working together. The strategy should answer the following questions[8]:

1. Why: the effect of the objective to be achieved
2. What: the activities required to achieve the objective
3. Who: the individuals responsible for each activity
4. When: the chronologic sequence of activities
5. How: the materials, media, methods, and techniques to be used
6. How much: a cost estimate of materials and time

For ease in addressing these questions, many community oral health programs begin on a small scale. Using a smaller population with the intent to expand later is called *pilot testing*. In a pilot test for a fluoride mouthrinse program, for example, only one school would be involved the first year and the program would be expanded to include two or more schools the following year. This implementation strategy allows for an opportunity to test the program's effectiveness and provides ease in control and monitoring of the program activities. A pilot program provides useful information and enables decisions to be made about the future of the program. Piloting is a form of evaluating the implementation.

Evaluation

Evaluation is a judgment of merit or worth of the program. The first step is to review the program goals and then to examine the specific measurable objectives. To evaluate the effectiveness of health programs, specific measurement instruments must be set up for collection of data on the attainment of each program objective. The data that are obtained through measuring the objectives are called *measurable outcomes*. Each objective should be reviewed to determine how well it meets the program goals. The bottom line in evaluation is accountability—to consumers, providers, and all involved agencies. Evaluation determines whether the program accomplishes what it was designed to accomplish (e.g., were the objectives of this study or program successfully met? If not, why not?). Summarizing what went well and what did not, or drawing conclusions based on intuition, is not adequate; the objectives themselves must be specifically addressed.

Inherent in this approach is the possibility of attaining a negative outcome, that is, the conclusion that the objectives have not been met. At the same time, however, this does not mean that the program has been a failure. If a program is evaluated properly so that negative outcomes become learning experiences and indicators of future programming and research, in some sense it has been a success.[7] Formative evaluation during the implementation process can point out problems and identify opportunities to correct program deficiencies early on. With ongoing evaluation and change, the summative evaluation (end result) may in fact measure a program with initial problems as successful.

Program evaluation is an example of applied research. Basic (clinical) research (see Chapter 7) involves inquiry into the truth about facts, behaviors, relationships, and principles. Applied research is concerned with these same concepts but emphasizes the application of the knowledge and developing solutions to problems. For example, a basic researcher would be concerned with the effectiveness of the fluoride mouthrinse on the teeth and which concentration to use. A program evaluator would be concerned with the effect of the program operation and its ability to meet the program objectives. The fundamental purpose of program evaluation is to assist in decision making on the effectiveness of the program in its entirety and to reassess the program and make necessary changes to make the program more effective.

Dental hygienists play a role in assessing, planning, implementing, and evaluating community oral health programs. The dental hygienists who have chosen careers as state dental directors, public health educators, or promoters have played an important role in the advancement of dental public health, but there is much more that can be accomplished by all of the dental hygiene profession. By knowing how to organize an effective community oral health program and becoming involved in its implementation, dental hygienists can have an impact in reaching the goal of optimal oral health care for all people.

PRIMARY PREVENTION PROGRAMS: FLUORIDES, SEALANTS, ORAL HEALTH EDUCATION

Community Water Fluoridation

Community water fluoridation is the addition of a controlled amount of fluoride to the public water supply with the intent to prevent dental caries in the population. Fluoridation has been recognized as one of the top ten public health measures of the twentieth century.

At the turn of the century, most Americans could expect to lose their teeth by middle age. That situation began to change with the discovery of the properties of fluoride and the observation that people who lived in communities with naturally fluoridated drinking water had far fewer dental caries than people in comparable communities without fluoride in their water supply.[2]

In the 1920s, Dr. Frederick McKay first noticed that people living in regions of Colorado had brown stains on their teeth (fluorosis, or mottled enamel) but few if any caries. In the 1930s, Dr. Trendley Dean conducted epidemiologic studies to prove the relationship of dental fluorosis, concentration of fluoride in the water, and reduction of dental caries.

Fluoride is the thirteenth most abundant natural element; it is found in rocks, soil, fresh water, and ocean water. Therefore trace amounts of fluoride are found in all natural water sources. As a result of the general availability of public water sources to most people, the adjustment of the natural fluoride content found in the water to levels optimal for combating oral disease has proved to be a successful public health measure. This approach provides fluoride to the population, with minimal regard to socioeconomic factors, in a passive vehicle for the consumer. Water fluoridation, accomplished in this manner, results in improved oral health, reduced expenditures for dental restorative procedures, and decreased absences from school and work resulting from oral pain, with a resultant increase in learning and productivity.

The first city in the United States to adjust the fluoride content in the community water supply was Grand Rapids, Michigan, in the 1940s. Subsequent studies of adjusted fluoridation demonstrated that 50% to 70% of caries were prevented in the permanent teeth of children. Today, decay reduction rates in fluoridated communities are approximately 8% to 37% for children and 20% to 40% for adults.[9]

Figure 6-1 correlates the percentage of the population residing in areas with fluoridated community water systems and the mean number of decayed, missing (because of caries), or filled permanent teeth (DMFT) among children aged 12 years in the United States from 1967 to 1992. The average number of DMFT steadily declined from 1967 to 1992 because of populations residing in fluoridated communities.[10]

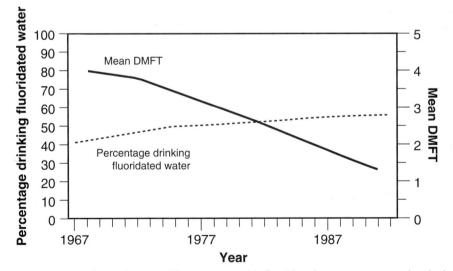

Figure 6-1 Percentage of population residing in areas with fluoridated water systems and with decayed, missing, or filled permanent teeth (DMFT) among children 12 years of age, 1967 to 1992. (Data from Centers for Disease Control and Prevention [CDC]. Fluoridation Census. Atlanta: CDC; 1993; CDC: Third National Health and Nutrition Examination Survey, 1988 to 1994; National Center for Health Statistics, 1974 and 1981; and National Institute of Dental Research, 1989.)

Fluoridated Communities

In the 1950s and 1960s, many states and cities were quick to implement fluoridation programs. In the next years, this trend began to level off. Fluoridation decisions are currently left to states and frequently to local governments and city councils. The expansion of fluoridation therefore is not easily accomplished and requires decisions at various levels. Recent increases in community water fluoridation can be attributed to the emphasis on its importance in caries prevention as discussed in the 2000 Surgeon General's report, *Oral Health in America* and its recognition in the *Healthy People 2010* and *2020* Objectives.[11]

The *Healthy People 2010* and *2020* objective for community water fluoridation is an increase in the proportion of the US population served by community water systems with optimally fluoridated water. The target goal provided in *Healthy People 2010* was 75% of the population. Every 2 years, the CDC releases statistics on the percentage of the US population on community water fluoridation. In 2006 that percentage was 69.2% or 184 million people. In 2008, 195.5 million people or 72.4% on public water systems had access to optimally fluoridated water. **Figure 6-2** shows the percentage of the US population on public water systems served by fluoridation in 2006. For updated maps on this information visit: www.cdc.gov/fluoridation/statistics. htm. **Box 6-5** shows the population in numbers served by water fluoridation in the United States, reported in 2008.[12,13]

Cost of Water Fluoridation

It has been calculated that the mean annual per capita cost of community water fluoridation ranges from 68 cents for systems with a population of more than 50,000 and 98 cents for systems with a population base between 10,000 and 50,000 to $3 for systems with fewer than 10,000 people[11] (**Table 6-1**). The lifetime cost of fluoridation per person is less than the cost of one dental filling. With the escalating cost of health care, community water fluoridation remains a preventive measure of minimal cost. In determining the economic importance of fluoridation, we should remember that the cost of treating dental disease is paid not only by the affected individual but also by the public through health departments, health insurance premiums, and federally supported programs such as Medicaid.

BOX 6-5 **Population Served by Water Fluoridation in the United States as of 2008**

Total US population	304,059,724
US population on public water systems	269,911,707
Total US population on fluoridated drinking water systems	195,545,109
% of US population on public water systems receiving fluoridated water	72.4%

Adapted from www.cdc.gov/fluoridation/statistics/2008stats.htm.

Table 6-1 **Estimated Annual Per Capita Cost for Community Water Fluoridation**

Community Size	Cost/Person
<10,000 (small systems)	$3.00
10,000-50,000 (medium systems)	$0.98
>50,000 (large systems)	$0.68

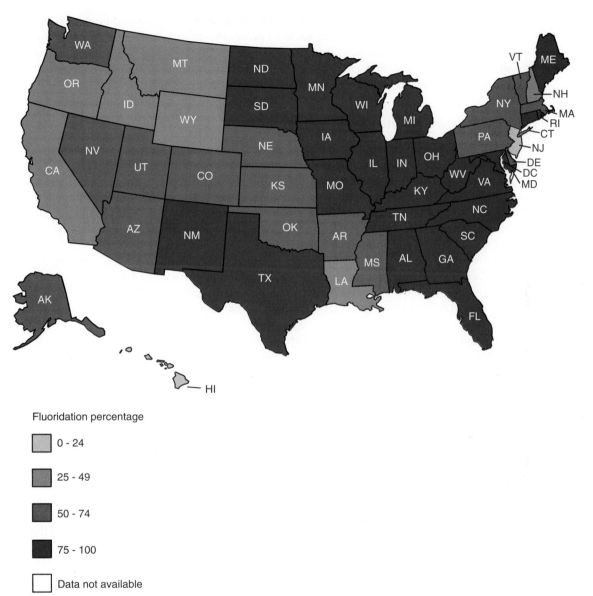

Fluoridation percentage

0 - 24

25 - 49

50 - 74

75 - 100

Data not available

Figure 6-2 Proportion of people who have public water systems served by fluoridation in 2006. (From Centers for Disease Control and Prevention [CDC] Fluoridation Census. Atlanta: CDC; 2006.)

Optimal Amounts of Fluoride

Several states have fluoridation projects that assist communities in their efforts to assess the need for fluoridation and to design and implement fluoridation of their public water systems. The state fluoridation staff also provides training and technical assistance for local water facility operators.

When the water supply is being fluoridated in a community, climatic temperature and consumption of water are taken into consideration. The recommended levels for water fluoridation in the US range from 0.7 to 1.2 parts per million (ppm) of fluoride, depending on the average daily temperature for that area. This range is based on the hypothesis that water consumption increases with increasing climatic temperature. This assumption may not be as accurate as earlier research indicates because of the increased use of air conditioning and the increased consumption of soft drinks and bottled water.[14]

Examples of Community Water Fluoridation Program

Indiana. An example of a state that has successfully adopted fluoride into its community water systems is Indiana. The Indiana State Department of Health has given community water fluoridation a high priority and reached the *Healthy People 2010* objective of 75% fluoridation in the 1970s.[15] Grant monies were applied for and secured from departments within the US Public Health Services. As a result of the efforts of dedicated professionals, including dental hygienists fulfilling the roles of educators and consumer advocates, the state of Indiana is 98% fluoridated.

The successful implementation of this program can be attributed to effective planning, implementation, and evaluation procedures. In the planning stage, assessment of the community needs and feasibility studies were conducted. The cooperative efforts of professionals, city officials, and citizens resulted in positive voluntary voting for the implementation of community water fluoridation.

Important evaluation measures of the program are the surveillance visits to monitor the amount of fluoride levels in the community drinking water. More than 1500 surveillance visits are conducted per year to ensure that optimal fluoride levels are maintained. Because of this monitoring, 98% of the 262 fluoridating Indiana communities and 92% of the 56 fluoridating Indiana schools routinely have optimal fluoride levels. Ongoing DMFS surveys convey the successful results of reduced dental decay.[15]

Other Fluoride Programs

Mouthrinse Programs. In communities in which a public water source is not available or community water fluoridation is undesired for various reasons, school-based fluoride mouthrinse programs have been implemented and offer the benefits of fluoride in a structured environment. Such programs are a popular and cost-effective means of providing fluoride benefits for children. Participation by children in a school-based program requires parental permission and oversight by a licensed dentist.

The mouthrinse program is administered by school personnel or volunteers on a weekly basis to participating children. The children rinse for 60 seconds with 10 ml of 0.2% sodium fluoride. The fluoride rinse is then expectorated into a paper cup, a napkin is placed inside the cup to absorb the solution, and the cup is discarded. The procedure takes less than 5 minutes.

Dietary Fluoride Supplements. The use of dietary fluoride supplements is another popular way of providing fluoride to children. These supplements are available only by prescription and are intended for use by children living in nonfluoridated areas to increase their fluoride exposure to a level equivalent to children who live in optimally fluoridated areas.

Supplements are available in two forms: (1) drops for infants aged 6 months and older and (2) chewable tablets for children and adolescents. To decrease the risk of dental fluorosis in permanent teeth, fluoride supplements should be prescribed only for children living in nonfluoridated

Table 6-2   Dietary Fluoride Supplement Schedule*

	FLUORIDE ION LEVEL IN DRINKING WATER (ppm†)		
Age	*<0.3 ppm*	*0.3-0.6 ppm*	*>0.6 ppm*
Birth-6 mo	None	None	None
6 mo-3 yr	0.25 mg/day‡	None	None
3-6 yr	0.50 mg/day	0.25 mg/day	None
6-16 yr	1.0 mg/day	0.50 mg/day	None

Copyright 2001 American Dental Association. Available at www.ADA.org.
*Approved by the American Dental Association, American Academy of Pediatrics, and American Academy of Pediatric Dentistry.
†1.0 part per million (ppm) = 1 milligram/liter (mg/L).
‡2.2 mg of sodium fluoride contains 1 mg of fluoride ion.

areas. The need for continuation of fluoride supplements should be reevaluated in the event of a child's change of residence.

The correct dosage is based on the child's age and the existing fluoride level in available drinking water sources (**Table 6-2**).[16] The water sources to be considered should include the following:

- Water in the home
- Bottled water
- Water at a school or a day care center
- After-school care sources

The need for compliance over an extended period of time is a major procedural and economic disadvantage of community-based fluoride supplement programs. This liability makes them impractical as an alternative to water fluoridation as a public health measure. Although total costs of the purchase of supplements and administration of a program are small, compared with the installation and startup costs associated with fluoridation equipment, the overall cost of supplements per child is much greater than the per capita cost of community water fluoridation. Additionally, community water fluoridation provides decay prevention and oral health benefits for the entire population regardless of age, socioeconomic status, educational attainment, or other social variables. This is particularly important for families and individuals who do not or cannot access regular oral health services.

Fluoride Varnishes.   Developed in Europe during the 1960s, **fluoride varnishes** were introduced to the United States in 1994 and remain in wide use in Europe and Canada. The varnish is applied by an operator, with a recommended twice-yearly reapplication for optimal benefit. The varnish is not intended to be permanent, like a sealant, but to hold the fluoride in contact with the tooth for a period of time.

Varnishes may be used to prevent root surface caries on adults with gingival recession. They offer easy applicability of fluoride for disabled children or hospitalized patients.[17] Studies in Europe have demonstrated their efficacy.[18] Fluoride varnish is being more widely used in the United States, especially with children at-risk for caries. It has been found to be an effective evidenced-based approach in preventing caries in permanent teeth and has been shown to prevent or reduce caries in primary teeth of young children.[19]

An example of using fluoride varnish to prevent early childhood caries is a program implemented by the Division of Dental Health, Virginia Department of Health. This program is funded by an HRSA Collaborative Systems Grant. The primary focus of the program is to train dental and nondental (medical) providers to use an oral health risk assessment tool and place fluoride varnish on the teeth of children younger than the age of 3 years. Grant funds are also supporting development of educational materials targeting the Medicaid eligible population. Other partners collaborating on the grant include the Division of WIC and Community Nutrition Services, Early Head Start, Virginia's Department of Education, University of Virginia School of Medicine, Department of Medical Assistance Services, and Virginia Commonwealth University School of Dentistry. The Division of Health, Virginia Department of Health, also provides other dental services for the residents of Virginia, including a school fluoride mouthrinse program and a statewide oral health education program.[20]

Additional Fluoride Sources

The introduction of systemic fluoride through water, vitamins, and tablets during the enamel formation phase of both primary and permanent teeth of children, in utero and postpartum, provides for optimal dental decay preventive benefits through fluoride ion exchange and the resultant denser enamel matrix. Fluoride is provided topically through toothpaste, mouthrinses, and professionally prescribed fluoride gels, pastes, rinses, and varnishes. The benefits associated with topical fluoride include the remineralization of early incipient lesions. The effectiveness of various fluoride sources in the reduction of dental caries is shown in **Box 6-6**.[21]

With all the additional sources of fluoride available today, the prevalence of caries has decreased, but the prevalence of dental fluorosis has increased in both fluoridated and nonfluoridated communities. Factors associated with increased fluorosis today are as follows[21]:
- Early use of fluoride toothpaste
- Use and misuse of dietary supplements
- Consumption of infant formula containing fluoride

Health care professionals, such as dentists, dental hygienists, and physicians, are important sources of information for patients regarding the use of fluoride-containing products, such as toothpaste, and may be able to help reduce the prevalence of enamel fluorosis by educating the public on the appropriate use of these products.

Even though other sources of fluoride are available and despite the increased risk of fluorosis, community water fluoridation remains the most cost-effective, the most practical, and the safest means of preventing tooth decay.

BOX 6-6 Community Water Fluoridation, Early Studies

- **Community water fluoridation:** Early studies: 50% to 70% reduction in caries, currently 20% to 40% reduction in caries in adults and 8% to 37% reduction in caries in children as the result of additional availability of other fluoride sources
- **Mouthrinses:** Studies in the 1970s and 1980s demonstrated a reduction in caries ranging from 20% to 50%
- **Fluoride tablet supplements:** Controlled trials in the United States in the 1970s indicated approximately a 20% to 28% reduction
- **Toothpaste:** In clinical trials done between 1945 and 1985, 23% to 32% reduction in caries

Data from Milgram P, Reisine S. Oral health in the United States: The post-fluoride generation, Annu Rev Public Health 2000;21:403.

Antifluoridationists

Antifluoridationists are opponents of community water fluoridation. Their reasons include individual rights, safety, government mistrust, and religious freedom. The arguments against fluoridation do not have any merit based on scientific knowledge. The economic and health benefits of fluoridation for millions of Americans have been confirmed in numerous studies by renowned scientists.[17,22]

Antifluoridationists attempt to appeal to people's emotions. They provide inaccurate, false information to the public and elected officials and attempt to link adverse health effects with fluoridation. Dental hygienists, in the roles of educators and resource persons, can influence the public knowledge about the benefits of fluoridation in their community and can provide scientific, accurate information to the community officials.

For antifluoridationists to be defeated, community education must be executed in a well-planned, unified manner. As active members of the American Dental Hygienists' Association (ADHA) and the local components, dental hygienists become an effective force that can have an impact on the community. An organized plan of action can make a difference. Being aware of the issues and being well-versed on fluoridation studies and cognizant of the political process are necessary steps in winning a fluoridation campaign. Dental hygienists also work as change agents in promoting the legislative approval of fluoridation.

Some states and cities have taken administrative action to implement fluoridation; this means that state legislatures and the city council or commission have voted for fluoridation because of the public health benefits. People usually prefer to have a voice in the decision-making process; however, if fluoride is on the ballot, people need to be educated on the issue to make a wise decision. Education is the key to the success in reaching the *Healthy People 2020* goal of increasing the proportion of the US population served by community water systems with optimally fluoridated water.

Dental Sealants

An effective primary preventive strategy, commonly used to protect permanent molars from decay, is the application of dental **sealants.** Although the percentage of school-age children with sealants has risen in recent years as the public and private sectors have been using the procedure, as dental insurance has paid for the sealants, and as parents have requested sealants for their children, little increase has occurred among children in low-income populations. One goal of *Healthy People 2010* was to have 50% of all children receive dental sealants on their permanent molars. According to the 1988–1994 baseline data, only 23% of 8-year-old children and 15% of 14-year-old adolescents had dental sealants on their permanent molars.[23]

To reach the *Healthy People 2020* goal of increasing the proportion of children who have received dental sealants on their molar teeth, many states have instituted school-based sealant programs (SBSPs). In some programs mobile dental vans are sent to schools and the sealants are applied in the van. In other programs, portable equipment is transported from school to school and is set up in available spaces. Students are then brought to the designated room for the procedure.

Sealant programs generally focus on 6- to 8-year-olds and 12- to 14-year-olds because the first and second molars usually erupt during these years. Placing sealants on these teeth shortly after their eruption protects them from development of caries in areas where food and bacteria are retained. The CDC reports that school-based pit and fissure sealant programs reduce dental caries as much as 60%.[24] If sealants were applied routinely to susceptible tooth surfaces in conjunction with the appropriate use of fluoride, most tooth decay in children could be prevented.

The Wisconsin Children's Dental Alliance partnered with the Wisconsin Department of Health Services to administer the state "Seal a Smile" program, which provides grants for school-based and school linked dental sealant programs. The Wisconsin Children's Dental Alliance facilitates the Wisconsin Oral Health Coalition whose mission is that no child in the state should go without adequate oral health care, preventive services, or education. The organization has developed a planning guide for communities wanting to set up a Seal a Smile Program. The guide is free of charge and provides a step-by-step plan for starting a sealant program.[25]

Table 6-3 provides the 2009 CDC recommendations for SBSPs. These recommendations, which were prepared by an appointed CDC-expert workgroup, and the accompanying report in Gooch and colleagues,[24] will increase practitioners' awareness of SBSPs as an important and effective public health approach that complements clinical care.

Oral Health Education

Health education is the process of teaching people about health. The scope of health education may include educational activities for children, parents, policymakers, or health care providers. Educational programs are developed and presented in many different formats and settings.

Oral health education is learning experience directed at helping people prevent oral disease. Oral health education can be presented directly to clients through individual or group activities, such as health fairs, or in school curricula (**Figure 6-3**). The intent of oral health education is to assist people in making decisions about their oral health and to choose behaviors conducive to maintaining this health.

For health education to be effective, the participant must be actively involved in the learning process. The cognitive model alone (attitude + knowledge = behavior change) has been ineffective

Table 6-3   CDC Recommendations for School-Based Sealant Programs

Topic	Recommendations
Indications for sealant placement	Seal sound and noncavitated pit and fissure surfaces of posterior teeth, with first and second permanent molars receiving highest priority.
Tooth surface assessment	Differentiate cavitated and noncavitated lesions: • Unaided visual assessment is appropriate. • Dry teeth before assessment with cotton rolls, gauze, or compressed air when available. • An explorer may be used to gently confirm cavitations. • Radiographs are unnecessary solely for sealant placement. • Other diagnostic technologies are not required.
Sealant placement and evaluation	Clean the tooth surface: • Toothbrush prophylaxis is acceptable. • Additional surface preparation, such as air or enameloplasty, is not recommended. • Use a four-handed technique when resources allow. • Seal the teeth of children, even if follow-up cannot be assured. • Evaluate sealant retention within 1 year.

From Gooch BF, Griffin SO, Gray SK, et al. Preventing dental caries through school-based sealant programs. J Am Dent Assoc 2009;140:1356.

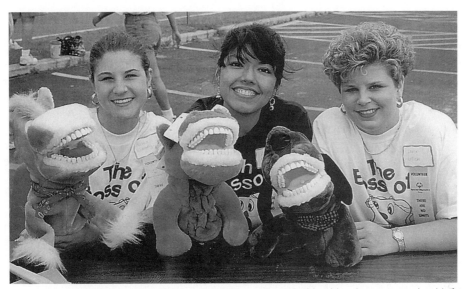

Figure 6-3 Dental hygiene students use puppets to present oral health education at a health fair.

BOX 6-7 Factors that Influence the Dental Education Process

Individual Factors (Internal)
- Education level
- Beliefs, values, perceptions
- Age, income, race, and other sociodemographic factors

Environmental Factors (External)
- Intrapersonal interactions with family and peers
- Community influences, including cultural norms and public policy
- Technology to deliver the information

in producing change. The educator must consider many factors that influence learners and their behavior. Both internal and external factors should be considered in developing an oral health educational program (**Box 6-7**). Patient attitudes and environment affect behaviors and the possibility of change. The outcome of the oral health education process will be successful only if all factors are considered.

With regard to the sociodemographic factor of age, most dental education programs have been implemented for children. Oral health education for children is a priority because of the high prevalence of dental caries in this group. If a society free of dental disease is the goal, educational programs must be targeted for the future of society—the children. The school system therefore continues to be the setting used to implement large-scale oral health education programs. The school-based oral health education program remains an important component of the goal of optimal oral health for all citizens. Oral health education should be an integral component of all school health education curricula.

Other opportunities for oral health education can be accessed through faith-based, community-based, and social service organizations such as the WIC Program, Head Start, Lions Clubs, and Rotary Clubs. These organizations present opportunities for oral health education on diverse topics such as the following:
- Prenatal and postnatal oral health education for parents, infants, and toddlers
- Oral health concerns of special care patients
- Oral health education for older adults
- Oral health effects of tobacco and oral cancer information

Oral health educational programs can be given through health care facilities, such as hospitals and clinics, and long-term care facilities, such as nursing homes and alternative care centers. Specialty groups such as 4-H Clubs, Future Farmers of America, sports clubs, and youth organizations welcome educational programs. See Chapter 8 for additional information on health promotion.

When planning to provide a presentation to a selected population, the first step would be to develop a lesson plan. A five-step lesson plan described by Gagliardi includes preparation, anticipatory planning, objectives, instruction/information, guided practice activities, and closure (**Box 6-8**).[26] An example of a lesson plan using the five steps can be seen in **Figure 6-4**.

State Oral Health Programs

Box 6-9 presents a synopsis of the most common oral health programs offered in various states. The most common programs are in the areas of fluoridation, sealants, early childhood caries, health education and promotion, and tobacco cessation.[27] Examples of successful programs in the fluoride arena and in the placement of sealants have been provided.

In the area of early childhood caries, the Texas Department of State Health Services has implemented an oral health education program called "Take Time for Teeth." In this program outreach workers, educators, and health care providers are taught a standardized oral health message that emphasizes preventive oral health practices at an early age. The people trained are chosen because they interact with the target population: children and families. Topics include the following:
1. Dental checkups for pregnant women
2. Recognition of "white spots" and how to prevent baby bottle tooth decay
3. The benefits of taking a child to the dentist every 6 months beginning at 6 months of age
4. The importance of dental sealants and fluorides in preventing tooth decay

---

BOX 6-8 Gagliardi's Five-Step Lesson Plan

Components of a Lesson Plan
1. Anticipatory planning (introduction of the lesson and materials needed)
2. Objectives (what the student will gain from this lesson)
3. Instruction/information (the bulk of the lesson that is new and exciting for the student)
4. Guided practice activities (to reinforce the information taught)
5. Closure (restatement of the objectives to test knowledge)

Adapted from Gagliardi L. Dental Health Education: Lesson Planning and Implementation. Norwalk, CT: Appleton & Lange; 2009.

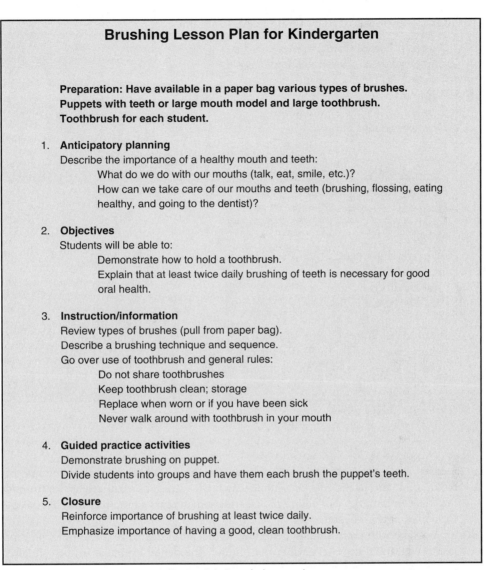

Brushing Lesson Plan for Kindergarten

Preparation: Have available in a paper bag various types of brushes. Puppets with teeth or large mouth model and large toothbrush. Toothbrush for each student.

1. **Anticipatory planning**
   Describe the importance of a healthy mouth and teeth:
       What do we do with our mouths (talk, eat, smile, etc.)?
       How can we take care of our mouths and teeth (brushing, flossing, eating healthy, and going to the dentist)?

2. **Objectives**
   Students will be able to:
       Demonstrate how to hold a toothbrush.
       Explain that at least twice daily brushing of teeth is necessary for good oral health.

3. **Instruction/information**
   Review types of brushes (pull from paper bag).
   Describe a brushing technique and sequence.
   Go over use of toothbrush and general rules:
       Do not share toothbrushes
       Keep toothbrush clean; storage
       Replace when worn or if you have been sick
       Never walk around with toothbrush in your mouth

4. **Guided practice activities**
   Demonstrate brushing on puppet.
   Divide students into groups and have them each brush the puppet's teeth.

5. **Closure**
   Reinforce importance of brushing at least twice daily.
   Emphasize importance of having a good, clean toothbrush.

Figure 6-4 Sample lesson plan.

5. The use of xylitol, a sugar alcohol found in snacks and food, that inhibits demineralization of enamel

The long-term goal of this statewide program is to have a positive impact on oral health status and to facilitate a positive behavioral change relating to oral health and prevention.[28]

A national tobacco cessation program is the National Spit Tobacco Education Program (NSTEP), funded by the Robert Wood Foundation and administered by the Oral Health America and supported by Major League Baseball. The goal is to educate young people on the dangers of using spit tobacco. Tobacco is presented as a potentially dangerous drug that can cause oral cancer. NSTEP and its partnerships with public, private, and voluntary groups, including the dental and

BOX 6-9 **Synopsis of State Oral Health Programs**

Access to Dental Care Programs
Children Forensic Identification Team
Community Dental Sealant Programs*
Community Oral Health Systems Development
Community Water Fluoridation*
Dental Screening Programs*
Early Childhood Caries and Baby Bottle Tooth Decay Programs*
Fee-For-Service Programs for Indigent Children
Fluoride Supplement Programs
Fluoride Varnish Programs*
Head Start Grantees Reviews
Mouth Guard and Injury Prevention Programs
Needs Assessment and Oral Health Surveys*
Old Age Pensioners Dental Program
Oral Health Assurance
Oral Health Education and Promotion Programs*
Oral Health for School Nurses Program
Prevent Abuse and Neglect through Dental Awareness (PANDA) Program
Private Well Water Testing Program
School Fluoride Mouth Rinse Programs*
Tobacco Cessation and Spit Tobacco Programs*
Treatment Clinics and Mobile Dental Units

*The most common programs.

medical professions, are helping Americans to stop using tobacco. The program uses television, radio, print, and public service announcements featuring baseball celebrities to send its message into the community.[29] For additional information on oral health programs, refer to the Additional Resources in this chapter.

As oral health professionals, dental hygienists are educated to incorporate prevention and oral health education into every patient encounter. The dental hygienist in the role of educator uses the knowledge of primary preventive measures (e.g., fluorides, sealants, and oral hygiene care) to inform people on how to improve their oral health. Keeping updated on available resources and health education programs for special populations in the community is important in providing the most current information to patients and assists the dental hygienist in making appropriate referrals for care.

School-Based Oral Health Program

A comprehensive school-based program such as "A Rural School-Based Oral Health Program for South Texas" provides services in the prevention, treatment, and education components. This program was formed as a collaboration with Methodist Healthcare Ministries, University of Texas Health Science Center at San Antonio (UTHSCSA), Texas Department of State Health Services, and two independent school districts and was funded in part through a grant from the Robert

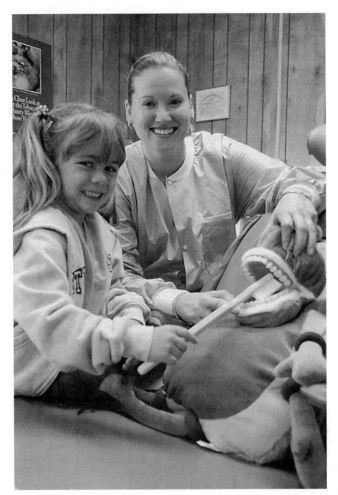

Figure 6-5 Dental hygiene student and first-grader practice oral hygiene skills.

Wood Johnson Foundation. The comprehensive model focuses on the prevention, treatment, and education needs of children as they relate to oral health. The prevention component includes annual assessments, sealants, fluoride treatments, mouth guard fabrication for sports, oral hygiene education, nutrition, tobacco use, and early intervention programs. The treatment component includes essential services such as emergency, diagnostic, preventive, and restorative care. Referrals are established for children requiring specialty care. Oral health education is incorporated into the curriculum at the schools. UTHSCSA dental hygiene faculty and students are helping to provide the treatment and educational services to children at the school-based health center (**Figure 6-5**).

The success of a school-based oral health program, such as "A Rural School-Based Oral Health Program for South Texas," depends on the integration of the program with other school health programs. The Division of Adolescent and School Health (DASH) has endorsed eight interactive components as essential elements of a coordinated school health program[30] (**Figure 6-6**). The

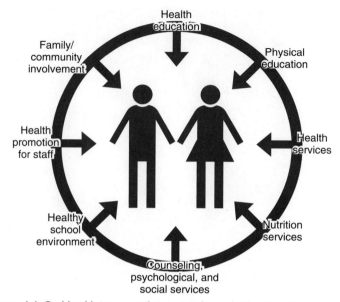

Figure 6-6 Oral health integrated into coordinated school health programs.

school can therefore be the facility where families, health care workers, youth organizations, and teachers can interact to maintain the well-being of young people.

SECONDARY AND TERTIARY PREVENTION PROGRAMS

Treatment Component

For a better understanding of the impact of public health on dental disease, one must remember that dental diseases become irreversible and are not self-curing. Although primary preventive procedures are very successful in reducing the prevalence and incidence of the major dental diseases, prevention has not been able to eliminate them. Approximately 60% of Americans visit a dental office yearly.[31] Cost is a major reason why people do not see a dentist. People often wait to visit a dentist only in emergencies. Financial barriers and geographic access become reasons why people do not receive primary prevention and are thus in need of secondary or tertiary treatment of dental disease. Therefore, in addition to a preventive component, a treatment component is an essential element of a public oral health program.

Delivery of dental care in public health dental clinics can include fixed dental clinics, which may be run by federal, state, county, city, or private, nonprofit organizations. The practice of clinical dentistry in the public health setting is also accomplished through mobile clinics (vans) or with the use of portable dental equipment (see Chapter 2). Secondary and tertiary levels of prevention include the treatment of dental disease for people of all ages and with diverse backgrounds.

Dental Home

"The **dental home** is the ongoing relationship between the dentist and the patient, inclusive of all aspects of oral health care delivered in a comprehensive, continuously accessible, coordinated, and family-centered way. Establishment of a dental home begins no later than 12 months of age and includes referral to dental specialists when appropriate."[32] The Texas Medicaid Program has implemented the First Dental Home Initiative to engage general and pediatric dentists to initiate preventive dental checkups for children enrolled in Early and Periodic Screening, Diagnosis, and Treatment (EPSDT) programs beginning at 6 months of age. Training to become certified First Dental Home providers is coordinated through the Oral Health Branch at the Texas Department of State Health Services. This certification allows providers to bill and receive enhanced reimbursement for preventive dental services for EPSDT children 6 through 35 months of age.[33] First Dental Home visits are directed not only at preventive dental services for the children but dental anticipatory guidance and oral health education for the parents/caregivers. Parents/caregivers are integrated into the dental checkup visit so that real time oral health information can be relayed to the parent/caregiver during the visit. Earlier oral evaluation allows for earlier identification of dental needs and the start of preventive dental services, including the application of topical fluoride varnish and therapeutic dental services as needed.

Services for Older Adults

An expanding population in need of both primary prevention and secondary and tertiary care is the elderly in our communities. Between 1900 and 1994, the number of older adults increased elevenfold (from 3 million to 33 million). These older adults are now the fastest growing segment of the US population. The US Census Bureau projects that the number of persons aged 65 and older will more than double by the middle of the twenty-first century to approximately 80 million. In 1994, 1 in 8 Americans was over 65 years of age; by the year 2030, 1 in 5 are expected to be in this category.[34]

The elderly not only are living longer but also are keeping their natural teeth and are therefore in need of dental services (**Figure 6-7**). The elderly are also in need of a means to pay for dental services as the incomes of older people decline with retirement, because insurance programs eliminate the dental component for persons older than 70 years, and Medicare does not cover dental services. In the role of change agent and consumer advocate, dental hygienists can actively participate in supporting legislation to include dental as a component of health care for the elderly.

An example of a program for elderly dental care at reduced cost is the "Apple Tree Geriatric Dental Program." Apple Tree provides both primary preventive services along with secondary restorative treatment and tertiary services that include making and fitting partials and dentures. This program began in Minnesota in 1986, when a few dental professionals recognized the problems of access to care in the aging population. The program was initiated in an effort to bring oral health to older adults. The program works with state and local authorities to establish mobile sites and to seek funding sources for dental care. The program has expanded to include patients with special needs, children with disabilities, and indigent families. Apple Tree Programs are located in Minnesota and in North Carolina. More than 95 locations are available where numerous dental professionals provide oral health care to persons with special needs.[35]

With the growing elderly population, it is apparent that there is a need for more community oral health programs similar to Apple Tree and a need for dental professionals to study the social, demographic, health, and economic characteristics of today's elderly citizens. The ASTDD developed a Basic Screening Survey (BSS) for use with the aging population. The purpose of the BSS is to collect reliable and valid data that can be used to document the need for policy changes and improved oral health programs for the aging population (see www.astdd.org).

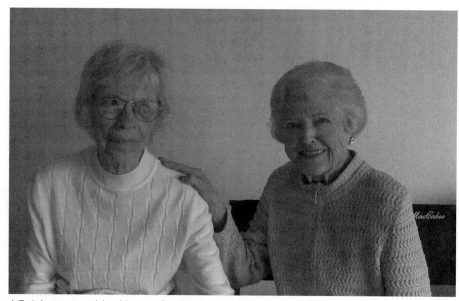

Figure 6-7 Adequate oral health care for the growing number of elderly patients is particularly important because more elderly persons are retaining their natural teeth.

FINANCING PROGRAMS

The financing of public oral health went through transitions during the 1990s and will continue to change in the future. Health care reform should include increased access to oral health services for various population groups.

At present, funding for programs addresses the health issues of women and children and is accomplished through numerous federal initiatives. These public programs are concerned with the health and well-being of pregnant women and children. They not only cut across multiple agencies but also have multiple federal and state funding streams. The private sector and the business community work with state governors on initiatives that strive to improve health status and strengthen families. Public financing programs for oral health care are defined in **Table 6-4**.[36]

Federal Initiatives

Federal initiatives that provide funding to states for programs addressing women and children's oral health issues include the following:
- Maternal and Child Health Services Block Grants (Title V)
- Special Supplemental Nutrition Program for WIC
- Children's Health Insurance Plan Reauthorization Act (CHIPRA) of 2009, formerly known as the *State Children's Health Insurance Program* (S-CHIP) through Title XXI
- Medicaid (Title XIX)
- Administration for Children and Families (ACF)

Block Grants

Maternal and Child Health Services Block Grants (Title V grants) provide funding to states for the provision of prenatal care for women, primary and preventive care for children, and health and supportive services for children with special health care needs.

Table 6-4   **Public Financing Of Oral Health Care**

Program	Explanation
Medicaid (funded jointly by federal and state governments)	Comprehensive dental services for children under the Early and Periodic Screening, Diagnosis, and Treatment (EPSDT) program.
Children's Health Insurance Program Reauthorization Act of 2009 (funded jointly by federal and state governments)	Provides direct legislative mandate for dental services in each state's program.
Medicare (funded by federal government)	Medical insurance program for the elderly that does not cover dental care except when dental services are directly related to the treatment of the medical condition.
Head Start (funded by federal government)	The dental component of Head Start includes mandated screening and referrals for necessary care. Some programs also provide fluoride treatments and pay for dental care for children who are not covered by Medicaid. All programs require that the children brush their teeth after eating meals provided by Head Start.

Women, Infants, and Children's Program

The WIC program provides grants for supplement foods, health care referrals, and nutritional education for low-income pregnant, breast-feeding, and non-breast-feeding women in addition to infants and children found to be at nutritional risk.

CHIPRA is a joint state-federal funded program through Title XXI grants to develop comprehensive health insurance coverage for children not covered by Medicaid or other third-party health insurance. CHIPRA mandates oral health services and traditional medical services. It also provides a wraparound benefit so that children who have medical insurance benefits are now eligible for dental benefits through CHIPRA. The CHIPRA (Public Law 111-3) reauthorized the Children's Health Insurance Program (CHIP). CHIPRA finances CHIP through fiscal year 2013. It will preserve coverage for the millions of children who rely on CHIP today and provide the resources for states to reach millions of additional uninsured children. This legislation will help ensure the health and well-being of our nation's children.

Medicaid, or Title XIX, is a joint state-federal financed program that is administered by the states to provide medical assistance for low-income individuals. For children enrolled in Medicaid, the EPSDT program provides comprehensive medically necessary services, including comprehensive dental services. In many states, the Medicaid program has ventured into the managed care health arena for both medical and dental services in an effort to reduce health care expenditures while maximizing preventive health measures. For more state-specific information about Medicaid and CHIPRA, see www.InsureKidsNow.gov.[37]

Administration for Children and Families

ACF, an agency of the DHHS, is responsible for 60 programs that provide assistance to needy children and families, including the administration of the Head Start program, which serves approximately 900,000 preschool children annually. Head Start provides medical and oral health screening and treatment of conditions identified for enrolled children. It also includes daily oral hygiene activities and weekly oral health curricula.

The provision of oral health services to individuals who fall outside the eligibility guidelines for entitlement programs, such as Medicaid, are often addressed through voucher or fee-for-service programs. These may be administered by state health departments, by state dental associations, or through private entities. Many of the fee-for-service programs provide emergency oral health services for school-age children. These programs use nominators, who are generally school nurses or social workers familiar with the economic status of the families seeking services. Although the initiation of the fee-for-service program is generally due to an emergent cause, providers are encouraged to try to meet all of the oral health needs of the patient within the guidelines of the program.

Federally Qualified Health Center

A federally qualified health center (FQHC) is a community health center that has been designated by the federal government as adhering to regulations pertaining to the scope and quality of health services provided to anyone, *regardless of ability to pay*. In 2006, there were 1200 community health centers across the United States serving more than 15 million patients. An FQHC "look alike" is a health center that has been identified by the HRSA and certified by the Centers for Medicare & Medicaid Services (CMS) as meeting the definition of "health center," although it does not receive grant funding from the federal government[38] (see www.chcact.org/Content/What_is_a_FQHC_.asp).

Donated Dental Services Program

The Donated Dental Services (DDS) Program also addresses the oral health needs of medically compromised, permanently disabled, or elderly people. This program is a joint effort of participating dentists, dental laboratories, and coordinating personnel. It provides one-time, comprehensive oral rehabilitation for qualifying individuals. Begun in Colorado, the DDS Program is branching out into other states as participating providers are identified.[39]

SUMMARY

The various community oral health programs introduced in this chapter offer practicing dental hygienists an extension of their private practice experience. Becoming acquainted with the oral health care needs of the community at large—in conjunction with an understanding of the available program and funding resources from the local, state, and national levels—provides an opportunity for dental hygienists to have a positive impact on the overall health of their communities.

Applying Your Knowledge

1. Research and prepare a report on fluoride concentration levels in existing water supply sources in your community.
2. Have a classroom debate on fluoridation. Appoint people to take pro and con positions, and research your position before the debate. Have a mock city council decide the outcome.

3. Develop a community oral health educational program. Write your goal and measurable objectives. Show all stages of development, including assessment, planning, implementation and evaluation of the program.
4. Discuss how you, as a private practice dental hygienist, might help implement the core essential public health functions and oral health services in your community.
5. Research the possibility of forming an oral health coalition in your community. Whom would you invite to join the organization? Decide on the goals and objectives of the organization.

Dental Hygiene Competencies

Reading the material in this chapter and participating in the activities of Applying Your Knowledge will contribute to the student's ability to demonstrate the following competencies:

Community involvement
CM.2 Provide screening, referral, and educational services that allow clients to access the resources of the health care system.
CM.3 Provide community oral health services in a variety of settings.
CM.5 Evaluate reimbursement mechanisms and their impact on the patient's or client's access to oral health care.
CM.6 Graduates will be able to evaluate the outcomes of community-based programs and to plan for future activities.

Health promotion
HP.1 Promote the values of oral and general health and wellness to the public and organizations within and outside the profession.
HP.2 Evaluate factors that can be used to promote patient or client adherence to disease prevention and/or health maintenance strategies.

Community Case

The dental hygiene school in your community has received a 3-year grant to establish an elementary school-based dental program that includes oral health education, disease prevention, and treatment components. You are the newly employed dental hygienist at the school and will supervise dental hygiene students on-site at the elementary school and in the clinic.
1. All of the following are components of establishing the oral health program except which of the following?
   a. Planning
   b. Assurance
   c. Evaluation
   d. Implementation
2. The program goal is to improve the oral health of the school-age children. Which objective that you have written for the second-grade class's educational component would be measurable?
   a. The students will completely understand the connection of oral health to general health.
   b. The students will label the parts of the tooth accurately on a diagram.
   c. The students will know how to brush and floss.
   d. The students will remember the cause of tooth decay.
3. Which preventive program would have the most benefit for all of the school-age children?
   a. School fluoride mouthrinse program
   b. Fluoride varnish program
   c. Sealant program
   d. Community water fluoridation

4. Which program would be able to provide funding for dental treatment in the school clinic?
   a. Medicaid
   b. Medicare
   c. Head Start
   d. WIC
5. Which dental hygiene service provided by the dental hygiene students is evidenced-based?
   a. A parent educational session at the PTA
   b. The development of brochures on good oral health practices
   c. The application of fluoride varnish on the teeth of the children
   d. The referral of children to the dental clinic for treatment

References

1. Institute of Medicine Committee for the Study of the Future of Public Health, Division of Health Care Services. A Vision of Public Health in America: An Attainable Ideal. In: The Future of Public Health. Washington, DC: National Academies Press; 1988.
2. Oral Health in America. A Report of the Surgeon General. Rockville, MD: US Department of Health and Human Services, National Institute of Dental and Craniofacial Research, National Institutes of Health; 2000.
3. Association of State & Territorial Dental Directors. Guidelines for State and Territorial Oral Health Programs. Sparks NV: 1997.
4. Washington State Department of Health. Child and Adolescent Health. Available at www.doh.wa.gov/cfh/oralhealth/docs/communityroots.htm. Accessed October 2010.
5. Zarkowski P. Community oral health planning and practice. In: Darby M, editor. Comprehensive Review of Dental Hygiene. 5th ed. St. Louis: Mosby; 2002.
6. Turnock BJ. Public Health: What It Is and How It Works. Gaithersburg, MD: Aspen; 1997.
7. Cormier PP, Levy JI. Community Oral Health. New York: Appleton-Century-Crofts; 1981.
8. Mann ML. Planning for community dental programs. In: Gluck GM, Morganstein WM, editors. Jong's Community Dental Health. 5th ed. St. Louis: Mosby; 2003.
9. Newbrun E. Effectiveness of water fluoridation. J Public Health Dent 1989;49:279.
10. Centers for Disease Control and Prevention. Achievements in public health, 1900–1999: Fluoridation of drinking water to prevent dental caries. MMWR Morb Mortal Wkly Rep 1999;48:933. Available at: www.cdc.gov/mmwr/preview/mmwrhtml/mm4841a1.htm. Accessed January 2010.
11. Community and other approaches to promote oral health and prevent diseases. In: Oral Health in America: A Report of the Surgeon General. Rockville, MD: US Department of Health and Human Services, National Institute of Dental and Craniofacial Research, National Institutes of Health; 2000.
12. Centers for Disease Controls and Prevention, Division of Oral Health. Water Fluoridation Statistics for 2006. Available at www.cdc.gov/fluoridation/statistics/2006stats.htm. Accessed January 2010.
13. Centers for Disease Control and Prevention, US Department of Health and Human Services. Water Fluoridation: National Fluoridation Report 2006. Available at http://apps.nccd.gov/gisdoh/waterfluor.aspx. Accessed January 2010.
14. Heller KW, Sohn W, Burt BA, et al. Water consumption in the United States in 1994–96 and indications for water fluoridation policy. J Public Health Dent 1999;59:3.
15. Indiana State Department of Health. Oral Health Programs. Available at www.in.gov/isdh/23287.htm. Accessed January 2010.
16. Fluoridation Facts. Dietary Fluoride Supplement Schedule, 1994. Available at www.ada.org/consumer/fluoride/facts/tables.html. Accessed January 2010.
17. Allukian M Jr, Horowitz AM. Effective community prevention programs for oral diseases. In: Gluck GM, Morganstein WM, editors. Jong's Community Dental Health. 5th ed. St. Louis: Mosby; 2003.
18. Helfenstein U, Steiner M. Fluoride varnishes (Duraphat): A meta-analysis. Community Dent Oral Epidemiol 1994;22:1.
19. Association of State & Territorial Dental Directors, Fluoride Varnish: An Evidenced-Based Approach Research Brief. September 2007.
20. Virginia Department of Health, Division of Dental Health Services. Available at www.vahealth.org. Accessed January 2010.

21. Milgram P, Reisine S. Oral health in the United States: The post-fluoride generation. Annu Rev Public Health 2000;21:403.
22. Horowitz HS. Why I continue to support community water fluoridation. J Public Health Dent 2000;60:67.
23. Healthy People 2010: National Health Promotion and Disease Prevention Objectives. Atlanta: Centers for Disease Control and Prevention, Health Resources and Services Administration, National Institutes of Health; 1999.
24. Gooch BF, Griffin SO, Gray SK, et al. Preventing dental caries through school-based sealant programs. JADA 2009;140:1356.
25. Wisconsin's Children's Dental Health Alliance, Seal-A-Smile Program. Available at www.chawisconsin.org/sas.htm. Accessed January 2010.
26. Gagliardi L. Dental Health Education: Lesson Planning & Implementation. Stamford, CN: Appleton & Lange; 1999.
27. Centers for Disease Control and Prevention. Synopsis of State Oral Health Departments. Atlanta: Centers for Disease Control and Prevention, Association of State & Territorial Dental Directors; 2000.
28. Texas Department of State Health Services. Take Time for Teeth, Oral Health Branch. Available at https://secure.thstepsproducts.com/default.asp. Accessed January 2010.
29. Oral Health America: National Spit Tobacco Education Program (NSTEP). Available at www.nstep.org/. Accessed January 2010.
30. Centers for Disease Control and Prevention, Division of Adolescent and School Health (DASH). Coordinated School Health Program. Atlanta: Centers for Disease Control and Prevention, Division of Adolescent and School Health; 2002. Available at www.cdc.gov/HealthyYouth/CSHP/index.htm. Accessed January 2010.
31. Centers for Disease Control and Prevention. National Center for Health Statistics. Fastats A to Z, updated January 19, 2000. Available at WWW.CDC.GOV/NCHS/FASTATS/DEFAULT.HTM. Accessed January 2010.
32. American Academy of Pediatric Dentistry. Dental Home Online Resource Center. Available at www.aapd.org/dentalhome/. Accessed August 2010.
33. Texas Department of State Health Services. First Dental Home, Oral Health Branch. Available at www.dshs.state.tx.us/dental/FDH.shtm. Accessed January 2010.
34. Hobbs FB. The Elderly Population. U.S. Census Bureau. Available at http://factfinder.census.gov/home/saff/main.html?_lang=en. Accessed January 2010.
35. Apple Tree Dental Program. Available at www.appletreedental.com. Accessed January 2010.
36. Bailit H, Edelstein B, Tinanoff N. Public financing of dental care: Impact and policy implications. J Dent Educ 1996;63:882-6.
37. Children's Health Insurance Program Reauthorization Act. Available at www.insurekidsnow.gov/. Accessed January 2010.
38. Community Health Center Association of Connecticut. What is an FQHC? Available at www.chcact.org/Content/What_is_a_FQHC_.asp. Accessed January 2010.
39. National Foundation of Dentistry for the Handicapped. Donated Dental Services. Available at http://nfdh.org/joomla_nfdh/content/view/16/37/. Accessed January 2010.

Additional Resources

Association of State and Territorial Dental Directors. 2010 Best Practice Approach Reports: Improving Children's Oral Health Through Coordinated School Health Programs and Prevention Control of Early Childhood Tooth Decay
www.astdd.org

Centers for Disease Control and Prevention. 2009 Frequently Asked Questions. Dental Sealants
www.cdc.gov/oralhealth/publications/factsheets/sealants_faq.htm

Centers for Disease Control and Prevention. Community Water Fluoridation
www.cdc.gov/fluoridation

7

Research

Stacy A. Weil, RDH, MS

Objectives

Upon completion of this chapter, the student will be able to:
- Differentiate between the hypothesis and the null hypothesis of a research study.
- Explain the importance of the scientific method in research.
- Define a population and a sample as related to research.
- Discuss sampling techniques and their uses.
- Discuss the difference between the independent and dependent variables.
- Use the terms *mean, median,* and *mode* to express the results of data collection.
- Define the terms *continuous data* and *discrete data* and their respective scales of measurement.
- Discuss the uses of various statistical techniques.
- Use different types of displays to exhibit data.
- Explain the difference between type I and type II errors.
- Define probability and statistical significance.
- Express the importance of evaluating dental literature.
- Explain the criteria for reviewing scientific literature.
- Review a scientific journal article relating to dentistry.

Key Terms

Hypothesis	Convenience sampling	Range
Null hypothesis	Experimental group	Variance
Calibrated	Control group	Standard deviation (SD)
Validity	Independent variable	Correlation
Reliability	Variable	Parametric
Interrater reliability	Dependent variable	Normal distribution
Intrarater reliability	Data	t-test
Population	Discrete data	Analysis of variance (ANOVA)
Parameter	Continuous data	Nonparametric
Target population	Nominal scales	Chi-squared test
Sample	Ordinal scales	Power analysis
Statistic	Interval scales	P values
Pilot study	Ratio scales	Type I alpha (α) errors
Random sampling	Descriptive statistics	Type II beta (β) errors
Stratified sampling	Inferential statistics	Refereed
Systematic sampling	Mean	Abstract
Purposive (judgmental)	Median	
sampling	Mode	

Opening Statements

Questions in Research

- How does a public health team decide that fluoridation in a community's water supply will reduce the incidence of new carious lesions?
- Exactly how much fluoride is required to add to the water to achieve a therapeutic effect without a toxic reaction?
- How would officials determine that dental hygienists might improve the quality of life in older people if they were able to work independently in extended-care facilities?
- How do communities decide to spend money on a program providing dental care to individuals with human immunodeficiency virus (HIV) infection instead of to children with special disabilities?
- Where can dental hygienists readily find employment, and what salary can they expect to earn?
- What is the effectiveness of school based sealants in managing caries?

QUESTIONS AND ANSWERS IN RESEARCH

Although dental hygienists may seek the answers to the questions in the Opening Statements, patients may have other concerns such as the following:

- Does a particular mouthrinse really reduce plaque buildup?
- Which brand of toothpaste is best?
- Can nonsurgical periodontal therapy provide results comparable to those of a surgical procedure?

Even though students may commonly learn the answers to these questions from instructors or colleagues, it is important to understand where to find reliable answers to these questions independently and to understand the process that provides these answers.

Research via the scientific method is the basis from which these answers are produced. Manuscripts published in reputable scientific journals disseminate the results of independent research. To determine whether the information contained therein is indeed reliable and valid, certain knowledge and skills must be a part of the repertoire of every competent dental hygienist practicing in the dental community. This chapter provides a basic outline of what research entails and a method of evaluating the results of that research.

THE SCIENTIFIC METHOD AND DEVELOPMENT OF A RESEARCH PROBLEM

Understanding the basics of research entails gaining an appreciation for the components of a good research study, that is, understanding how a research idea is formulated, how a study is designed and executed, and how the resulting data are critically evaluated so that one can infer appropriate conclusions. Research can be thought of as a search for truth and the knowledge gained from this search. A true definition of research is a systematic inquiry that uses orderly scientific methods to answer questions or solve problems.[1]

The discoveries provided by research may lead to new knowledge or to the revision of existing knowledge. Dental research involves a systematic search for knowledge about issues relevant to the profession. To increase the chance that research will be valid, reliable, and relevant, the scientific method—a series of logical steps starting with the formulation of a problem—is employed (**Box 7-1**).

BOX 7-1 The Scientific Method

- Formulation of a problem (asking the question)
- Formulation of a hypothesis (a proposed answer to the question)
- Collecting the data (finding existing information related to the question, as well as gathering of your own information)
- Analysis and interpretation of the results
- Presentation of the results
- Formulation of conclusion (relationship of results to hypothesis)

Formulation of a Problem (Asking the Question)

The first step in beginning a research study is the formulation of an idea. The idea is usually formed from a question that has been raised by a researcher. The question may arise from a very simple observation or thought. For example, during the clinical phase of dental hygiene education, participants might debate about the following:

1. Which areas of the mouth are most difficult to probe accurately?
2. What are the effects of diet on periodontal disease?
3. How can adequate oral health care be maintained by physically and mentally challenged people?

From simple notions such as these, a research question or problem can be formulated.

Examples of a research problem formulated from the previous questions might be as follows:

1. Which quadrant in the human dentition is least accurately probed by the second-year dental hygiene student at University X when using the Periodontal Screening Record (PSR) method of probing?
2. What is the percentage of calories from carbohydrates in the diet of patients exhibiting class II periodontal disease?
3. What effect does modifying the brushing techniques of disabled patients in long-term care facilities have on the gingival bleeding index of these patients?

The research problem should be kept as simple and concise as possible. A successful study often depends on an uncomplicated research design, which results from simple questions.

Formulation of a Hypothesis (a Proposed Answer to the Question)

After a research question is formulated, the next step is the development of a **hypothesis,** a statement that reflects the research question. The hypothesis is stated in positive terms that represent the researcher's prediction or opinion. An example of a hypothesis for the question "Which quadrant in the human dentition is least accurately probed by the second-year dental hygiene student at X University when using the PSR method of probing?" would be as follows: Second-year dental hygiene students at University X using the PSR method are most inaccurate when probing the distal lingual surface of teeth in the upper right quadrant of the mouth.

The research statement is often expressed as a **null hypothesis,** which assumes that there is no statistically significant difference between the groups being studied. An example of a null hypothesis for the preceding question would be as follows: Second-year dental hygiene students at University X show no difference in the accuracy of probing any tooth in the mouth when using the PSR method.

Once the hypothesis has been formed, data can be collected to prove or disprove the statement.

Collecting Data (Finding Existing Information and Gathering Information Independently)

After a research idea and a hypothesis are initially identified, the relevant available literature is reviewed. By examining an area of general interest, the researcher may be inspired to create a research question to resolve unknown or unexplained portions of the area of interest. Alternatively, when a general topic has been selected, a literature review may help to bring the topic into sharper focus. Emulating the accepted research designs that have been previously validated by others, the researcher can then design a study to evaluate the idea. Analysis of the literature is described later in this chapter.

After review and analysis of the available literature, the researcher can plan how the study will be conducted and how the data will be collected. Many different techniques can be used to collect data (see Chapter 3). During data collection, it is important to use **calibrated** instruments that are both valid and reliable. When examiners are involved in data collection, it is imperative that they be calibrated (i.e., in agreement with a set standard of performance for the data collection). For example, if one examiner notes caries on the occlusal surface of a first molar, a second examiner should also be able to note caries on the occlusal surface of the same first molar.

Validity is concerned with gathering data that have been intended to be collected. For example, if two calibrated dentists are examining children for occlusal caries on first molars, both dentists must examine and record caries only on the occlusal surfaces and only on first molars. They are examining the correct surfaces and collecting data that were intended to be collected.

Reliability refers to the consistency and stability of the data. The data are reliable if the examiners are calibrated and can reproduce the results. Both examiners must find the same three occlusal caries on first molars in child No. 1. If they examine child No. 1 an hour later, they should still find the same three occlusal caries as detected previously.

A rater is the person who is collecting the data or making an assessment during a research experiment. The reliability of the data is important, and raters must be consistent both with their own findings, as well as each other's assessment of the same situation. The terms **interrater reliability** and **intrarater reliability** are used to describe this consistency between and within each rater. Interrater reliability refers to the extent that two or more raters obtain the same result when using the same instrument to measure a concept. Intrarater reliability or consistency refers to the same rater making the same assessment on two or more occasions.

In developing the plan for conducting the study, it is important to identify the characteristics of the group involved in the study. Group characteristics are defined by such terms as population, sample, experimental, and control. The term data, or information, collected from the study group is defined and used in different ways. These terms and their relationship to the collection of research data are explained next.

Population and Sampling

Population. **Population** can be defined as the entire group or whole unit of individuals having similar characteristics from which the results of an investigation can be inferred.[2] In regard to numeric characteristics of the population, the term **parameter** is used.

Populations can be very large or very small, depending on the topic to be studied. For example, in the first research question (which quadrant in the human dentition is least accurately probed by second-year dental hygiene students at University X using the PSR method of probing?), one can infer that the total population consists of second-year dental hygiene students. It would be optimal to examine each of these students to arrive at the answer. The second-year dental hygiene students are also known as the **target population,** or the population from whom the information is being collected. Because of time constraints, lack of resources, or financial issues, however, it may be decided that a smaller group within this group can provide the researchers with a significant result.

Sampling. Taking a portion of the population is known as *sampling*. A **sample** is a portion or subset of the entire population that, if properly selected, can provide meaningful information about the entire population. When one is discussing numeric characteristics of samples, the term **statistic** is used.

Samples can be large or small and are chosen to most appropriately reflect the research being done. A large sample usually provides the most accurate representation of the population and increases the exactness and accuracy of the data collected. Occasionally a small sample may be used, as in the case of data collection for a **pilot study,** or trial run, done in preparation for a major study.

The importance of using a sample becomes obvious in regard to our research question. Suppose there is an urgent need to refine teaching techniques for probing and there is not enough time to adequately assess each second-year dental hygiene student's probing at University X. The researcher may thus decide to use only a portion, or sample, of the first-year class.

If it is decided that a sample of the population is to be used, different techniques are used to choose the sample. There are several types of sampling.

Random Sampling. The method of sampling that provides the most external validity, or degree to which the results of the study can be generalized to settings other than the one included, is called **random sampling.** This method provides a sample in which each member of a population has an equal chance of being included and is the procedure of choice because it prevents the possibility of selection bias by the researcher.

As an example, assume that all second-year dental hygiene students at University X have been given a number. There are 50 students in the second-year class, and it is determined that a sample of 10 students will participate in the research. Numbers 1 to 50 would be written on separate slips of paper and placed in a container. From the container a number is drawn. The number is noted as one of the 10 students to be used in this sample. That number is then placed back in the container, and another selection is made until the list of 10 numbers is complete. The importance of placing each number selected back into the container is to preserve a true random selection from 50 numbers. Numbers that are drawn more than once are put on the list only once and are again placed back in the container.

Stratified Sampling. What if probing discrepancies are unique to the university's dental hygiene program? A random sample may not accurately assess the problem for all second-year dental hygiene students; it may be necessary to include students from other universities as well in a method called **stratified sampling.** Subdivisions of a population with similar characteristics, such as second-year dental hygiene students attending different dental hygiene programs, are called *strata.* The random selection of subjects from two or more strata of the population is another way of defining stratified sampling.

Systematic Sampling. Another form of sampling, **systematic sampling,** involves the selection of subjects by including every *n*th person in a list. For example, if a researcher had a list of second-year dental hygiene students by number and chose every odd-numbered person, he or she would be sampling the population systematically. In this case, unless the list is in random order, not every person may have an equal or random chance of being selected; thus systematic sampling may not be considered a true random sample.

Purposive (Judgmental) Sampling. If an instructor who most often works with students who are learning probing techniques chooses the sample, it is easy to imagine that a great deal of bias may be introduced into the study. **Purposive** or **judgmental sampling** provides a sample, through personal judgment, of subjects who would be most representative of the population.

Convenience Sampling. A convenience sample may also introduce bias. Selection of a sample through **convenience sampling** provides a group of individuals who are most readily available to be subjects in the study. For example, a researcher conducting the probing study might enroll only individuals from the researcher's university as subjects.

Experimental and Control Groups and Variables

Experimental and Control Groups. After the sample population is selected, subjects may be divided randomly into experimental and control groups, which are used to answer a research question posed when an experimental treatment or manipulation is imposed on the research setting. The **experimental group** is the sample group in a study that receives the experimental treatment or intervention. The **control group** is the group in a study that does not receive the experimental treatment or intervention. The control group provides the baseline against which the effects of the intervention on the experimental group can be measured.

For example, assume that the study on probing accuracy found an area of the mouth in which inaccuracy predominated. At this point, one might choose to conduct another research study, introducing a new method of probing instruction that would focus on the area of the mouth in which most inaccuracies occur. This new method of teaching would be administered to the experimental group, whereas the control group would continue to receive the traditional method of instruction.

Variables. The experimental treatment or intervention that is imposed on the experimental group can also be called the **independent variable.** A **variable** is a characteristic or concept that varies, or is different, within the population under study. The independent variable is controlled or manipulated by the researcher and is believed to cause or influence the **dependent variable.** The dependent variable is thought to depend on or to be caused by the independent variable. It is the outcome variable of interest.

In the case of the research question, which involves teaching a new probing technique to the experimental group, the dependent variable would be probing accuracy. The independent variable would be the probing technique that is being taught. Other variables not related to the purpose of the study are *uncontrolled variables* and may influence the relationship between the independent and dependent variable. To increase internal validity, it is important to control for extraneous variables. *Internal validity* refers to the fact that it is the experimental treatment or independent variable that is responsible for the observed effects and that these effects are not due to extraneous variables. A good research study controls for extraneous variables through research design or through statistical procedures.[3] By understanding the previous terms and definitions, one can implement a method of data collection, or the gathering of information, to address a research problem.

Data

Pieces of information, such as numbers collected from measurements and counts obtained during the course of a research study, are known as **data.** Although the concept of data itself may seem fairly straightforward, there are different types of data and different ways to measure data (**Table 7-1**). Two types of data are as follows:

1. **Discrete data** have only one of a limited set of values and are counted only in whole numbers. Discrete variables may include things like hair color, gender, political preference, and number totals, such as how many times a person brushes his or her teeth or the number of decayed, missing, or filled teeth. These data are considered to be qualitative in nature.
2. **Continuous data** are measurements made from a particular value within a defined range. Variables along a continuum, such as temperature, scores on a test, and time, are continuous data. These data are considered to be quantitative in nature.

Different scales of measurement are used for discrete and continuous data. Discrete data can use nominal or ordinal scales of measurement. Continuous data use interval and ratio scales of measurements.

Nominal scales of measurement consist of named categories with no order. For example, females may be placed in category A and males in category B.

Ordinal scales of measurement consist of categories of variables in which the categories are in order, but there is no equal or defined distance between them. For example, cancer staging for tumors is grouped into four stages designated by Roman numerals I to IV. In general, stage I cancers are small localized cancers that are usually curable, whereas stage IV usually represents inoperable or metastatic cancer. Stage II and III cancers are usually locally advanced and/or with involvement of local lymph nodes. It is known that type II is worse than type I and that type III is worse than type II, but each type of cancer is slightly different, making it difficult to define precisely for all cancers.[4]

Table 7-1   Types of Data

Types of Data	Characteristics	Examples	Related Scales of Measurement	Appropriate Data Display
Discrete	Limited set of values, represented as whole numbers, qualitative	Hair color, number of times a person brushes, DMF teeth	Nominal (named categories; e.g., male or female) Ordinal (same as nominal but categories in order; e.g., stages of cancer)	Bar graph
Continuous	Particular value within a range, variables along a continuum, quantitative	Temperature, test scores, time	Interval (same as ordinal plus equal distance between variables but no zero; e.g., Fahrenheit) Ratio (same as interval plus equal distance between variable with zero; e.g., height, weight)	Histogram

DMF, Decayed, missing, filled.

Interval scales of measurement have equal distance between variables, but there is no true zero point (i.e., temperature on a Fahrenheit thermometer).

Ratio scales of measurement have equal intervals between the variables, but there is a meaningful zero point (i.e., height and weight).

As listed in the following, each scale of measurement takes on the characteristics of the previous one, making ratio the most powerful measurement:

Nominal: Named categories only

Ordinal: Same as nominal plus categories are in order

Interval: Same as ordinal plus equal intervals between categories

Ratio: Same as interval plus meaningful or true zero point

After the data have been collected from a chosen population and variables have been defined and measured, it is time to proceed to the next step of the scientific method, presenting and interpreting the data and presenting the results.

Data Analysis and Presentation of Results

Statistics

Statistics is a science that provides a way of processing numbers or analyzing the data that have been collected. Statistics may be used to describe, analyze, and interpret the numbers collected in the data. The purpose of statistical analysis is to make an inference or an assumption about a population.[5] Two types of relevant statistics are as follows:

1. **Descriptive statistics** are used to describe and summarize data. Their objective is to communicate results, without generalizing beyond the sample, to any population. Some ways in which results are communicated are through (1) measures of central tendency (mean, median, and mode) and (2) measures of dispersion.
2. **Inferential statistics** (see later section) are used to apply information from the sample to a larger population.

Measures of Central Tendency

Measures of central tendency are used to describe the sample based on the data gathered. They include components such as the mean, median, and mode.

The **mean** is the average of the group. It is a sum of all the values divided by the number (n) of items and is statistically noted as $\bar{x}$. The mean is calculated in the following manner:

$$\text{mean} = \frac{\sum \bar{x}}{n}$$

The positive aspect of the mean is that it includes the value of each score; the negative aspect is that it can be affected by any extreme scores and may not give a true average. For example, a test is administered; 10 people in the class score an 85 and 2 people score a 30. The class average becomes approximately 76, which is not a true representation of the class scores.

The **median** represents the exact middle score or value in an ordered distribution of scores; it is the point above and below which 50% of the scores lie. When the total number of scores is even, the sum of the two middle scores, divided by 2, provides the median.

Unlike the mean, extreme scores do not affect the median. In the previous example, the median score would be 85. However, it is not difficult to imagine what would happen if scores were not evenly distributed and the median were used as an example of the middle score. The information provided in this case may not demonstrate a true midpoint for the class.

The **mode** is the score or value that occurs most frequently in a distribution of scores. Once again, the mode for the preceding example would be 85. The distribution of scores may be unimodal, bimodal, or multimodal, or there may even be no mode.

Figure 7-1 presents the mean, median, and mode of a group of test scores. **Figure 7-2** illustrates a symmetric distribution in which the mean, median, and mode are the same; it also shows skewed curves, where the mean and median are located to the left and right of the mode.

Measures of Dispersion

In addition to the measures of central tendency (mean, median, and mode), measures of dispersion (also known as measures of variation) may also be used to describe data. Measures of central tendency provide a first step in the measure of distributions. Occasionally, however, a measurement is also desired to determine how far scores differ from the mean.

The most obvious way of measuring the dispersion of data is the **range,** which measures the difference between the highest and lowest values in a distribution of scores. If the median is defined as the point where 50% of the scores are lower and 50% of the scores are higher, the location of the 0 and 100th percentile would define the range. More commonly, the value of the range is used to define the 5th and 95th percentiles. These are the points that 5% of the subjects may be below or 95% of the people may be below. If a person has taken a test and is in the 95th percentile, 95% of the people have scored lower than that person has.

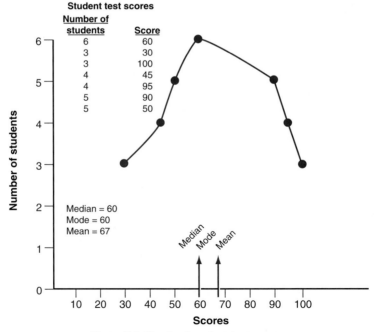

Figure 7-1 Graph of student test scores.

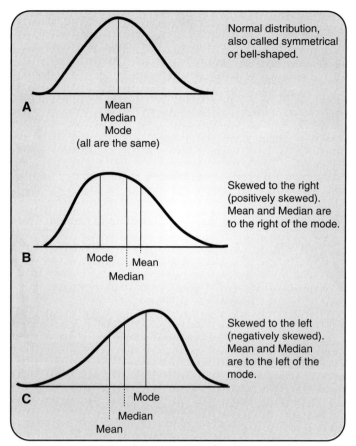

Figure 7-2 Graphing measures of central tendency.

Another measure of dispersion, called **variance,** is a method of ascertaining the way individual variables are located around the mean. Variance is most often used to measure interval and ratio variables.

A first step in the calculation of variance is to determine the average deviation, which can be derived through calculating the difference between each point of data and the mean, adding the answers together, and dividing by the total amount of data points. The main problem with calculating the average difference is that there are as many negative data points as positive; this situation ultimately results in an answer of zero.

A way around this problem is to square each data point so that all terms are positive. Therefore the difference between each data point and the mean squared, summed, and divided by the total amount of data points results in the average squared deviation, also known as variance.

Variance is simply a step in determining the **standard deviation (SD)** and is equal to the square of the SD. The formula for the SD is as follows:

$$SD = \sqrt{\frac{\text{sum of } (\text{data point} - \text{mean})^2}{\text{No of values}}}$$

It makes sense, then, that the farther away the data points are from the mean, the greater the variance and SD. **Box 7-2** presents the calculations to find the range, variance, and SD of student test scores.

Box 7-3 demonstrates the calculations from data collected in a community research project involving unwed teenaged mothers and their knowledge of baby bottle tooth decay. Twelve mothers are in this study group. The mothers' scores from the pretest range from a low score of 25% to a high score of 70%.

Correlation

After we determine the previous information about our data, we may want to next determine whether any **correlation** exists between the variables. Correlation is a statistical method for

BOX 7-2 Range, Variance, and Standard Deviation of Student Test Scores

Student Test Scores

Number of Students	Score
6	60
3	30
3	100
4	45
4	95
5	90
5	50

Range is the difference between highest and lowest score: 100 – 30 = 70.

Variance is the average deviation or spread of scores around the mean.

The variance is calculated as (individual score – mean)^2/# of scores.

$(60 - 67)^2 = 49$
$(30 - 67)^2 = 1369$
$(100 - 67)^2 = 1089$
$(45 - 67)^2 = 484$
$(95 - 67)^2 = 784$
$(90 - 67)^2 = 529$
$(50 - 67)^2 = 289$

49 × 6 (# of scores of 60) = 294
1369 × 3 (# of scores of 30) = 4107
1089 × 3 (# of scores of 100) = 3267
484 × 4 (# of scores of 45) = 1936
784 × 4 (# of scores of 95) = 3136
529 × 5 (# of scores of 90) = 2645
289 × 5 (# of scores of 50) = 1445

All above summed = 16,830

16830 ÷ 30 (total number of scores) = 561
561 is the variance
Standard deviation is the positive square root of the variance: $\sqrt{561}$
The square root of 561 = 23.7 (standard deviation)

BOX 7-3 Calculations of Test Scores on Baby Bottle Tooth Decay

Subject (mother)	Score	
1	45	
2	45	
3	45	
4	30	
5	35	Median = 45%
6	25	Mode = 45%
7	40	Mean = 48%
8	50	
9	60	Range = 70 − 25
10	65	= 45
11	70	Variance = $\dfrac{\text{sum of (individual scores} - \text{mean})^2}{\text{\# of scores}}$
12	70	Variance = 210
		Standard deviation = $\sqrt{210} = 14$

Table 7-2 Correlation of Test Scores and Hours of Education

Group Number	Group Type and Pretest Scores	Hours of Education	Average Posttest Score Increase (Points) %
1	Four mothers with an average pretest score of 50	2	60
2	Four mothers with an average pretest score of 50	4	70
3	Four mothers with an average pretest score of 50	6	80
4	Four mothers with an average pretest score of 50	8	90

determining whether a variation in one variable may be related to a variation in another variable. For example, height and weight often show a correlation because taller people usually have a higher weight than shorter people. Age and periodontal disease may have a correlation because older people may have higher incidence of periodontal disease than younger people.

The technique used to determine correlation depends on the type of variable being explored. Different techniques are used for discrete or continuous variables. The measurement scale may also influence the technique. For example, nominal, ordinal, interval, and ratio scales of measurement are all calculated slightly differently.

The results of the calculation for correlation show either a negative or positive relationship. When the relationship is *positive,* it is predicted that as the value of one variable increases, the other also increases. Perfect positive correlation is shown by +1.0. An example would be the finding that, in the research with unwed mothers, the more time the examiner spends with them on patient education, the greater the increase in the mothers' knowledge. **Table 7-2** presents a correlation of increased education with increased knowledge. **Figure 7-3** demonstrates a graphic display of the same positive correlation of the two variables.

In contrast, a *negative* correlation shows an inverse relationship between variables. Perfect negative correlation is shown by −1.0. **Figure 7-4** shows that a diet including six servings of fruits and vegetables each day *decreases* the incidence of certain cancers.

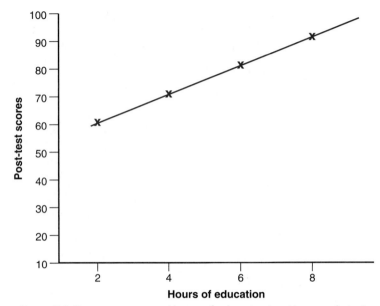

Figure 7-3 Post-test scores and hours of education (positive correlation).

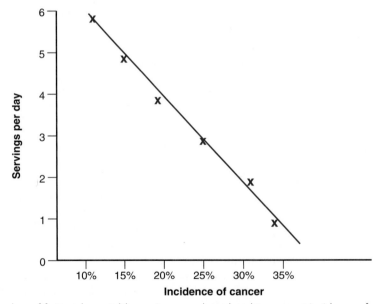

Figure 7-4 Number of fruit and vegetable servings per day related to percent incidence of cancer (negative correlation).

In review, a perfect positive correlation is noted as +1.0 and a perfect negative correlation showing an inverse relationship is noted as −1.0 Although a perfect positive or perfect negative correlation may occur, it may be possible to find no relationship at all; this instance is noted as 0.0. Some literature states that generally a correlation coefficient above .70 is considered satisfactory.[1] In each study, the nature of the variables and the numbers involved in the comparison must also be considered along with the correlation coefficient in determining what is a significant relationship. The closer the relationship is to +1.0 or −1.0, the more perfect, or stronger, the correlation.

Presentation of the Data

In addition to the data displayed in the previous graphs, other types of data display include the following:

A *bar graph* is most often used to display nominal or ordinal data that are discrete in nature. With the use of data that may be gathered from the study on teenaged mothers and baby bottle tooth decay, one can create a bar graph to present the data pictorially (**Figure 7-5**).

A *frequency polygon* is used to represent data that are continuous in nature. An example from the study with teenaged mothers is depicted in **Figure 7-6**. The figure contains dots connected to straight lines to present the frequency distribution of the data. In this case the frequency polygon demonstrates how many times per week the mothers brush their children's teeth.

A *histogram,* although a type of bar graph, is used most often to represent interval or ratio scaled variables that are continuous in nature (**Figure 7-7**). The bars in a histogram are of equal width and touch each other to indicate that the data are being presented on a continuum.

Inferential Statistics

In addition to including descriptive techniques to describe data, inferential statistics may also be used. Whereas descriptive statistics are used to determine information only about the sample being studied, inferential statistics seek to determine a generalization between the sample studied and the actual population. The larger the sample size, therefore, the greater the number of generalizations that can be made regarding the population. Depending on the type of data collected,

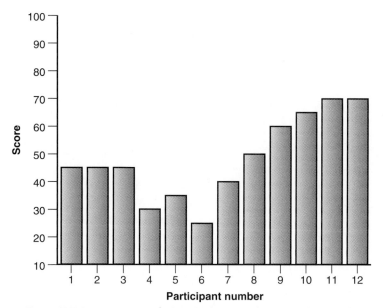

Figure 7-5 Pretest scores of 12 participants as shown in a bar graph.

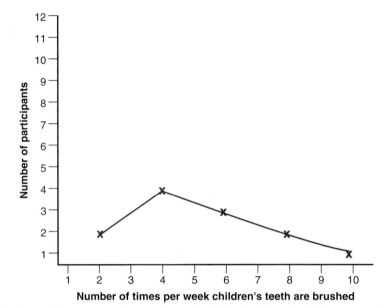

Figure 7-6 Number of times per week participants brush their children's teeth as shown in a frequency polygon.

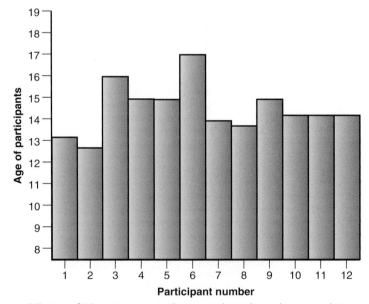

Figure 7-7 Age of 12 participants in the research study as shown in a histogram.

the use of inferential statistics may include either parametric or nonparametric statistical techniques. Inferential statistics are based on the assumption that sampling is conducted randomly, although that is not always the case.

Parametric Inferential Statistics

Parametric statistics are used when the data include interval or ratio scales of measurement. Parametric techniques work best when the sample is large and randomized and the population from which the sample is taken is normally distributed. In a normal distribution, 50% of the values lie on the left half of the distribution, and 50% lie on the right half. A **normal distribution** assumes that approximately 68% of the population fall within one SD of the mean, approximately 95% fall within two SDs of the mean, and 99% lie within three SDs from the mean.[6] The plotting of these data on a graph results in a bell-shaped curve (**Figure 7-8**).

t-Test. Parametric statistics are calculated by means of several different methods or tests. One of the most common is the **t-test,** or Student's t-test, so named for the man responsible for development of this technique. The t-test is used to analyze the difference between two means. It provides the researcher with the difference between treatment and control groups or groups receiving treatment A versus treatment B.

When the test is used on a single group that yields pretreatment and post-treatment scores, it is known as a *t-test for dependent samples.* This test analyzes data when only one independent variable is tested. For example, a researcher may want to examine the difference in blood glucose levels of diabetic subjects before and after treatment with a new diet. Assuming that all of the subjects were the same age and had the same degree of disease present, the t-test for dependent samples can be used to determine pretreatment and post-treatment scores.

The independent t-test determines differences in the mean between two independent groups such as an experimental and control group or males versus females. This test is used when only one or two independent variables are tested. Most often, data involving interval or ratio scales of measurement are statistically analyzed with an independent t-test. For example, a study might investigate the effect of a new toothbrushing method on gingivitis. The subjects would be randomized into two groups: (1) a control group receiving no instruction and asked to use their normal brushing method and (2) an experimental group asked to practice a new method of toothbrushing. The instrument may be a gingival bleeding index that is conducted before the start of the

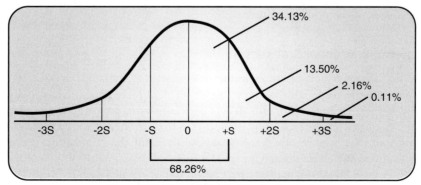

Figure 7-8 Normal distribution (bell curve).

Table 7-3   Data Used in Analysis of Variance (ANOVA) Testing

Patient Number	TP 1	TP 2	TP 3	TP 4	TP 5
1	6.0	5.0	4.0	5.0	2.0
2	5.0	5.0	3.0	4.0	3.0
3	7.0	5.0	4.0	5.0	3.0
4	5.0	4.0	4.0	3.0	4.0
5	6.0	5.0	5.0	4.0	4.0

TP, Toothpaste brands 1 to 5.
Key: 1.0-10 = pain relief (10 is maximum relief).

study and again 8 weeks later. The hypothesis is that the new method of toothbrushing will decrease the gingival bleeding index of patients with gingivitis.

Analysis of Variance. Another commonly used test for parametrics is **analysis of variance,** or **ANOVA.** This test allows comparison among more than two sample means and compares interactions among the variability in the multiple sample groups with the variability within the groups.

A simple example is the comparison of the many brands of desensitizing toothpaste. Five brands of toothpaste that claim relief of tooth pain caused by sensitivity have been located. A group of subjects is assembled, and each subject is given a different toothpaste disguised in a plain white tube. Each subject is asked to use this tube and is given other tubes to use until all of the various toothpastes are used. Subjects are asked to rank pain relief from tooth sensitivity on a numeric scale of 1 to 10 for each toothpaste used. The scale may look like the one in **Table 7-3**.

ANOVA allows the dental hygienist to compare each toothpaste used and the pain relief experienced by the patients. It also allows a comparison of the different responses from each patient for each individual toothpaste brand. ANOVA may yield information about which of the brands is actually more effective and how each brand compares with another. In essence, ANOVA compares variability within groups with variability between groups.

The t-test, or Student's t-test, and ANOVA are just two of many tests that may be used in statistical analysis of data. These tests are perhaps the most common parametric inferential statistical techniques.

No matter which technique is chosen, the sample should be randomly and independently selected from normal populations. Although these tests provide more detailed information of the interaction of variables, the research should include means and SDs in the report for accurate assessment of the tests' magnitude.

Nonparametric Inferential Statistics

Besides parametric tests, **nonparametric** inferential statistical techniques may be selected. Nonparametric techniques are most useful for data to be measured on the nominal or ordinal scale. Remember, nominal or ordinal data are "qualitative," and although numbers may be included, these numbers are derived more subjectively than numbers associated with quantitative data. Nonparametric tests involve fewer assumptions about the population. The sample size may be small, and variables are discrete.

The most commonly used nonparametric test is the **chi-squared test**. This test may be used to analyze questionnaire data and to determine whether a relationship exists between two variables. The chi-squared test is used to examine the differences between observed and expected frequencies.

Determining Statistical Significance

Statistical tests provide researchers with an idea of what the data they have collected say about the sample and perhaps what the data imply about the population from which the sample was drawn. An important factor in research is determining the statistical significance of the data. Statistical significance is a way of indicating that the results found in an analysis of data are unlikely to have been caused by chance; more likely, the results have been caused by the independent variable. Using too small or too large a sample may influence the statistical significance. Typically, the use of too small a sample (less than 30) provides too little information to make generalizations about the populations and to create any significance of results.

Power Analysis. Determining how many subjects are needed to provide significance is called a **power analysis,** which is calculated according to a specific statistical formula based on what the researcher hopes to observe in most of the subjects. The power of a study, or its ability to detect relationships among variables, is directly related to sample size, the definition of the independent variable, and the precision with which the study is planned and conducted.[7] When too large a sample is used, the effects may be statistically significant but clinically of no consequence.

The true importance of determining statistical significance is that the greater the significance, the more statistical inference can be made regarding the population from whom the sample was taken. That is, statistical significance reinforces our ability to generalize the conclusions we make about our study population to a larger population, perhaps even to the "general population."

A major issue in regard to statistical inferences is that every measurement taken from the sample being researched has some degree of error. Researchers may describe the possibility of error or lack of error in various ways.

Confidence Intervals. The term *confidence interval* refers to how researchers describe the probability of the statistical results being correct. A confidence interval indicates a range of values within which the parameters of the population have a probability of lying. Researchers usually use a 95% to 99% confidence interval. A 95% confidence interval indicates a probability that the researcher is wrong 5 times in 100. By using a 99% confidence interval, the researcher may be wrong 1% of the time; however, increasing the confidence interval also decreases the specificity of the data. Therefore, when the confidence interval is 95%, there is a 5% chance that the observed results or differences between study and control groups are due purely to chance and not a true difference caused by the independent variable.

P **Values.** Researchers also use ***P* values** to describe statistical significance. The *P* value states how likely it is that the study could have come to a false scientific conclusion. *P* values are calculated according to the sample size, the difference between the means of the control and experimental group, and the SD of the distribution. The smaller the *P* value, the more significant the findings of the study are considered.

A normally acceptable *P* value is $P < .05$. Results with a *P* value at less than .05 are generally considered statistically significant and provide the basis for rejection of the null hypothesis. $P < .05$ means that the results were due to chance only 5 times in 100. *P* values of approximately .01, .001, and lower increase the significance of the study.

Table 7-4   Types of Statistics

Types of Statistics	Characteristics	Consider	Measurement/Statistical Techniques
Descriptive	Describe and summarize data in sample being studied, no generalization	Mean, median, mode	Measures of central tendency, measures of dispersion
Inferential	Used to generalize, apply information from sample to population, includes parametric and nonparametric	Confidence intervals, normal distribution	Nonparametric: t-test, analysis of variance (ANOVA) Parametric: Chi-square

Table 7-5   Null Hypothesis

Null Hypothesis Is Actually ...	Null Hypothesis Is Accepted	Null Hypothesis Is Not Accepted
True	No error	Type I α (alpha) error
False	Type II β (beta) error	No error

Descriptive or Inferential?

- Last semester, the heights of students at the college ranged from 5 feet to 6 feet.
  - This is an example of a *descriptive statistic* because the data from the sample is exact (height of students) and there is no generalization applied to the group.
- Flossing can help prevent periodontal disease.
  - This is an example of an *inferential statistic* because the statement is a generalization of a larger population based on an interpretation of research data from a smaller study.

  Table 7-4 compares descriptive statistics with inferential statistics.

Formulation of a Conclusion and Relationship of Results to the Hypothesis

Based on the statistical results of the data analysis, the researcher determines whether the study shows significance. Whether it shows much, little, or no significance, a conclusion can be formulated. From the results discovered, the researcher decides to either accept or reject the null hypothesis of the study. Occasionally, when formulating a conclusion, a researcher may make an error. Errors within research are of two types:

Type I alpha (α) errors occur when, according to statistical results, the researcher rejects the null hypothesis when it is true. The researcher's conclusion states that a relationship exists when it does not. Most statistical analyses use a level of .05, which means that there is a 1 in 20 chance that a conclusion will state that a difference exists when there is no difference.

Type II beta (β) errors occur when the null hypothesis is accepted but is actually false. The conclusion states that no relationship exists when one actually does (**Table 7-5**).

ANALYSIS OF THE LITERATURE

A thorough review of the literature is often completed to begin development of an adequate plan for collecting the data. Being informed and up to date not only are professional responsibilities but also serve a purpose in each of the roles of the dental hygienist: clinician, educator, advocate, administrator, and researcher.[8] The assimilation of information requires more than listening to colleagues and attending occasional Continuing Education programs. An excellent source of information is dental and other scientific literature.

A literature analysis, besides helping the dental hygienist to develop a data collection plan, provides valuable information about theories, methods, and products that are available. Reviewing the literature is an important step in remaining current within the field of dentistry and provides information used to intelligently answer many questions posed by patients. Scientific literature contains information that can help one to maintain competency and helps to set the exceptional practitioner apart from others in the field of dentistry.

Not all dental hygienists receive regular subscriptions to scientific magazines or have access to Internet services. Although these are the most common ways to obtain information about literature, a trip to a local library with a scientific collection can provide essential information. Becoming skillful at obtaining scientific information is not as easy as might be expected. However, it is a skill worth cultivating because it provides a valuable tool for researchers and for practicing dental hygienists.

The topic described next presents an overview of what is available in the form of written resources, how to choose the best sources of this information, and how to critically review this literature. Although a critical analysis of the scientific literature is ideal, it is best to remain open-minded when inquiring about new products, services, and techniques.[9]

Finally, keeping focused on the research or specific information to be reviewed should help to provide simple yet intelligent answers to the question at hand.

Selection of Literature

To begin a literature review, the dental hygienist or researcher must select appropriate journals. The scientific writing to be reviewed should be comprehensible to the average dental hygienist who is knowledgeable about the topic area. The selection of literature that is pertinent to the field of dental hygiene will allow the researcher to obtain a complete understanding of the research topic while focusing the research on issues important to dental hygiene. Because of the technicality and intricate scientific detail of its topics, the *Journal of Biochemical Research* might not be an ideal place to start looking for information on periodontal host factors, whereas the *Journal of Periodontology* and *Journal of Dental Hygiene* might be preferable choices. Although both journals publish in-depth scientific literature, the material is tailored to the dental field and thus is relevant and understandable to the average oral health researcher.

Equally important is the selection of a reputable journal. Several aspects lend credibility to a reputable source, including an editorial review board that evaluates each contributed article for accuracy, relevancy of content, and issues involving style and method of scientific writing. This is also known as a "**refereed**," or a *"peer-reviewed,"* journal. Individuals who are considered experts on the article's content review the articles submitted with a peer review board. A refereed journal ensures that an article is written in appropriate scientific style and that the data published therein reflect current knowledge. A reputable journal is commonly affiliated with a professional group or society, a specialty group, or a reputable scientific publisher. A reputable scientific journal is not a journal that is a popular magazine or published by a commercial firm.

Examples of poor choices for scientific literature include any of the typical newsstand health and recreation journals and glamour and beauty magazines. Professionals should appreciate the fact that although many attractively presented dental publications exist, many are simply glorified advertising brochures and do not represent an acceptable source of scientific material. When selecting a journal article, the reader should be careful to note that the author has the appropriate qualifications. (An attorney writing an article about orthodontics, for example, might not be the most credible source of information.) Authors should also possess experience or a current relationship with the field about which they are writing. If the written work is a research study, there should be evidence of facilities in which to conduct the research and financial support for the project.

Readers usually find a tremendous amount of available information. Although older information may be considered classic and therefore occasionally useful in conducting a review, most often readers want to research the most current information. One classic study was the Vipeholm study, conducted in Sweden in the 1950s.[10] The study investigated the incidence of decay in relation to sugar intake and is often mentioned in scientific writing. Although the information from this research has proved valuable, this study was conducted in a disadvantaged population and by today's standards would not have received approval because of ethical considerations. One of the most often cited concerns about the Vipeholm study was whether the subjects enlisted possessed the mental capacity to give their consent for the research.

Information is usually considered current if it has been published within the last 3 to 5 years. References cited in journal articles should be carefully screened to validate their relevancy and age. Sometimes only a limited amount of information is available on a given topic, and this is reflected in the article. An example is the lack of true research involving herbal or alternative dental therapies.

Current Topic of Interest Example: Bisphosphonate-Related Osteonecrosis of the Jaw

Dental hygienists working in the community, particularly in association with research institutions such as Veterans Affairs hospitals, often come across topics of interest to the profession affecting patient treatment options to which the community at large has not yet been exposed. Participation in the research related to these topics and publication of the research along with development of subsequent treatment options is often an opportunity for dental hygienists. Review of research is essential in determining not only treatment options but also consideration of patient health outcomes during dental treatment. A current example is the evolution of the diagnosis of bisphosphonate-related osteonecrosis of the jaw (BRONJ). The original research article on the topic appeared in the *Journal of Oral and Maxillofacial Surgery* in 2004,* and the disease was subsequently detailed in the position paper by the American Association of Oral and Maxillofacial Surgery (AAOMS) in September 2006.† The position paper includes oral hygiene recommendations relevant to the practice of dental hygiene in controlling the disease. After further research on the topic within and outside the dental field, recent treatment options were refined and related oral hygiene considerations were continued to be noted as important in the treatment of the disease. A literature search and review shows several current publications available for dental hygienists review and consideration. Based on the new original research recently conducted, the AAOMS updated its position paper in January 2009.‡

---

*See Rugierro SL, Mehrotra B, Rosenberg TJ, et al. Osteonecrosis of the jaws associated with the use of bisphosphonates: A review of 63 cases. J Oral Maxillofac Surg 2004;62:527.
†Available at www.aaoms.org/docs/position_papers/osteonecrosis.pdf.
‡Available at www.aaoms.org/docs/position_papers/bronj_update.pdf.

Evaluation of the Selected Literature

After a journal and the information relevant to the reader's goals are selected, the reader can pursue a comprehensive evaluation of this literature. Various types of journal articles undergo different types of review. For example, a review article may examine an assortment of studies that have already been conducted and provides an overview of the research that has already been done. A review article can help one formulate an idea or a new research question and can help direct the reader to other sources of information through references cited within the article. Validation of a good review article should follow all of the practices stated earlier, including author expertise, accurate and recent references, and review from a refereed journal.

The Primary Research Manuscript

Perhaps the most useful type of journal article and truly the archetypal "research paper" is the primary research manuscript (**Box 7-4**). A primary research study describes the original research,

---

BOX 7-4 **What to Look for in a Research Study Manuscript**

A. Abstract
- Contains 200 words or less.
- Clearly states purpose of study in the first few sentences.
- Includes brief description of the following: population, type of research, overview of statistics, results, and conclusions.

B. Introduction
- Review of the supporting literature.
- Statement of hypothesis (null hypothesis).
- Reason for study.

C. Methods and Materials
- Appropriate selection of instrument.
- Appropriate method of conducting research (i.e., prospective, retrospective, randomized, etc.).
- Descriptive enough that reader can replicate the study.

D. Results
- Appropriate statistical tests.
- Appropriate display of data.
- Clear and understandable presentation of the data.
- Correct interpretation of data.

E. Discussion
- Conclusions are based on fact.
- Results are tied into previous research discussed in introduction.
- Inferences and opinions are stated as such.
- Future plans are included for further research

including its methods, materials, results, and conclusions. When one is considering a primary research article, the practice of checking author expertise, accurate and recent references, and peer review from a refereed journal still applies; additionally, other steps are to be followed. The first step is often an assessment of the paper's abstract.

Abstract

A relevant **abstract** is usually confined to approximately 200 words and concisely defines the study's purpose, methods, materials, and results. The abstract, a brief description of the research, appears at the beginning of the manuscript and is designed to provide the reader with an overview of the study. Although it may present an idea of what the study involved, the abstract may not always paint an accurate picture of the study and the results. The only way to truly assess a scientific article is to read the content within and critically examine each piece for information.

A primary research article begins with a review of the current literature and an introduction to the study. Within this section, an accurate and complete description of the research problem is given and the purpose of the study is clearly stated. The research question can be stated as a hypothesis and may include objectives to be accomplished.

Materials and Methods

The next section of the primary research manuscript, materials and methods, describes the population or sample and the techniques used to gather information about the population studied. One of the primary reasons for disseminating results in peer-reviewed journals (in addition to sharing the results) is so colleagues might duplicate the experiment to validate the results or might modify it in some respects to further refine the conclusions implied in the study. Toward that end, the materials and methods text should be complete enough so that other readers might reasonably expect to recapitulate the experiment and verify the results.

The reviewer will want to determine whether the researcher has selected an appropriate group to test and whether it is one that is relevant to the reviewer's needs. This necessity for appropriateness applies whether the "group" in question is a population of laboratory animals, human subjects, or tissue culture cells. For example, if reviewers are looking for information regarding nonsurgical periodontal therapy, they should ensure that the study has used a similar population or sample relative to their needs.

The number of subjects in the group is also important. Has the study included enough subjects so that readers can generalize the findings to their group of interest? If the subject is a 35-year-old woman and the research involves men older than 50 years of age, the results may not necessarily be relevant to the reader's cause; if the subject is a 35-year-old woman but only one or two subjects are involved, the information might also be irrelevant.

Ensuring that no author bias has been introduced is very important. Bias may be defined as any influence that produces a distortion in the results of a study.[1] Here are some considerations:

- Is the subject a patient of the researcher, who also happens to be the one who developed the new technique?
- Are all variables in the study controlled for (e.g., diet, standard of living, gender, age, dental history)?
- Is there a control group and an experimental group?
- Is one group receiving the standard treatment and the experimental group receiving the new therapy?

An example of a research study may be the evaluation of the efficacy of sealants in caries prevention. The study design may consist of a group of test subjects (the experimental group) who are to receive sealants and are then to be monitored for a number of years to determine the caries rate. Because reference data are essential, a control group (the group without sealants) is compared with the group with sealants.

Readers must also consider the following issues when evaluating research design:

- If an instrument (e.g., a questionnaire) is to be part of the study, have validity and reliability been previously established?
- Are the conditions under which the treatment is accomplished similar and completely described?
- Are both groups monitored for an adequate period of time to assess long-term results of the therapy?

Results

After the methods and materials are described, the results section, including a statistical analysis, follows. The results text should detail how the hypothesis of the study has been tested. Statistical tests should be appropriate for the study and should be described. Tables and graphs may be included to provide a visual representation of the results, but they should be clear and understandable to the reader. The author should justify the statistical method used.

Discussion

Finally, a discussion of the conclusions and the inferences drawn from the results of the research is presented. The conclusions are also used to define outcomes of the research.

The conclusion should clearly state the rejection or acceptance of the null hypothesis. It may discuss facts derived from the research but may also include investigator speculation on what the results mean. The conclusion usually discusses the research study's strengths and weaknesses and may mention further research necessary to obtain the desired results.

Complications observed during the research should also be presented. The results of the study are related to the literature cited. Most important, the conclusions are a direct reflection of the findings. Although speculation may be appropriate, it should be stated as such. It is never appropriate to make statements that are not based on fact or that are not derived from study results.

SUMMARY

This chapter provides an overview of the basics of research, including the steps in the scientific method, the steps in analyzing the literature, and the components of a primary research manuscript.

Although all research should be conducted according to the scientific method to provide results with a measure of validity and reliability, scientific research remains an inexact science. However, when studies are properly designed and accurately analyzed with the use of the appropriate statistical design, the information obtained not only will be new but also may serve as a springboard for further studies. The inventive and inquisitive practitioner will seek to discover information that enhances the practice of dental hygiene and all its contemporary roles and keeps the profession moving in a forward direction.

Applying Your Knowledge

1. Formulate a research problem based on a question you have that is related to the field of dentistry.
2. Develop a hypothesis and a null hypothesis for the research problem.
3. Considering your research problem, define the following:
   a. Population
   b. Sample
   c. Experimental group
   d. Control group
   e. Independent variable
   f. Dependent variable
4. Determine whether the data collected from your study will be continuous or discrete. Will nominal, ordinal, interval, or ratio scales of measurement be used?
5. Complete a literature review for the research problem formulated in No. 2, and write an abstract for one of the journal articles examined during your literature review.
6. Using data that you have reviewed or collected, determine the mean, median, and mode.
7. Give five examples of positive and negative correlations. Compare variables related to dental hygiene or to data from articles you have read.
8. Using one of the research studies from your literature review, describe the statistical analysis. Were the statistical techniques used appropriate? Were the data displayed in an appropriate manner?
9. Design and complete a research study or community project following the steps listed in Box 7-1 (the scientific method). Complete your study by creating a poster presentation using appropriate displays of data and the description of your study.

Dental Hygiene Competencies

Reading the material in this chapter and participating in the activities of Applying Your Knowledge will contribute to the student's ability to demonstrate the following competencies:

Core competencies
C.4 Assume responsibility for dental hygiene actions and care based on scientific theories and research as well as the accepted standard of care.

Community involvement
CM.6 Evaluate the outcomes of community-based programs, and plan for future activities.

Patient/client care
PC.1 Systematically collect, analyze, and record data on the general, oral, and psychosocial health status of a variety of patients or clients using methods consistent with medicolegal principles.
PC.3 Collaborate with the patient, client, or other health professionals to formulate a comprehensive dental hygiene care plan that is patient-centered and based on scientific evidence.

Community Case

Allison is a registered dental hygienist who has spent the last 10 years working in a periodontal practice that treats clients referred from several different dental practices in town. Most of the clients present with moderate-to-advanced periodontal disease. Allison has been intrigued by the different information she has seen in several professional journals regarding the link between periodontal disease and heart disease. Allison is also interested in a nutritional supplementation plan she read about that provides protection from inflammation and facilitates wound healing. Allison remembers that much of the information linking periodontal disease and cardiac health indicates inflammatory factors may be a possible culprit. Allison hypothesizes that she can take the relatively small sample her client population provides and make some generalizations regarding oral health as related to cardiac health. After speaking with her employer and gaining regulatory approval for her project, Allison consents and enrolls 100 subjects into her study. Allison enrolls subjects diagnosed with moderate periodontal disease and randomly assigns half into a group treated with standard therapy and the other half into a group treated with standard therapy plus the nutritional supplement purported to provide antiinflammatory and wound-healing benefits. Allison hypothesizes that the group treated with standard periodontal therapy plus the nutritional supplemental will present with a lower incidence of cardiac risk at the end of her study. Allison's subjects will be followed over the next 5 years. At the end of the study she plans to compare prestudy laboratory and physical analysis with poststudy laboratory and physical analysis to provide information determining whether an increase or decrease in cardiac risk factors occurred in the experimental group. Allison feels she will be able to then generalize her results to other clients in different practice settings who are treated with a similar protocol.

1. The experimental group in this study is which of the following?
   a. All the subjects Allison enrolls
   b. The subjects receiving standard care
   c. The subject receiving standard care plus the nutritional supplement
   d. All the subjects Allison attempts to recruit for her study
2. The independent variable in this study is which of the following?
   a. The standard periodontal therapy provided to each subject
   b. The nutritional supplement
   c. The cardiac status of subjects at the end of the study
   d. The laboratory tests
3. The data that Allison is collecting to perform her analysis include laboratory parameters (hematology and chemistry). An example of one test result would be a cholesterol level valued at 350. The type of data collected and the scale of measurement most applicable to these data would be which of the following?
   a. Continuous and interval
   b. Discrete and nominal
   c. Continuous and ratio
   d. Discrete and ordinal
4. For her data analysis and presentation of results, Allison considers several types of statistical analyses. Allison intends to follow her original plan of applying the information she has collected to patients outside of her study. Which of the following would be the best choice?
   a. Descriptive statistics
   b. Inferential statistics
   c. Nonparametric statistics
   d. Power statistics
5. To strengthen her argument and reduce the amount of bias introduced in her study, Allison had planned for some additional data analysis involving laboratory values compared to physical parameters such as age and weight of her subjects. On review of a subset of her data, Allison notices that regardless of the group the subjects were randomized to, as the weight of the subjects increases, a known biomarker for heart disease, the triglyceride level, also increases. When Allison plots out this data she becomes aware of a relationship between her subjects' weight and triglyceride levels. The information Allison has collected shows which of the following?

a. A positive correlation between the laboratory value and subject weight
b. A negative correlation between the laboratory value and subject weight
c. A positive correlation between the experimental treatment and heart disease
d. Both a and c

References

1. Polit D, Hungler B. Nursing Research Principles and Methods. 5th ed. Philadelphia: JB Lippincott; 1995.
2. Monsen E. Research: Successful Approaches. Chicago: American Dietetic Association; 1992.
3. Norman G, Streiner D. PDQ Statistics. Philadelphia: BC Decker; 1986. p. 15-18.
4. Cancer Facts and Figures 2004. Cancer Basic Facts: How is cancer staged? Available at www.cancer.org. Accessed November 2004.
5. Zarkowski P. Community oral health planning and practice. In: Darby M, editor. Comprehensive Review of Dental Hygiene. 5th ed. St Louis: Mosby; 2002.
6. Rose L. Overview of biostatistics. In: Gluck GM, Morganstein WM, editors. Jong's Community Dental Health. 5th ed. St Louis: Mosby; 2003.
7. Potter P, Perry A. Research in nursing care. In: Contemporary Nursing: Dimensions and Dynamics. St Louis: Mosby; 1993.
8. Darby M, Walsh M. Dental Hygiene Theory and Practice. 2nd ed. St Louis: Saunders; 2003.
9. Hittleman E, Afes V. Accessing and reading dental public health research: Evidence-based dental practice. In: Gluck GM, Morganstein WM, editors. Jong's Community Dental Health. 5th ed. St Louis: Mosby; 2003.
10. Gustafsson BE, Quensel CE, Swenander LL, et al. The Vipeholm Dental Caries Study: The effect of different levels of carbohydrate on caries activity in 436 individuals observed for five years. Acta Odont Scand 1954; 11:232.

Bibliography

Armstrong RL. Hypothesis formulation. In: Krampitz SD, Pavlovich N, editors. Readings for Nursing Research. St Louis: Mosby; 1981.
Campbell JP, Draft RL, Hulin CL. What to Study: Generating and Developing Research Questions. Beverly Hills, CA: Sage Publications; 1982.
Huff D. How to Lie with Statistics. New York: WW Norton; 1954.
Kleinbaum DG, Kupper LL, Morganstern H. Epidemiological Research. Belmont, CA: Lifetime Learning Publications; 1982.
Kraemer LG. Research and theory development in dental hygiene. In: Darby ML, Walsh MM, editors. Dental Hygiene Theory and Practice. Philadelphia: WB Saunders; 1995.
Norman GR, Streiner DL. PDQ Statistics. Philadelphia: BC Decker; 1986.
Pagano RR. Understanding Statistics in the Behavioral Sciences. 9th ed. Belmont, CA: Wadsworth Publishing; 2008
Polit DF, Hungler BP. Nursing Research: Principles and Methods. 5th ed. Philadelphia: JB Lippincott; 1995.

Additional Resources

American University literature review tutorial
    www.library.american.edu/Help/tutorials/lit_review/index.html
Guidelines for reading/reviewing scientific research papers
    www.unm.edu/~lkravitz/UNM%20Pages/readingreseach.html
Journal of Dental Hygiene online articles
    http://oberon.ingentaconnect.com/vl=949594/cl=25/nw=1/rpsv/cw/www/adha/15530205/
National Dental Hygiene research agenda
    www.adha.org/downloads/Research_agenda%20-ADHA_Final_Report.pdf

Health Promotion and Health Communication

8

Beverly Isman, RDH, MPH, ELS

Objectives

Upon completion of this chapter, the student will be able to:
- Apply various health promotion strategies and theories to situations for promotion of oral health.
- Follow a sequence of steps in the health communication process when developing a health communication project.
- Discuss the distinctions among "generic," "targeted," "personalized," and "tailored" health messages.
- Discuss ways to assess needs of diverse populations before designing health communication strategies.
- Identify strategies for delivering health information to consumer groups by using materials, activities, and evaluation methods that are culturally sensitive and linguistically competent.
- Outline the basic components, advantages, and limitations of poster presentations, oral papers, and roundtable discussions as methods for communicating scientific information to health professionals.
- Identify and take advantage of opportunities for personal growth and development in health promotion and health communications.

Key Terms

Health promotion	Diffusion of Innovations	Focus groups
Theories	Theory	Health literacy
Stages of Change Theory	Organizational Change: Stage	Learning styles
Health Belief Model	Theory	Quantitative evaluation
Social Learning Theory	Health communication	Qualitative evaluation
Community Organization	Health marketing	Poster presentation
Theory	"Framing" health messages	Oral paper
	"Tailoring" messages	Roundtable discussion

Opening Statements

Challenges to Promoting Oral Health
- Despite years of research on prevention of oral diseases, very little is known about how best to promote oral health.[1]
- More community-based participatory research, in which community members are involved at all stages, and more interdisciplinary research, with nondental behavioral scientists, might shed more light on effective strategies.
- More evidence is needed to document that changes in attitudes and beliefs about oral health lead to improved oral health outcomes.

- Improved knowledge levels alone rarely translate into healthy behaviors, so approaches need to be designed around proved behavioral theories.
- Most behavioral change that occurs after oral health education or promotion is short term and not sustained without periodic reinforcement. What does it take to create sustainable changes?
- Today, dental hygienists have unique and unlimited opportunities to become involved in community health activities and research and to contribute to the development of a better understanding and application of effective oral health promotion and communication approaches.

The main goal of this chapter is to help dental hygienists incorporate a thought process for assessing needs, forming evaluation questions, and planning communication strategies before jumping to implement what seems like a "good idea."

HEALTH PROMOTION

The World Health Organization defines *health* as a state of complete physical, mental, and social well-being and not merely the absence of disease or infirmity. Health is a personal resource that permits people to lead productive lives.[2] **Health promotion** is a broad concept that refers to the process of enabling people and communities to increase their control over various determinants of health (see Chapter 3) and therefore to improve their own health. Health promotion introduces the role of behaviors, not just attitudes and knowledge, into the health equation and goes beyond a focus on individual behavior toward a wide range of social and environmental interventions. Health promotion goes beyond health education and links oral health to other health issues. Thus this chapter focuses on the concepts of oral health promotion, strategies to effect behavioral and community changes, and the dental hygienist's role in communicating health messages to other health professionals and the public.

The Ottawa Charter, a global health promotion imperative, identifies three basic health promotion strategies: (1) advocating for health, (2) enabling people to achieve their full health potential, and (3) mediating different societal interests in pursuit of health. The following five action steps can help achieve these strategies:

- Build healthy public policy (e.g., tobacco-free restaurants and bars)
- Create supportive environments for health (e.g., exercise rooms in work places)
- Strengthen community action for health (e.g., support for local farmers markets)
- Develop personal skills (e.g., healthy meal planning and cooking)
- Reorient health services (e.g., provider incentives for keeping people well)[2]

All of these steps have direct relevance to oral health, the health promotion theories enumerated in this chapter, and health care reform efforts in the United States and other countries.

Oral health promotion efforts can increase use of oral health and wellness services and preventive self-care measures. The anticipated outcome of these efforts is a reduced incidence and severity of oral diseases with improved oral health and overall health. Yet, as we see in the challenges in the Opening Statement, applied research relating to oral health promotion is still in its infancy and not yet well integrated or coordinated with research and theories developed by other health disciplines.

Health Promotion Theories

When promoting health and preventing disease, **theories** help us analyze and interpret health problems and then plan and evaluate interventions. What is a theory? A theory is a set of interrelated concepts, definitions, and propositions that present a systematic view of events or situations by specifying relations among variables to explain and predict the events or situations.[3]

A theory is an abstract notion that comes to life only when it is applied to specific topics and problems. Sometimes, theories are called *conceptual frameworks* or *models*. The best way to remember each theory is to focus on key concepts such as readiness to change, susceptibility to health risks, or how innovations are adopted.

How can theories be applied to dental hygiene practice and public health practice? Every day, dental hygienists face challenging situations that result in oral health problems such as families who feed their babies cariogenic liquids in baby bottles, athletes who sustain oral injuries because they refuse to wear a mouth guard, adults who say they are too busy to follow oral care recommendations, or administrators who eliminate school-based dental sealant programs but retain orthodontic screening programs. Theories can help us analyze these situations and apply solutions that have been effective in similar circumstances.

Traditionally, dental hygienists have viewed oral health problems primarily as the "patient's" problem and have proceeded to "educate" the patient about how to improve oral health. This approach is doomed to failure because it skips directly to a generic intervention and does not assess or validate the patient's point of view or health beliefs and does not consider the environmental, literacy, or cultural circumstances that have influenced the person's attitudes, beliefs, or health practices. It is important to analyze oral health problems from more than one perspective and to understand how each perspective affects the others.

Behavior that leads to improved oral health can be affected at three levels:
- Intrapersonal (within the individual)
- Interpersonal (between people)
- Community (including institutional or organizational change and public policy)

The following section describes selected health promotion theories that relate to these three levels and that have the most relevance to oral health issues. An overview of the six selected theories is provided in **Box 8-1**. A narrative of each theory, including an oral health example, is accompanied by a table that contains key concepts, definitions, and general applications. For easier reading and to select theories that are most relevant to situations you may encounter, there is an overview table of additional theories with their focus and key concepts in Glanz and Rimer, which is available online.[3]

BOX 8-1 Overview of Health Promotion Theories

Intrapersonal Level
- Stages of Change Theory
- Health Belief Model

Interpersonal Level
- Social Learning Theory (Social Cognitive Theory)

Community Level
- Community Organization Theory
- Diffusion of Innovations Theory
- Organizational Change: Stage Theory

Intrapersonal Level

Stages of Change Theory (Transtheoretical Model)

Initially developed by Prochaska and DiClemente, the **Stages of Change Theory** views change as a process or cycle that occurs over time rather than as a single event. This theory allows the dental hygienist to assess a person's readiness to change a behavior toward a more healthful lifestyle such as daily brushing to prevent gingivitis. The theory assumes that at any point in time everyone is at a different stage of readiness to make lifestyle changes and that people cycle through the various stages over time, depending on the behavior to be changed and whether the environment is supportive. The major stages of this model with definitions and applications are outlined in **Table 8-1**.

Oral Health Example. The cycle starts by increasing one's awareness of a problem (e.g., a person has gingivitis) to initiating behavior change (brushing effectively and using antimicrobial rinses) and progresses to maintaining motivation to continue preventive actions (returning in 3 months to check progress). To be effective in changing behavior, health messages and programs should be matched to an individual's current stage of readiness to change.

Health Belief Model

Originated by Rosenstock and others in the 1970s to explain people's use of preventive health services, the **Health Belief Model** allows us to assess perceptions of how susceptible one is to a health risk and whether one believes that recommended preventive behaviors will result in less susceptibility.

One application of the Health Belief Model is to develop messages that are likely to persuade people to make decisions to improve their oral health. The components of the model and some applications are shown in **Table 8-2**. The primary hypothesis is that increased perception of severity and susceptibility to a disease results in an increased probability of taking action. Perceived ability to take action and cues to action are important factors.

Table 8-1   Stages of Change Theory (Transtheoretical Model)

Concept	Definition	Application
Precontemplation	Being unaware of problem; not having thought about change.	Increase awareness of need for change; personalize information on risks and benefits.
Contemplation	Thinking about change in the near future.	Motivate and encourage to make specific plans.
Decision/ determination	Making a plan to change.	Assist in developing concrete action plans or setting gradual goals.
Action	Implementing specific action or plans.	Assist with feedback, problem solving, social support, and reinforcement.
Maintenance	Continuing desirable actions or repeating periodic recommended steps.	Assist in coping, using reminders, finding alternatives, avoiding slips or relapses.

Adapted from Glanz K, Rimer BK. Theory at a Glance: A Guide for Health Promotion Practice. Bethesda, MD: National Institutes of Health; 2005.

Table 8-2   **Health Belief Model**

Concept	Definition	Application
Perceived susceptibility	One's opinion of chances of getting a condition	Define population at risk and risk levels; personalize risk based on a person's features or behavior; heighten perceived susceptibility if too low.
Perceived severity	One's opinion of how serious a condition and its sequelae are	Specify consequences of the risk and the condition.
Perceived benefits	One's opinion of the efficacy of the advised action to reduce risk or seriousness of impact	Define action to take: How, where, when; clarify the positive effects to be expected.
Perceived barriers	One's opinion of the tangible and psychologic costs of the advised action	Identify and reduce barriers through reassurance, incentives, and assistance.
Cues to action	Strategies to activate readiness	Provide how-to information; promote awareness, send reminders.
Self-efficacy	Confidence in one's ability to take action	Provide training and guidance in performing action.

Adapted from Glanz K, Rimer BK. Theory at a Glance: A Guide for Health Promotion Practice. Bethesda, MD: National Institutes of Health; 2005.

Oral Health Example. Does your father think that he is at risk for development of oral cancer because he smokes a pipe? Does he believe that limiting use of the pipe would reduce his oral cancer risk? The model also looks at perceived severity of a disease threat, benefits of taking a particular health action, and barriers to completing the action. Does your father believe that the effects of quitting pipe smoking are worse than the effects of oral cancer? Does your father believe he can quit smoking his pipe? What types of support does he need to succeed?

Interpersonal Level

Social Learning Theory

The **Social Learning Theory** posits that people learn primarily in the following four ways:
1. Direct experience
2. Vicarious experience such as reading or viewing or listening to various forms of mass media
3. Judgments voiced by others such as testimony or promotions by experts
4. Inferred knowledge

The basic premise of this theory, developed by Bandera and sometimes known as the *Social Cognitive Theory*, is that people learn through their own experiences, by observing the actions of others, and by the results of these actions. Behavioral change is accomplished through the interaction of personal factors, environmental influences, and individual behaviors. Self-efficacy and self-confidence are important concepts. **Table 8-3** lists the relevant definitions and applications of the major concepts.

Oral Health Example. Consider helping a single mother to feel confident about performing toothbrushing for her young child by using techniques such as demonstration, watching a video, providing ongoing encouragement, and giving periodic feedback. When the mother gains some

Table 8-3   Social Learning Theory (Social Cognitive Theory)

Concept	Definition	Application
Reciprocal determinism	Behavioral changes result from interaction between the person and the environment; change is bidirectional	Involve the individual and relevant others; work to change the environment, if warranted.
Behavioral capability	Knowledge and skills to influence behavior	Provide information and training about action.
Expectations	Beliefs about likely results of action	Incorporate information about likely results of action in advance.
Self-efficacy	Confidence in ability to take action and to persist in action	Point out strengths; use persuasion and encouragement; approach behavioral change in small steps.
Observational learning	Beliefs based on observing others like oneself and/or visible physical results	Point out others' experience and physical changes; identify role models to emulate.
Reinforcement	Responses to a person's behavior that increase or decrease the chances of recurrence	Provide incentives, rewards, praise; encourage self-reward; decrease possibility of negative responses that deter positive changes.

Adapted from Glanz K, Rimer BK. Theory at a Glance: A Guide for Health Promotion Practice. Bethesda, MD: National Institutes of Health; 2005.

confidence in her skills, she can then assist the child care workers and other parents at the day care center in learning these skills so that they can support each other and so that oral hygiene care becomes a daily activity for all of the children.

Community Level

Community Organization Theory

Community Organization Theory is the process of involving and activating members of a community or subgroup to identify a common problem or goal, to mobilize resources, to implement strategies, and to evaluate their efforts. People usually refer to this process as empowerment. This is a grassroots approach to health promotion, rather than an effort that is initiated and conducted by health professionals. **Table 8-4** outlines the key components.

Oral Health Example. Consider the role of a church pastor and a congregation in oral health promotion. Church members notice that many of the elders have stopped coming to church suppers because they have lost their teeth and are embarrassed to eat in public. The pastor calls the dental school for help, and the congregation raises money to help defray the cost of examinations and dentures for the elders. Dental and dental hygiene student teams work together to assess each elder's needs and to fabricate and fit the dentures. They also discuss oral health, denture care, and the challenges of eating with dentures. Gradually, the elders become comfortable eating and speaking with the dentures, and they resume their attendance at church suppers. The following year, the church leaders continue to work with the student teams to promote oral health to people of all ages within their parish.

Table 8-4 **Community Organization Theory**

Concept	Definition	Application
Empowerment	Process of gaining mastery and power over oneself or one's community to produce change	Give individuals and communities tools and responsibility for making decisions that affect them.
Community competence	Community's ability to engage in effective problem solving	Work with community to identify problems, create consensus, and reach goals.
Participation relevance	Learner should be active participant and work starting "where the people are"	Help community set goals within the context of preexisting goals, and encourage active participation.
Issue selection	Identifying winnable, simple, and specific concerns as focus of action	Assist community members in examining how they can communicate the concerns and whether success is likely.
Critical consciousness	Developing understanding of root causes of problems	Guide consideration of health concerns in broad perspective of social problems.

Adapted from Glanz K, Rimer BK. Theory at a Glance: A Guide for Health Promotion Practice. Bethesda, MD: National Institutes of Health; 2005.

Table 8-5 **Diffusion of Innovations Theory**

Concept	Definition	Application
Relative advantage	The degree to which an innovation is seen as better than the idea, practice, program, or product it replaces	Point out unique benefits such as monetary value, convenience, time saving, prestige, etc.
Compatibility	How consistent the innovation is with values, habits, experience, and needs of potential adopters	Tailor innovation to the intended audience's values, norms, or situation.
Complexity	How difficult the innovation is to understand or use	Create a program, idea, or product to be easy to use and understand.
Trialability	Extent to which one can experiment with the innovation before a commitment to adopt is required	Provide opportunities to try on a limited basis (e.g., free samples, introductory sessions, money-back guarantee).
Observability	Extent to which the innovation provides tangible or visible results	Ensure visibility of results through feedback or publicity.

Adapted from Glanz K, Rimer BK. Theory at a Glance: A Guide for Health Promotion Practice. Bethesda, MD: National Institutes of Health; 2005.

Diffusion of Innovations Theory

Developed by Rogers, the **Diffusion of Innovations Theory** helps us assess how new ideas, products, or services spread within a society or to other groups (i.e., how innovations are adopted). During the assessment, attention is directed to the characteristics of the innovation, the communication channels, and the social systems. **Table 8-5** displays the components.

Oral Health Example. Researchers found that despite numerous clinical trials showing their effectiveness in caries prevention, adoption of dental sealants by practitioners proceeded slowly.

Adoption occurred much sooner in public health clinics, where there was a critical need for effective caries-preventive measures and strong advocacy for the procedure, than in private dental offices, where patients had low caries rates, some insurance companies did not reimburse for the service, and practitioners were wedded to the use of amalgams for managing rather than preventing dental caries. Over time, caries rates in occlusal surfaces declined dramatically in children who received regular care and sealants at the clinics, whereas caries rates remained stable in the children visiting private or public dental practices that did not apply sealants. Major educational efforts, policy changes regarding reimbursement, and advocacy efforts were used to eventually change attitudes and patterns of practice in the private sector, thus resulting in reduced rates of dental caries in all children in the community who received sealants.

Organizational Change: Stage Theory

Organizations pass through a series of four stages as they initiate change (**Table 8-6**). For the **Organizational Change: Stage Theory** to be complete all stages must be implemented including new policies being integrated within the organization.

In addition, organizational structures and processes influence workers' behavior and motivation for change.

Oral Health Example. Consider a situation in which health educators asked the cafeteria staff in a hospital to offer healthier foods. A number of stages were involved in instituting the change (e.g., pricing different food items, buying from local farmers, reviewing sample menus, or announcing the new food items). Eventually, a larger percentage of employees began to select the new food options, thus eating healthier lunches. Soon they asked for a larger selection of these foods. The health educator and the cafeteria staff then worked together to host a weekly onsite farmers market and to distribute health-promoting recipes so that employees also were encouraged to prepare healthy meals at home. This process not only resulted in institutional change but also created healthier lifestyles in the employees' families.

Table 8-6   Organizational Change: Stage Theory

Concept	Definition	Application
Definition of problem	Problems recognized and analyzed; solutions sought and evaluated	Involve management and other personnel in awareness-raising activities.
Initiation of action	Policy or directive formulated; resources for beginning change allocated	Provide process consultation to inform decision makers and implementers of what adoption involves.
Implementation of change	Innovation is implemented; reactions and role changes occur	Provide training, technical assistance, and aid in problem solving.
Institutionalization of change	Policy or program becomes entrenched in the organization; new goals and values internalized	Identify high-level champion, work to overcome obstacles to institutionalization, and create structures for integration.

Adapted from Glanz K, Rimer BK. Theory at a Glance: A Guide for Health Promotion Practice. Bethesda, MD: National Institutes of Health; 2005.

EXPANDING DENTAL HYGIENE KNOWLEDGE AND STRATEGIES

To use these theories effectively, dental hygienists need to acquire new knowledge and approaches for assessing and changing health behaviors and systems of care. In addition, dental hygienists need to keep abreast of innovative programs occurring in other professions and ways that other health care systems and countries address health problems. The Guiding Principles include examples of knowledge and approaches needed to assess and change behaviors and systems.

GUIDING PRINCIPLES

Knowledge and Strategies Needed to Assess and Change Behaviors and Systems[4]
- Knowledge of factors that are considered a risk for development of oral diseases and those factors that can be modified through preventive efforts at the primary, secondary, and tertiary levels
- How to assess a person's risk for development of oral diseases and other health problems
- The level of scientific evidence for and the extent of certainty of the effectiveness of various preventive measures
- Which categories of interventions yield the desired impact (e.g., personal behaviors, programs, societal and environmental modifications, policies)
- Effective oral, written, and electronic communication skills
- Appropriate and effective communication methods and channels
- Ways in which innovations are diffused and ways of bringing about organizational change
- Ways to motivate people to access services and return for continuing care
- The structure of various health care systems and community-based organizations
- How to deliver effective services and education
- How to evaluate efforts (e.g., effectiveness, costs, access, quality, outcomes) using both qualitative and quantitative methods

Some of the information may be learned during the dental hygiene educational process, with additional strategies acquired through experience, research, and professional development. Resources for professional development are discussed later in the chapter. The next section examines how to design health messages, specifically, how to frame and tailor them.

HEALTH COMMUNICATION AND HEALTH MARKETING AS NEW FIELDS

Health communication emerged as a separate Focus Area in the national *Healthy People 2010* Objectives and will have increased focus in the new *Healthy People 2020* Objectives. Health communication encompasses the "study and use of communication strategies to inform and influence individual and community decisions that enhance health."[5] **Figure 8-1** demonstrates important stages of the health communication process.[6] One of the challenges in designing health communication programs is to identify the most effective channels, context, and content that will capture people's attention and then motivate them to use health information. Research on strategies to address these challenges is becoming more widespread, sophisticated, and cross-cutting, with results that are applicable to oral health.

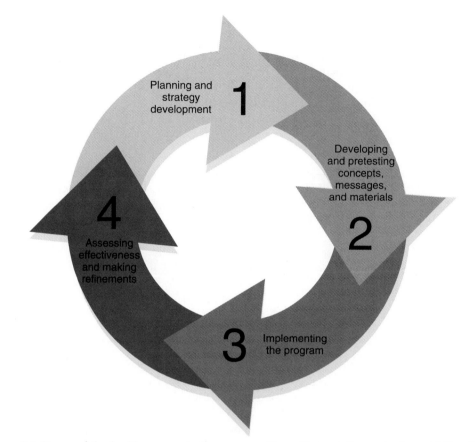

Figure 8-1 Stages of the health communication process. (From National Cancer Institute. Making Health Communication Programs Work. Bethesda, MD: National Cancer Institute; 2002.)

The multidisciplinary field of **health marketing** grew out of the need to advance the science of health communication. Health marketing involves creating, communicating, and delivering health information and interventions using customer-centered and science-based strategies to protect and promote the health of diverse populations.[7] Within the past decade, health communication and health marketing research have increased exponentially. Dental hygienists might take advantage of opportunities for graduate study, national credentialing through the National Commission for Health Education Credentialing, or continuing education in these fields to help advance the science of oral health promotion.

FRAMING HEALTH MESSAGES

New forms of technology are changing our options for framing, delivering, and evaluating health messages for the public. The concept of **"framing" health messages** relates to the cues (e.g., sounds, symbols, words, pictures) that signal how and what to think about an issue. In the process of framing messages, an attempt is made to connect to people's values, beliefs, knowledge levels, and emotions. **"Tailoring" messages** relates to the specific cues used to make messages meaningful for a specific individual.

A fundamental error in many oral health education efforts is the assumption that increased knowledge will result in meaningful changes in behavior. Traditionally, oral health messages have been packaged as "generic" messages that cover a number of concepts and try to appeal to the greatest number of people. A typical brochure would cover brushing and flossing and the use of fluorides, sealants, antimicrobials, and other preventive measures. It might also describe various diagnostic procedures such as radiographs, periodontal probing, and microbial tests. This type of brochure is based on the assumption that dental hygienists should provide as much information as possible and that people will sort through the information to select the pieces that apply to them. Numerous research studies have shown that this assumption is not valid; overwhelming people with information is not effective for changing behaviors, particularly when people are busy, they are low-level readers, or when only some of the information is immediately relevant.

With the use of a more focused approach, health professionals have begun using "targeted" materials intended to reach a specific subgroup or population, usually based on demographic characteristics (e.g., older adults, African Americans). The assumption that underlies this approach is that a large number of people still can be reached and that homogeneity exists in the group to justify the messages and formats used. Subgroups, however, often represent very heterogeneous groups, thus reducing the effectiveness of this approach in some situations.

Another approach is to "personalize" messages. One way to personalize information (e.g., in a brochure) is to highlight only the information and key messages that apply to the person who receives it. Mobile technologies and social media, such as Facebook or Twitter, create unique opportunities for delivering personal messages. For example, individuals receive messages that allow them to find where H1N1 vaccinations are being given by entering their zip code. The Internet promotes individualization by allowing people to search for and discuss information that applies to their particular situation or answers their specific questions. With such a proliferation of information, however, it is often difficult for consumers to determine its validity, especially if there are conflicting viewpoints or statistics. The *Healthy People 2020* Objectives particularly emphasize increasing individuals' access to the Internet, especially to quality health-related Web sites.[8]

The most effective way to reach individuals to increase their knowledge or to change behavior is to "tailor" messages.[9] These messages or strategies are intended to reach a specific person on the basis of characteristics unique to that person that were discovered through an assessment process. This is the basis of many computerized risk assessment/risk reduction programs in health care (e.g., heart disease, diabetes). The technique can be applied to formation of an individualized oral health plan based on risk assessment and primary prevention measures. The assumption is that tailored messages provide a more meaningful and motivating strategy built on a person's specific input. The use of personal trainers for health improvement through exercise is an example of this strategy. Professionals sometimes try to tailor messages without going through the essential assessment process, only to find that their messages are ineffective, or they do not adjust the messages based on an individual's gains or lapses.

SELECTING AND EVALUATING COMMUNICATION FORMATS FOR DIFFERENT AUDIENCES

Consumer-Oriented Communication

Before providing health information to an individual or group, an assessment and planning process is crucial. Depending on the audience and topic, a needs assessment can be accomplished through a literature review, informal observations or conversations, surveys, in-depth interviews, **focus**

groups, or situation analyses. A needs assessment reveals important cultural beliefs, health practices, **health literacy,** and knowledge levels that can result in misconceptions, barriers to care, or stumbling blocks to behavioral change. The Surgeon General's "A National Call to Action to Promote Oral Health" emphasizes the need to develop messages that are culturally sensitive and linguistically competent.[10] This means that language and graphics should be inclusive, not promote stereotypes, and be easy to understand for any reader or listener. Special considerations are needed when designing or translating materials for non-English speakers.[11] **Box 8-2** lists some problems associated with translating materials and suggestions for preventing or overcoming these problems. These should be considered during any needs assessment and when field testing materials.

A variety of resources are available for dental hygienists to use when selecting communication formats and designing and evaluating health messages. Examples of formats for presenting information are included in **Box 8-3**. References and resources listed in this chapter describe the benefits and limitations of these various formats.[6,9,11,12] Some of the formats can be combined to allow for differences in **learning styles** of the audience. Assessing learning styles of individuals is much easier than planning messages to reach a diverse group of people. As a guide, people usually remember:

- 10% of what they read
- 20% of what they hear
- 30% of what they see

BOX 8-2 Translation Barriers and Suggestions for Overcoming Them

Problems with Translating Materials
- Medical and dental terms may not be understood or may have different meanings, or may not be directly translatable in another language. Even within languages such as Spanish, people from different nations or regions may use different words for a term such as *x-ray* or *baby teeth*.
- Literally translating word for word often is confusing because there may be no direct translation or a variety of phrases may be used, depending on the person's age, gender, social standing, or other characteristics. Literal translations without considering local language patterns and word usage may be annoying to the intended audience, causing them to ignore the information or reducing its credibility.
- Some people may speak a language that does not have a written equivalent, or they may speak one language but not be able to read the language.

Suggestions for Overcoming Translation Barriers
- Use materials originally developed in that language or have new materials developed in the target languages rather than translating them from English.
- Field test the materials with a variety of members from the intended audience. Some researchers recommend two-way translation—one person translates the text from English to the other language and a second person translates it back to identify any inconsistencies or mistranslations. It is best to use translators who are both bilingual and bicultural.
- Use only trained translators who are familiar with low literacy readers, as well as more sophisticated ones.
Some educational materials are produced in a dual language format so that both English and the other language are included. This can be useful for both print and video productions.

BOX 8-3 Formats for Presenting Oral Health Information to the Public

Visual Displays
Posters, bulletin boards, fotonovelas, models, information kiosks

Written Media
Newsletters, newspaper articles, fact sheets, booklets, storybooks, blogs

Audiovisual Materials
CD and DVDs, public service announcements, websites, TV, streaming video

Interactive Formats
Songs, role playing, storytelling, gaming, theater or puppet shows, demonstrations, interactive computer programs, science experiments or science fairs, debates, simulations, text messages, widgets, social media

- 70% of what they see and hear
- 90% of what they see, hear, and do

Hands-on, interactive, multimedia formats are usually more effective for retaining knowledge than simply reading or listening to a message. This is true whether one is presenting information to the general public or to other health professionals.

The use of focus groups is one effective method for an intermediate level of assessment Focus groups are particularly useful for determining whether messages are at the appropriate language and literacy levels and whether they are culturally acceptable to the people in the group. Information about the appearance and appeal of materials can also be gathered.[6] Group interviews are conducted with 5 to 10 members of the intended target audience and last approximately 30 to 60 minutes. A moderator uses structured questions to guide the discussion. When developing or testing health messages or materials, the moderator can use one or more versions of the materials to ask questions. For example, in field testing a public service announcement (PSA) about dental sealants, you might ask the following:

- What is one message you remember from the PSA?
- Were there any messages that were confusing?
- Did you relate to the people in the video? How were they like you? Different from you?
- Was the PSA too short, just right, or too long?
- Should the PSA list more resources for those who want more information on dental sealants?
- Would this PSA motivate you to ask about dental sealants for your child's teeth?

The participants' responses are summarized and analyzed to help make decisions on final content and format before release to the public.

On the basis of the findings from a needs assessment (baseline information), the objectives, and the methods selected for health promotion activities, an evaluation plan should be designed that includes evaluation methods, measures and anticipated outcomes before any interventions are started. Evaluation measures should be linked directly to health promotion objectives, and both short-term and long-term outcomes should be considered, if possible (see Guiding Principles).

GUIDING PRINCIPLES

Questions to Determine the Effectiveness of Interventions
- Has the intervention achieved the desired results? If not, why not?
- Should this intervention be continued in its current form?
- What messages or activities produce the best results?
- How can the intervention be improved?
- Can it be replicated successfully in other settings?
- Are the resources (e.g., people, money, materials) that were used reasonable and cost-effective?

Evaluation can occur both during (formative evaluation) and after interventions (summative evaluation). Measures can be **quantitative** (e.g., how many people increased their knowledge of the causes of early childhood caries) or **qualitative** (e.g., why did people participate in the activity and how do they intend to change their parenting behaviors?). Evaluation plans do not always have to be complicated and do not always have to use sophisticated statistical analysis. The key is to try to evaluate your efforts and document the outcomes. Examples of simple evaluation strategies include the following:

1. Ask five questions to assess parents' knowledge and attitudes about sealants before and after a school-based sealant program.
2. Provide healthy snack recipes to a day care center; follow up after 2 months to determine which snacks have been made for the children and which snacks the children seem to like the best.
3. Survey school soccer coaches before and after initiating an oral injury or mouth guard campaign to determine use of mouth guards during practices and games, changes in policies on athletic equipment, and barriers that have been (or have not been) overcome in the attempt to implement the campaign.
4. Survey members of a community to identify how many heard the radio PSA about oral cancer prevention, what the key messages were, and whether they followed any of the recommendations.
5. Use a consumer satisfaction questionnaire in a clinic to determine whether the patients are receiving all of the health information they want and need in formats that answer their questions or concerns in a clear and culturally appropriate manner.

Presentations to Health Professionals

The purpose of professional presentations is to deliver thought-provoking information to a group of health professionals in a short period of time in a clear, concise, and visually appealing format. The same principles and processes that apply to communicating with the general public also apply to communicating with other health professionals. Although direct needs assessment of the audience may not be possible before the presentation, acquire some background information from the organizers. Presentations generally focus on new research, programs, theories and ideas, clinical techniques, products or materials, career opportunities, educational techniques, policies or legislation, health care systems, or methods for disease prevention or detection. The information covers a specific topic with key messages highlighted and sources documented. Presentations can be made to small groups, to large groups at conferences, via webinars, podcasts or other online learning formats.

Specific guidelines for presentations may vary by the sponsoring organization. Various online resources and organizational handouts provide tips.[13,14] When selecting a topic and format for a presentation, consider the following five questions (see Guiding Principles):

GUIDING PRINCIPLES

Five Questions for Selecting a Topic and Format
- Who will be the audience? How large a group do I want to address?
- What is their level of knowledge or interest in my topic?
- What questions might they ask? Will I be able to learn new information related to my topic from some members of the audience?
- How much time will I need to cover my key points?
- What audiovisual materials will most enhance my key points?

Most presentations follow a sequence, such as the following:
1. Introduction and background
2. Methods and materials
3. Findings/results or key points
4. Discussion and significance
5. Summary and conclusions

Three common types of presentations at dental or public health meetings are now compared.

Presentation for a Poster Display

Note: The **poster presentation** display format (**Figure 8-2**) is becoming popular because of the number of presentations that can be accommodated in a specified time frame and no audiovisual equipment is needed. A variety of examples are included in an online tutorial on Advice on Designing Scientific Posters.[13]

Time: Session lasting 1 to 2 hours; discussion time varies by number and type of questions asked

Format: Presenter discusses visual display with people who stop to look; posters lined up next to each other; poster usually attached by pushpins to a board or other backing material

Size of Audience: Varies greatly; some people "cruise by" quickly, some just pick up handouts, others stop to read display and discuss topic

Appropriate audiovisuals: Text, data, artwork, or photographs on paper or poster backing or printed as one large banner; audio or video applications not allowed; handouts encouraged

Benefits and limitations: Opportunity to discuss topic, share ideas, and acquire additional ideas; unpredictable attendance (sometimes crowded and noisy but at other times nobody comes by); not appropriate for topics that require videos or other types of media

Tips: Use color to attract attention and highlight key points; use large, readable print and catchy title; use outline form; intersperse categories of information with charts, graphics, and photos; consider this format for easy setup and transport; include copy of abstract, which is also printed in the program

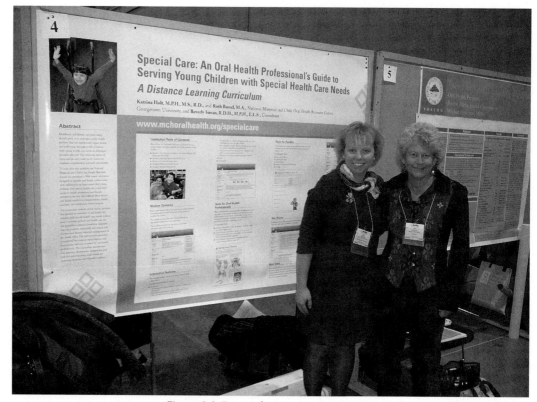

Figure 8-2 Format for poster presentation.

Presentation for an Oral Paper

Note: The **oral paper** format usually is part of a session with a theme or a panel. Advice for creating this format is included in an online tutorial on Preparing Oral Presentations.[14]

Time: 10 to 15 minutes, including time for questions

Format: Oral presentation of information (using notes), accompanied by audiovisuals

Size of Audience: Usually more than 30 people but suitable for hundreds of people, especially if part of a satellite session broadcast to many sites.

Appropriate audiovisuals: PowerPoint slides, short videos, other computerized applications; Internet connectivity may be available, especially if free wireless

Benefits and limitations: Large group can be reached; presenter can speak from printed notes or directly from slide notes on computer; room lighting sometimes fairly dark; interaction with audience often limited; vast array of knowledge in audience

Tips: Try to maintain some eye contact and do not read the paper; use uncomplicated and effective audiovisual materials that highlight important information rather than detract from or repeat information you give orally; practice delivery, timing, and use of audiovisuals before the presentation; decide what information to delete if you are running over time allowance; include transitions between sentences and sections; upload your presentation per the sponsor's directions and check computer controls and room environment before your session

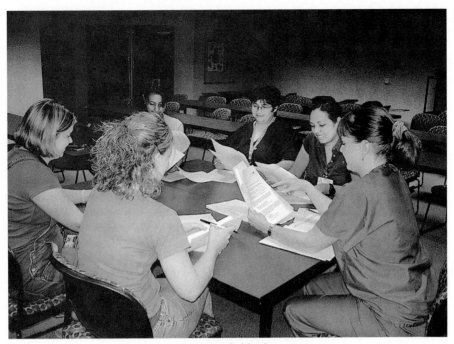

Figure 8-3 Roundtable discussion.

Presentation for a Roundtable Discussion

Note: The **roundtable discussion** format (**Figure 8-3**) is gaining in popularity for a more informal presentation.

Time: 30 to 60 minutes, presentation sometimes repeated to a new group

Format: Oral presentation and discussion supplemented by audiovisuals to people seated at a table or in a circle.

Size of Audience: Usually 8 to 10 people

Appropriate audiovisuals: Handouts, materials, or products; can use laptops with video application; usually Internet connectivity is too expensive unless free wireless is available

Benefits and limitations: Format allows interactive discussion; participants can introduce themselves and share information with whole table; good for controversial topics or new ideas and programs; limited number of people hear the topic

Tips: Speak from notes, handouts, or laptop; facilitation skills and ability to refocus group are needed if discussion is off-track or is monopolized by an individual

The effectiveness of professional presentations can be assessed through the use of course and conference evaluation forms completed by attendees or by asking the audience directly for some immediate feedback. Evaluation measures usually address the presenter's organization of information, effective use of audiovisuals, accuracy and relevancy of content, relation of theory to practice, knowledge of subject area, introduction of new information and ideas, and presentation style.

RESOURCES FOR PROFESSIONAL DEVELOPMENT

What avenues are available to dental hygiene students and practitioners to develop skills in health promotion and health communication? Chapter 7 outlines the importance of continual review of the scientific literature to keep abreast of new research and trends in dental hygiene and public health research and practice. Because public health covers such a broad array of topics, hygienists would benefit by reading literature from other subject areas such as health education/health promotion, health communications, injury prevention, cancer prevention and early detection, maternal and child health, geriatrics, and school health, to name a few. The many Internet sites devoted to health topics facilitate quick perusal of information on any topic. Self-study continuing education courses on a variety of topics are now more available online and via CD-ROM/DVD. **Box 8-4** includes useful resources on health promotion, health communication, health literacy, and health marketing.

Another avenue for updating knowledge, practicing presentation skills, or networking with other professionals is attending professional association meetings. Many of these organizations promote student involvement through reduced membership rates and special contests and awards. Broaden your dental hygiene horizons by attending general public health or health communication meetings or those of the Society for Public Health Education or the American Association for Health Education. In addition, the Centers for Disease Control and Prevention (CDC) and

BOX 8-4 Resources for Health Promotion and Health Communication

- CDC and ATSDR: *Simply put, testing for readability,* ed 2, 1999. Available at www.cdc.gov/healthmarketing/pdf/simply_put_082010.pdf
- Center for Health Promotion, University of Texas: *The six steps to planning a health promotion program.* Available at www.thcu.ca/infoandresources/publications/planaagtablev0.3.pdf
- Center for Health Promotion, University of Texas: *The twelve steps to developing a health communication strategy.* Available at www.thcu.ca/infoandresources/publications/actionsummariesv3.3.jan.05.pdf
- Center for Health Promotion, University of Toronto: *The eight steps to developing a health promotion policy.* Available at www.thcu.ca/infoandresources/publications/policyaagtablev0.3.pdf
- Center for Health Promotion, University of Toronto: *The ten steps to evaluating a health promotion program.* Available at www.thcu.ca/infoandresources/publications/evalaagtablev0.4.pdf
- Centers for Disease Control and Prevention, National Center for Health Marketing. Available at www.cdc.gov/healthmarketing
- Glanz K, Rimer BK: *Theory at a glance: A guide for health promotion practice,* ed 2, Bethesda, MD, 2005, National Institutes of Health, National Cancer Institute. Available at www.cancer.gov/PDF/481f5d53-63df-41bc-bfaf-5aa48ee1da4d/TAAG3.pdf
- Harvard School of Public Health: *Chart of health literacy–related health activities, materials and tasks,* Available at www.hsph.harvard.edu/healthliteracy/overview/#chart
- Oral Health America: *Communications guide for state oral health programs,* Media Outreach Materials, 2006. Available at www.oralhealthamerica.org/pdf/MediaTipsFinal2006.pdf
- The Cochrane Collaboration reviews and library. Available at www.cochrane.org/reviews/clibintro.htm

other groups sponsor annual learning institutes on topics such as health literacy, health communication, and evaluation.

SUMMARY

We live in a multicultural, global society in which some people are bombarded with health information, whereas others are isolated from scientific advances, new communication technologies and health information. In an attempt to create a more equitable distribution of resources and information, dental hygienists must broaden their perspectives on how to acquire and provide health information in a credible, appropriate, efficient and effective manner. Ways to accomplish this may include (1) applying well-researched health promotion and communication theories to oral health programs, (2) assessing people's learning styles, preferences, and information needs, (3) tailoring information in a culturally and linguistically appropriate manner based on needs assessment data, and (4) evaluating the impact of the activities.

Opportunities for using new communication modalities in a variety of settings outside the traditional clinical private practice setting are endless. Online courses and professional associations can be valuable resources for preparing dental hygienists to meet today's health promotion and health communication challenges.

Applying Your Knowledge

1. Create a game based on various health promotion theories. You can use the format of well-known games (e.g., Trivial Pursuit, Jeopardy) or a simple matching or fill-in-the-blank format. Students can also work in groups to design role-playing scenarios based on the types of behaviors described in the theories.
2. Choose a topic and audience for designing an oral health fact sheet. Describe how you would vary the design and frame the messages according to the following types of communication: (a) generic, (b) targeted, (c) personalized, and (d) tailored.
3. Choose an oral health topic for designing a health promotion activity for consumers (non-health professionals). Each student should select a different audience (e.g., age group, ethnicity) for the materials. The assignment is to (a) describe how you would conduct a needs assessment, (b) select an appropriate educational format, and (c) evaluate the impact of your approach.
4. Choose a topic for a 10-minute presentation. Describe how you would present this topic as (a) a scientific poster, (b) an oral paper, and (c) a roundtable discussion.
5. Brainstorm ideas for service-learning opportunities, and assume that appropriate resources are available. After the session, check off which ones already are offered to students. Now choose one or two of those not offered and discuss which issues should be considered and which resources would be needed to offer these options. (This activity could lead to a class-initiated project to develop and implement a new service-learning opportunity.)
6. Acquire information, copies of journals and newsletters, calls for abstracts/presentation proposals and agendas of annual meetings from various professional associations. Include at least one dental related group, one public health group and one health promotion or communication group. Compare the organizations for similarities and differences, including the potential for student presentations.
7. Select three online or print journals that focus on health promotion or health communications research or programs. Compare the journals in terms of target audience, array of topics, and frequency of publication. Discuss which publications you think will be most useful to you in your career.

8. You are asked by a local community clinic for your opinion on how to reach their adult African-American clients with preventive messages about oral cancer. Provide at least two suggestions for key communication strategies and messages, noting the rationales for your selections.

Dental Hygiene Competencies

Reading the material within this chapter and participating in the activities of Applying Your Knowledge will contribute to the student's ability to demonstrate the following competencies:

Core competencies
C.5 Continuously perform self-assessment for lifelong learning and professional growth.
C.8 Communicate effectively with individuals and groups from diverse populations both verbally and in writing.

Community involvement
CM.4 Facilitate client access to oral health services by influencing individuals and/or organizations for the provision of oral health care.

Health promotion
HP.4 Identify individual and population risk factors, and develop strategies that promote health and quality of life.

Community Case

You are a dental hygienist who has been working in clinical private practice for 3 years and now wants to work part-time in a public health setting. The local health department has hired you to work on a project to help mothers of children aged 0 to 5 years learn about: (1) the relationship between consumption of sugar, including sweetened beverages, and dental caries, (2) how to determine the amount and type of sugar from food labels, (3) how to select food low in refined sugars, and (4) how to use these foods to create healthy snacks for young children.

Your target population is approximately 2000 low-income women whose children are eligible for Medicaid benefits and services from the Women, Infant, and Children (WIC) program, and whose children attend Early Head Start or Head Start programs. According to the most recent health department data, 50% of the women are Caucasian, 25% Hispanic, 10% African American, 10% Asian, and 5% other ethnic background.

1. Your first task is to review the various health promotion theories and determine which one(s) might be useful for this project. You decide that you need to assess whether the women in the target population perceive that their children are given food high in sugars and whether that makes them at risk for dental caries. Which one of the following theories might be best to use for this?
   a. Social Learning Theory
   b. Stages of Change Theory
   c. Health Belief Model
   d. Organizational Change Theory
2. Your next task is to select and frame the health messages you want to include in your health communication approaches. Which one of the following approaches is an example of "tailoring" messages?
   a. Separate brochures for each ethnic group
   b. Learning modules that focus on the women's roles as mothers
   c. Short learning modules geared to what level of risk for dental decay they perceive their child to be in during the assessment process
   d. Short booklet that leaves a blank place to write the child's name

3. Research shows that people learn in different ways. Which one of the following statements generally is NOT true?
   a. Asking people to demonstrate a skill helps reinforce written instructions.
   b. People usually remember more of what they read than what they see or hear.
   c. Being asked to repeat instructions in their own words helps people remember information.
   d. Hands-on, interactive, multimedia approaches are most effective for retaining knowledge.
4. You decide that the project materials need to be available in at least English and Spanish. Which of the following approaches is LEAST likely to result in effective and culturally relevant materials?
   a. Use translators who are bilingual and bicultural.
   b. Test the materials in three focus groups: one for English only readers, one for Spanish only readers, and one for women who read some things in both languages.
   c. Do a literal translation from the English version to Spanish.
   d. Create the materials in dual-language format.
5. During the project you have an opportunity to present information on the project at a statewide public health association meeting. You are most interested in discussing and getting feedback on ways to improve the materials and messages. The presentation format that would allow you the best opportunity to accomplish this at a large professional meeting is:
   a. Roundtable discussion
   b. Poster presentation
   c. Oral presentation
   d. Informal networking with individuals.

References

1. Kay E, Locker D. Effectiveness of Oral Health Promotion: A Review. London: Health Education Authority; 1999.
2. Ottawa Charter for Health Promotion. Geneva: World Health Organization; 1986. Available at www.who.int/healthpromotion/en/index.html. Accessed February 2010.
3. Glanz K, Rimer BK. Theory at a Glance: A Guide for Health Promotion Practice. 2nd ed. Bethesda, MD: National Institutes of Health; 2005. Available at www.cancer.gov/PDF/481f5d53-63df-41bc-bfaf-5aa48ee1da4d/TAAG3.pdf. Accessed February 2010.
4. An Inventory of Knowledge and Skills Relating to Disease Prevention and Health Promotion. Washington, DC: Association of Teachers of Preventive Medicine; 1994.
5. US Department of Health and Human Services. Health Communication. In Healthy People 2010 (Chapter 11). 2nd ed. Washington, DC: US Government Printing Office; 2000. Available at www.healthypeople.gov/Document/tableofcontents.htm#Volume2. Accessed February 2010.
6. US Department of Health and Human Services, Public Health Service, National Institutes of Health, National Cancer Institute. Making Health Communication Programs Work. Bethesda, MD: National Cancer Institute; 2002. Available at www.cancer.gov/pinkbook. Accessed February 2010.
7. National Center for Health Marketing Web site. Available at www.cdc.gov/healthmarketing. Accessed February 2010.
8. Healthy People 2020 Health Objectives. Available at www.healthypeople.gov/hp2020. Accessed February 2010.
9. Kreuter M, Farell D, Olevitch, et al. Tailoring Health Messages: Customizing Communication with Computer Technology. London: Lawrence Erlbaum Associates; 2000.
10. US Department of Health and Human Services. A National Call to Action to Promote Oral Health. Rockville, MD: US Department of Health and Human Services, Public Health Service, Centers for Disease Control and Prevention, National Institutes of Health, National Institute of Dental and Craniofacial Research; NIH Publication No 03-5303, 2003. Available at www.surgeongeneral.gov/topics/oralhealth/nationalcalltoaction.html. Accessed October 2010.
11. DeSouza MB, Kressin NR. Dental health education. In: Gluck GM, Morganstein WM, editors. Jong's Community Dental Health. 5th ed. St Louis: Mosby; 2003.
12. Dickinson AO. Community oral health education. In: Mason J, editor. Concepts in Dental Public Health (Chapter 9). 2nd ed. Philadelphia: Lippincott Williams & Wilkins; 2010.

13. Parrington, C. Advice on Designing Scientific Posters. Available at www.swarthmore.edu/NatSci/cpurrin1/posteradvice.htm. Accessed October 2010.

14. Radel J. Preparing an Oral Presentation. Available at www.kumc.edu/SAH/OTEd/jradel/preparing_talks/TalkStrt.html.

Additional Resources

Healthy People 2010. Table of Contents for chapters in Vol 1 and 2
www.healthypeople.gov/Publications/

Sheiham A, Watt RG. The common risk factor approach: A rational basis for promoting oral health. Community Dent Oral Epidemiol 2000;28:399
www.ucl.ac.uk/dph/PDF%20Pubs/40cdoe2000.pdf

World Health Organization. Health Promotion Glossary
www.who.int/hpr/NPH/docs/hp_glossary_en.pdf

World Health Organization. The Bangkok Charter for Health Promotion in a Globalized World, 2005
www.who.int/healthpromotion/conferences/6gchp/bangkok_charter/en/

Social Responsibility

Diane Brunson, RDH, MPH

9

Objectives

Upon completion of this chapter, the student will be able to:

- Define the terms *social responsibility* and *professional ethics.*
- Discuss the various opinions surrounding health as a right or a privilege.
- Explain how the current delivery of oral health care services affects access.
- Identify how the concept of need versus demand affects allocation of resources and the hygienist's role as consumer advocate and educator.
- Explain the roles of the dental hygienist as they relate to community education, risk communication, and leadership.
- Explain the process for formulating oral health policy, informally and formally (legislative process).

Key Terms

Social responsibility	Professional ethics	Health security
Ethics	Access	Health equity

Opening Statement

Status and Future of Health Care

- The health care system in the United States is in crisis.
- The public health system in the United States is fragmented and insufficient.
- Oral health is a component of overall health, and access to health care services should be a right guaranteed to everyone.
- Human rights should be the foundation of public health practice, research, and policy in every country in the world.
- Perceived risks of health care interventions increase when the public receives contradictory opinions from responsible sources.
- Comprehensive oral health benefits for adults are often excluded in health care reform efforts.

SOCIAL RESPONSIBILITY AND PROFESSIONAL ETHICS

Social Responsibility

The following questions are often asked in relation to the responsibilities of the dental hygienist:

- What are the hygienist's responsibilities to the profession of dental hygiene, to the patients in the dental practice, and to society as a whole?

- Do these responsibilities entail taking a leadership role in a professional organization?
- Do they include maintaining competency in clinical skills and currency in dental science so as to provide the best possible care for the patient?
- Do they look beyond the patients of record in a practice to individuals and communities that lack access to needed oral health care?
- Do they embrace the art of communication to assure the public that it has the knowledge to improve its own oral health?

Certainly, the responsibilities of the dental hygienist include all of these and more. **Social responsibility** is a broad term that encompasses professionalism, personal and professional ethics, and the role of a profession in the context of the greater society.[1] It includes the concepts of a person's right to health care, the profession's obligation to raise the "dental IQ" of the community, and ensuring the health and well-being of the public. In this chapter, by necessity, more questions are asked than answered, but the stage is set for critical thinking and further discussion about individual and collective hygienists' roles, values, and beliefs. The dental hygienist is encouraged to share thoughts and to discuss personal answers and ideas with colleagues.

Professional Ethics

A term often equated with social responsibility is **ethics,** commonly defined as the general science of right and wrong conduct.[2] Add to this the concept of moral action, and discussions emerge regarding which moral principles should govern a particular action. So intertwined and abstract is this concept that the terms *ethics* and *morals* are often used interchangeably.[3]

Professional ethics is the code by which the profession regulates actions and sets standards for its members, with the recognition that professionals are accountable for their actions.[4] This code serves as a guide to the profession to ensure a high standard of competency, to strengthen the relationships among its members, and to promote the welfare of the entire community.[5] The Code of Ethics of the American Dental Hygienists' Association (ADHA) provides this guidance for the dental hygiene profession.

By virtue of the education, the written and clinical board examinations, and subsequent state licensure, dental hygiene is a profession, and dental hygienists are professionals and thus are required to make choices in practice that necessitate ethical decision making. Disagreements occasionally arise from different interpretations of the "proper" roles, responsibilities, and level of decision making of professionals involved in patients' oral care.[6] Often, these discussions take precedence over and are counterproductive to the larger issues of serving the needs of the public. Examples include whether dental hygienists should be able to (1) determine which teeth would benefit from sealant placement and (2) practice unsupervised in public health settings.

The Code of Ethics and Standards of Professional Conduct, adopted by the American Association of Public Health Dentistry, provides guidance for dental public health professionals through six basic principles, which may be summarized as follows:

Dental public health professionals have the following responsibilities:

1. Inform individuals and community organizations about health issues and options available for correcting oral health problems and inequities; facilitate health care decisions; ensure individual patient confidentiality; and respect individual and community customs, beliefs, and other cultural variations *(autonomy)*.
2. Provide individual and community services in a socially responsible manner while maintaining respect for the value of the services received and conservation of individual, private, and public resources *(nonmaleficence)*.

3. Provide the best care possible, but with the constraint that care should be equitable, that is, the best possible care that helps the largest number of people for the longest period of time *(beneficence).*
4. Not engage in acts of discrimination; but rather, promote policies that ensure equitable distribution of available resources and ensure that spokespersons for the public are included in the health policy development process *(fairness).*
5. Abide by their written, verbal, direct, and implied agreements; respects copyrights; and does not engage in activity in which there is real, or potential for, appearance of conflict of interest *(truthfulness).*
6. Participate in professional and community meetings; share knowledge and skills with colleagues and public; and recognize an obligation to protect the public *(professionalism).*[7]

Another set of debates arises in the attempt to define the term *public,* for instance:

- Does the word mean only those individuals who seek dental care? Are they the only ones the dental profession has "responsibility" for?
- What is the responsibility of the dental hygienist to the broader group of "public," which includes people without access to oral health care services, culturally diverse populations, and people with special health care needs?
- Do people have a right to receive quality dental health care at a cost they can afford?
- What is a fair, or just, distribution of limited dental health care resources?

It is imperative that these questions be seriously considered because the dental hygiene profession's commitment to ethical conduct is the foundation of society's trust and confidence.[8]

This ethical conduct is not confined to a particular practice setting. "Ethical leadership" is knowing one's core values and having to live them in all aspects of life in serving the common good.[9] This encourages dental hygienists to be involved in their communities.

A SYSTEM IN CRISIS

These questions, to which answers are as diverse as populations themselves, point to the need for a broader look at the general health care system in the United States. Many journals and newspapers report that health care in the nation is in a state of "crisis." Although this statement is resounding in many private and public health circles, it is controversial in the face of the technologic advances in medicine and dentistry that have been responsible for improved health standards not only in the United States but also in many countries of the world. Technology has allowed delivery of advanced surgical and cosmetic dental services to one segment of the population even while significant barriers to accessing even preventive and basic restorative care still exist for others.[10]

It is also apparent that the health care crisis has been recognized, reported, discussed, and debated for more than 50 years, with minimal progress made. The Surgeon General's report on oral health specifically quantifies the disparities in oral health status among underserved populations and the barriers many people face in obtaining care.[11] The health professions, including private- and public-delivery systems, national and state governments, public apathy, and a general lack of social responsibility on the part of society as a whole all have contributed to the failure of each attempt to render health care accessible to everyone. In one form or another, health reforms have been recommended for several decades with little success, and in most cases, oral health care services have not been included.

However, with the passing of health care reform legislation (Patient Protection and Affordable Care Act) in March 2010, significant oral health provisions were included. A few of these provisions are listed in the following:

1. Through the new insurance plans, oral health benefits for children are mandated with no out-of-pocket costs for preventive services.
2. Oral health surveillance is to be improved in all states.
3. Grants to school-based health centers, including oral health services, are available.
4. An evidence-based public education campaign is established to promote oral health, including a focus on early childhood caries, prevention, oral health of pregnant women, and oral health of at-risk populations.
5. Grant funding for school-based sealant programs is increased.
6. An alternative dental provider demonstration project is established.
7. Training, workforce development, and loan repayment provisions are established.[12]

There are increased expectations of the public health system and as work begins to appropriate funding for these provisions, there will undoubtedly be questions as to what constitutes public health and what the minimum standards for delivery of services should be.[13]

HEALTH CARE: A PRIVILEGE OR A RIGHT?

Health Care as a Privilege

The crux of the debate is the question of whether health care, including oral health care, is a "right" or a "privilege."[14] Who is responsible for "health?"

GUIDING PRINCIPLES

Who Has a Right to Health Care?
- Should the person who smokes have access to the same level of health care as the nonsmoker?
- Should children who are not eligible for Medicaid and who are living in poverty have access to after-hours treatment for ear infections and prescriptions for antibiotics?
- Should the senior citizen on a fixed income have equal access to properly fitting dentures?
- Should the immigrant female of childbearing age have access to culturally appropriate examinations and treatment?

Depending on your answers, who is responsible for delivering the health care and who is responsible for paying for it? Many would argue that it should not be only private providers offering reduced fees or donating their services. Additional publicly funded programs with acceptable reimbursement rates and dollars sufficient to serve the needs of the population are also needed. The following questions relate to whose responsibility it is to provide health care services and to pay for them:

- Should taxes be increased to support these programs or incentives implemented to increase provider participation?
- What is the responsibility of the patient seeking care?
- Should access to health care be a privilege of productive members of society who have the ability to pay for that health care?
- Are rights automatic, or are they "earned" as a reward for being socially responsible?

WHAT IS THE ROLE OF GOVERNMENT IN PAYING FOR AND ASSURING SERVICES?

These questions have no clear answers, and they challenge the individual provider's values and sense of social responsibility.

Health Care as a Right

The United States Constitution does not specifically guarantee a "right to health" because "health" is a dynamic, continually changing state, unique to each individual.[15] One interpretation is that health and access to health care are not so much a legal right; rather, they are a "moral" right and as such, the obligation of society as a whole is to provide care in response to that right, with providers playing an important role.[2] "The duty to ensure basic oral health for all Americans is a shared duty that includes federal, state, community, public, and private responsibilities. The dental profession, as the moral community entrusted by society with knowledge and skill about oral health, has the duty to lead the effort to ensure access for all Americans."[16] Society, however, has not universally accepted that responsibility despite several key events that have attempted to highlight the relationship among individual rights, human dignity, and the human condition.[17]

In 1946, the Constitution of the World Health Organization (WHO) defined health as "a state of complete physical, mental, and social well-being" (see Chapter 1). This was reiterated in the Universal Declaration of Human Rights adopted by the United Nations General Assembly on December 10, 1948 (Article 25):

> Everyone has the right to a standard of living adequate for the health and well-being of himself and of his family, including food, clothing, housing and medical care.[18]

An amendment to the Public Health Service Act, passed by Congress in 1966, states that "promoting and assuring the highest level of health attainable for every person serves the nation's best interests."

The fundamental basis of human rights is the recognition of the equal worth and dignity of everyone and implies that individuals, institutions, and society as a whole should protect and promote health and should ensure that health is neither impaired nor at risk. When the health of people has been left solely to the current health services system, many population groups have been left without access to health care and with little or no constituency advocating for their right to that care. Increasingly, this system has not been able to keep pace with the number of uninsured patients, expanding populations, shifts in demographics, degradation of the environment, and changes in lifestyles and value systems. This discussion becomes pertinent in the field of dental public health, which focuses on the prevention of oral diseases and promotes population-based health activities to ensure the oral health of all people.

POLICY DEVELOPMENT

As mentioned in Chapter 1, "policy development" is one of the core functions of public health and is often intertwined with promotion of oral health activities. Policy may be achieved through formal decisions (as in a school district decision), rules (as with a state dental board), or legislation at the national, state, or local level. To be successful, all policy initiatives should involve collaborative efforts between partners and stakeholders, including professionals, community leaders, coalitions, and the public.

Understanding the policy-making process is crucial to serving the needs of the public. Policy is used to connect the results of community "assessment" to "assuring" the oral health needs of the public are addressed. Regardless of the level of policy desired, the order of procedures is nearly identical, as follows:

- Develop personal and professional relationships with policy and decision makers.
- Collaborate with partners to identify data needed.
- Assess and quantify oral health needs and existing resources (see Chapter 3).
- Share data with partners and identify possible strategies and solutions.
- In a *succinct* and *clear manner*, share data and desired solutions with policymakers.
- Be available to policymakers for questions at all stages of the process and to provide information and testimony.
- Thank the policymaker, regardless of the outcome and continue to maintain the relationship for future efforts. Consider supporting other health policy initiatives supported or sponsored by this policymaker that may not have an oral health focus.

Examples of formal decisions include a determination by a school district to participate in a school-based sealant program; a process to assure nursing home residents receive daily oral hygiene care; a decision by a large employer to offer dental benefits; and a community water board decision to fluoridate their drinking water. Examples of rules include temporary dental hygiene licenses for Mission of Mercy projects and work with migrant and seasonal farm workers; and a process to certify mobile dental practices serving elementary schools.

In nearly all 50 states, state legislatures are bicameral (two houses). Nebraska is the only state currently with a unicameral legislature. Policy initiatives become "bills" and must pass both houses before going to the governor. Most state legislatures meet annually for a specified number of days, whereas other states meet every other year. **Figure 9-1** is an illustration of how an idea (bill) becomes policy (law) in most state legislatures.

It is during the committee hearings that testimony from interested members of the public may provide statements. In an ideal situation, the dental hygienist will have an established relationship with the bill sponsor (policymaker) and be available to provide testimony and answer questions. The status of bills may be tracked online through the state's government website.

At the federal level, bills may be tracked through the congressional website (http://thomas.loc.gov/). The process is the same, although the federal calendar is different. The dental hygienist's responsibility includes knowing who their state and congressional legislators are. Most state government websites have links to identify legislators based on zip codes. The ideal time to meet congressional leaders personally is when they are in their home offices. Establishing this relationship is beneficial when the time comes to contact them in their Washington office. The ADHA will occasionally send out "action alerts" to the membership because a piece of legislation is coming up for a vote that will impact oral health and the practice of dental hygiene. In the role of advocate, the dental hygienist can influence the opinion of his or her legislator by responding to these alerts, thereby improving the oral health of the public.

ACCESS TO ORAL HEALTH CARE

It is essential to understand the term **access** and its relationship to social responsibility. Access is assuring that conditions are in place for people to obtain the care they need and want.[19] The key

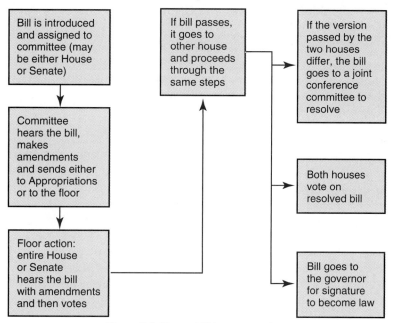

Figure 9-1 How a bill becomes a law.

word here is *assuring*. Many lawmakers and health providers feel that their responsibility is not to provide but to make sure that services are provided through different means and combinations with other partners. Herrell and Mulholland have termed this latter form of assurance **health security.**[20]

WHO further defines health security in terms of "the rights and conditions that enable individuals to attain and enjoy their full potential for a healthy life." However, some practitioners and lawmakers do not want the obligation of providing universal and comprehensive health services and do not want any resemblance to *socialized medicine*, a system in which the means of funding and distributing health care is centralized, usually with a government entity.

As a result, in the United States, a pluralistic system has evolved in which numerous, distinct health care delivery systems coexist simultaneously.[14] In dentistry, this translates to private offices, community health centers, Medicaid-only and nonprofit clinics, mobile vans, school-based health centers, and hospital clinics and emergency departments, each with set criteria determining which patients will receive services according to socioeconomic, geographic, age, and cultural variables. In some cases, this pluralistic system works well, but it is also easy to see how many populations are confused by the complexity of the system, thus "falling through the cracks" and not receiving any dental services. However, insurance does not necessarily equate access. **Table 9-1** shows the sources of payment for 18- to 44-year-old patients for dental care compared with office-based medical care.

Nearly twice as many dental costs are paid out-of-pocket as medical costs (43% versus 26%, respectively).[21] Oral health professionals, who are members of a society that relies on a moral infrastructure for its existence, are expected to contribute to causes that improve all of society rather than acting only out of self-interest.[16]

Table 9-1 Health Expenditures and Distribution by Source of Payment for 18 to 44 Year Olds: 1996

	Dental Provider Services (%)	Office-Based Medical Provider Services (%)
Out-of-pocket	42.9	26.4
Private insurance	51.7	55.5
Medicare	0	1.3
Medicaid	3.3	9.8
Other	2.1	7.0

DISTRIBUTION OF HEALTH RESOURCES

Shortage of Dental Professionals

The result of the health services system's inability to keep pace with a rapidly changing society is a maldistribution—and, in some instances, a "shortage"—of health care providers; such conditions have a direct impact on access to services. Many might convincingly argue that there was a shortage of dental hygienists in the 1990s and predict an even greater shortage of dentists and hygienists by the year 2015.

However, the shortage is a complicated phenomenon. It includes the closure of several dental and dental hygiene schools in the past several years, the varied length of time dental professionals remain in clinical practice, and part-time versus full-time employment opportunities. The shortage is particularly evident in the fields of dental education and dental public health, in which salaries and benefits have not kept pace with those available in private practice settings.[22] Finally, insufficient numbers of culturally diverse dental professionals are being trained and entering the workforce to provide care to underserved populations (**Figure 9-2**). This has resulted in a renewed interest in a dental mid-level provider (see Chapter 2).

Need Versus Demand

With the ratio of providers to population decreasing, who determines who receives what level of services? The concept of *need versus demand* enters the discussion. Briefly defined, need refers to those services deemed by the health professional to be necessary after a variety of assessment and diagnostic tools, and perhaps past experience, have been employed. The disproportionate burden of oral diseases indicates that some population groups are in greater need of oral health care. Demand refers to the health care services desired by the individual or community. The extent of oral health disparities among select population groups illustrates that many people in need of oral care do not demand services.[16]

When tremendous differences exist between need and demand in a community, however, it is imperative that health care providers educate the public and policymakers regarding what is needed to bring public demand as close to what is needed as possible for optimal use of scarce resources. Herein lies a major social responsibility of dental hygienists and other health care providers: education and communication.

As an example, in state programs, such as Children with Special Health Care Needs (CSHCN), limited funding is available for orthodontic services for low-income children with severe malocclusions. The qualifying malocclusions are usually due to skeletal malformations, resulting in

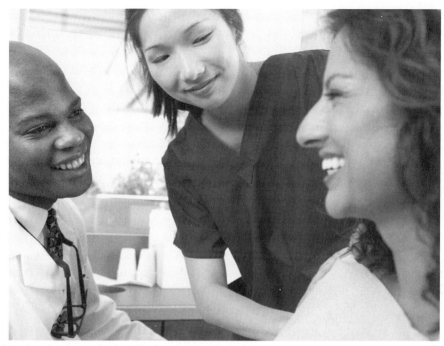

Figure 9-2 The shortage of culturally diverse dental professionals has contributed to the inability to keep pace with a changing society.

impaired speech and chewing ability, and facial asymmetry (as in cleft lip and palate) and are not due simply to an overbite or overjet, malalignment of several teeth, or cross-bite. The difference is often difficult for families desiring aesthetically appealing smiles for their children to understand why funds are going to other children for the restoration of functional occlusion. Educating families of children, public health providers, and lawmakers becomes as important as paying for needed services.

An important component and a useful tool in reconciling need and demand is the use of dental indices (see Chapter 4). Using Dean's Fluorosis Index, the Basic Screening Survey (BSS), Periodontal Screening and Reporting (PSR), and data from the Behavioral Risk Factor Surveillance Survey (BRFSS) gives health care professionals objective data to use when communicating to policymakers and individuals about the oral health care needs in their community and provides the basis for decisions and ongoing evaluation of programmatic activities.

PATIENT RESPONSIBILITY

An earlier question in this chapter concerned the patient's role in accessing health care. In a society in which a pluralistic health system exists, greater emphasis is placed on individual responsibility for health; however, when we look at the significant advances in any nation's health to date, personal lifestyle has not been the most important factor.[23] This is particularly true for improvements in overall oral health status, which can certainly be attributed to community water fluoridation, fluoride toothpaste, sealants, and better restorative materials.

Three factors have been associated with health care inequalities and increased burden of disease: (1) education, (2) housing, and (3) nutrition. Each of these factors is recognized by society as primarily the responsibility of government and publicly funded programs.[23] Those in favor of multiple oral health service delivery systems claim that increased patient responsibility would reduce the demand for oral health services. This would be easier than manipulating the way in which oral health services are provided, thereby helping to resolve the health care access dilemma.[24] Although prevention would go a long way toward reducing the need for emergency and episodic care, when we consider the 10 greatest public health achievements of the twentieth century (see Chapter 1), very little individual patient responsibility was involved. Some historians point out that most of these significant advances occurred during that century's infectious disease era; in today's information age, however, perhaps increased personal responsibility is appropriate as chronic diseases are responsible for greater morbidity and mortality.

Particularly difficult is assigning personal responsibility to children whose dental caries experience, for example, reflects the socioeconomic and educational constraints of their parents and caregivers, or to the elderly, who experience increased periodontal disease, decay, incidence of oral cancer, and tooth loss as income becomes fixed or decreases. Some believe that this type of health status data provides an important indicator of the degree to which human rights are enjoyed or denied as a result of inequity and discrimination. The inequality comes around full circle as declines in dental health and overall health perpetuate the inability to improve socioeconomic status. This inequality is really an example of disparities in **health equity**, or avoidable disparities in health and their determinants based on underlying social status, wealth, ethnicity, geographic location, etc.[25] In other words, not all people have opportunities for the same health outcomes due to barriers imposed by society.

This is not to say that individuals should not have responsibility for improving their own oral health and participating in conscientious brushing, flossing, and regular dental visits. According to the results of the BRFSS, one of the top responses adults give for not seeing a dentist in the past year is that they "did not see a reason to go." The dental hygienist, in the role of educator and consumer advocate, is in an ideal position to communicate the importance of regular oral health care and the relationship to general health and systemic disease, not only to patients but also to the public as a whole. Although this propels oral health into the forefront in patient and policymakers' eyes, it also implies the need for improved interprofessional communication. Currently, the patient has the primary responsibility for assuring the transfer of personal health information between providers as the Health Information Portability and Accountability Act (HIPAA) laws have been enacted to protect patient privacy. HIPAA may be seen as a step backward in interprofessional communication, but the emerging emphasis on health information exchange (HIE) and electronic health records (EHR) is assisting providers in the sharing of crucial information for the purpose of improving health outcomes.[25]

PATIENT CONFIDENTIALITY

Besides the dental professional's responsibilities in respecting cultures, maintaining patient confidentiality is paramount. The rights of the patient and maintaining patient confidentiality in private practice settings are emphasized throughout the dental hygiene student's clinical education; however, it is often forgotten that the same principles apply in dental public health practice.

In public health settings, which may include clinics, schools, and health fair screenings, the atmosphere is often less structured and more chaotic at times, thus necessitating greater attention to patient confidentiality. Ensuring a patient's right to privacy during screenings and treatment, protecting records (signed consents and medical histories), and refraining from sharing personal patient information (e.g., human immunodeficiency virus [HIV] status) with school personnel, policymakers, and other patients are part of the social and ethical responsibilities of the dental professional.

Community groups commonly want to highlight their successful projects by inviting media from newspapers and television to showcase their efforts. However, it is prudent to gain permission from patients if they are going to be in any photographs or film coverage. Many schools require signed permission forms from parents if their child is to be photographed. Inclusion of as many partners in the community as possible in the planning process helps avoid these social mishaps and ensures program visibility and success.

RISK COMMUNICATION

Understanding Risk

Inherent in the increase in interprofessional information sharing is an increased responsibility for risk communication. Health education, oral hygiene instruction, and posttreatment instructions and follow-up are of paramount importance and so is the communication of risk. It is the responsibility of the dental profession, including dental hygienists, to know what the public perceives as risk and to be able to assist in bringing to light peer-reviewed research to reduce public misperceptions.

For example, a segment of the general public perceives inherent risks in radiographs, amalgam restorations, biofilms in dental unit water lines, instrument sterilization techniques, transmission of disease (e.g., HIV infection, hepatitis) in dental offices, and fluoridation of community water supplies. It is the dental hygienist's responsibility to become knowledgeable about current research regarding these issues for ensuring compliance with recommended protocols, regardless of the practice setting, to minimize these risks. The next task is to communicate pertinent information to the public to reduce the spread of misinformation.

Communication

The messages obtained by the public regarding oral health issues are judged, primarily, not on their content but on whether the person providing the information is someone who inspires trust.[26] As a group, dentists and hygienists are regarded as very trustworthy, but this trust is understandably shaken when a member of the profession openly opposes water fluoridation, advocates removing amalgam fillings for reasons other than recurrent decay or fracture, or blatantly dismisses current infection control guidelines.

Communication is a two-way process, and to fully understand a community's concerns, the professional responsible for communicating risk must take these concerns seriously while providing sound scientific evidence. This is where the hygienist's role in staying abreast of current research and using skills in critically evaluating scientific research and literature not only is important but also is a component of the profession's social responsibility.

Comparative Analysis

Communicating risk is not an easy task. Many professionals use "comparative" risk analyses, which are not always effective and may be a hindrance in conveying trust.[26] Following are a few examples of potential risks in dentistry:

1. For the patient concerned about a full set of radiographs, x-ray exposure is explained as being comparable to 1 hour out in the sun at high altitude.
2. For the patient hesitant to accept amalgam fillings as part of a treatment plan because of the mercury content, the mercury level is considered comparable to that in common foods.
3. For the community resident fearful of 1 part per million (ppm) of fluoride in the water supply, the amount is said to be comparable to one drop of water in a bathtub half-full.

Providing these comparisons is not necessarily incorrect, but whether such information can succeed in allaying the concerns of the individual is unpredictable. Herein lies another key point: Scientists and professionals tend to define risk in terms of entire populations; laypeople are concerned with the risk to themselves. Each person approaches risk from a different frame of reference based on past experience, culture, and the media.

PERCEIVED RISK

In addition to the problems of comparisons, according to Peter Bennett, are "fright factors."[26] Popular antifluoridation arguments and the perceived risks based on these fright factors are outlined in **Table 9-2**.

Antifluoridation arguments include claims that the presence of fluoride in community water makes consumption of fluoride "involuntary and inescapable" and that some "at-risk" individuals have adverse reactions to fluoride (e.g., allergies, cancer), which remain unsubstantiated; however, adding to the difficulty is the fact that some arguments against fluoridation are true. For example, fluoride chemicals are a byproduct of the fertilizer industry, there is a printed warning on fluoride toothpaste tubes about not swallowing the paste, and the prevalence of dental caries is declining in nonfluoridated communities. However, these statements are used inappropriately and incorrectly when one is discussing fluoridating community water supplies at optimal levels.

The public does not always understand the differences. It is evident why some perceived risks, such as fluoridation, trigger so many more alarms than other health interventions, regardless of the scientific basis or evidence to the contrary. The right column of **Table 9-2** can easily be changed from "fluoridation" to "amalgam," "irradiated foods," "immunizations," etc., for other illustrations of why perceived risk is a communication challenge.

Responsibility in Communication

Risks not only are dependent on the context in which they are presented but also are intertwined with personal values; thus it becomes difficult to dismiss the antifluoridation arguments as "unreasonable." Attitudes about certain risks are often influenced by how people believe society should be; their relationship with nature; the benefits and disadvantages of technology; cultural influences; and occasionally, religious beliefs. Understanding a message regarding health risk is not the same as knowledge. People may understand a message perfectly but still maintain their own opinions.[27] It would be easier if strong beliefs could be altered with presentation of information and education programs. However, people's beliefs change very slowly, even when factual information is presented.[28]

Table 9-2   Perceived Fluoridation Risks

Factors that Heighten Perceived Risk	Population Antifluoridation Arguments to Illustrate Perceived Risk
1. Exposure is involuntary versus voluntary.	1. Fluoride in community drinking water is unavoidable.
2. Risk is unevenly distributed (some people have problems; others do not).	2. People with suppressed immune systems may be adversely affected by fluoride.
3. Risk is inescapable despite personal precaution.	3. Fluoride is in nearly all foods and beverages.
4. Source is unfamiliar.	4. Fluoride chemicals are a byproduct of fertilizer industry.
5. Fluoride is human-made rather than natural.	5. Chemicals used in the process include sodium fluoride, which is different from the calcium fluoride occurring in nature.
6. Hidden and irreversible damage may result.	6. Overexposure in the young results in fluorosis in permanent teeth.
7. Particular danger may be posed to children or pregnant women.	7. Warning on toothpaste tube cautions against swallowing the paste.
8. Illness, injury, or death is possible.	8. Chronic overexposure may result in crippling skeletal fluorosis.
9. Damage occurs to real people, not anonymous victims.	9. Fluoridated water is not used in kidney dialysis because of possible overdosing of fluoride, resulting in death.
10. Fluoridation is poorly understood by science.	10. Caries have decreased in nonfluoridated communities.
11. Statements from responsible sources have been contradictory.	11. Some health professions are opposed to fluoridation.

Successful risk communication raises the level of people's understanding of relevant issues and reassures those involved that they are adequately informed within the limits of available knowledge.[29] It is a social responsibility of the dental professional to communicate risk. Successful communication depends on respecting beliefs, gathering information consistent with the public's point of view, and then providing a professional account of the evidence underlying sound health decisions and treatment modalities.

DOMESTIC VIOLENCE

In the dental hygienist's role in helping promote the health and well-being of the public, difficult situations sometimes arise that test social and ethical principles and values. In many states the dental hygienist is a mandated reporter of suspected cases of domestic violence, including child abuse and neglect, and elder abuse. This means that the hygienist is required by law to report to the appropriate authorities any information regarding a patient whom the hygienist suspects is a victim of abuse or neglect. Prevent Abuse and Neglect through Dental Awareness (PANDA) programs provide training to dental professionals on recognizing and reporting suspected cases of domestic violence, including child abuse and dental neglect.[31]

As a mandated reporter, the dental hygienist should be alert for the following signs of abuse:
- Bruises, particularly around the areas of the head and neck
- Bruises of various colors, which indicate multiple stages of healing
- Injuries inconsistent with stories of how they occurred
- Inappropriate clothing for the temperature (long-sleeved sweaters in hot, humid climates)
- Unusual shyness or withdrawal or a reaction to oral procedures

These signs should raise questions as to whether abuse may have occurred. Parental disregard of or refusal to follow through on a child's needed dental treatment may be an indication of dental neglect. Unexplained injuries and bruising in an elderly patient may signal elder abuse. It is the professional responsibility of hygienists to know the legal requirements in the community, the agency to call to report gathered information, and the steps to take to ensure safety for themselves and for the patient.

LEADERSHIP

For every child without medical insurance, 2.6 children are without dental insurance, and for every adult with medical insurance, 3 adults are without dental insurance.[10] With the increasing number of people without health or dental insurance, continued leadership on the part of dental professionals to eliminate oral health disparities and to ensure access to oral health services for all is needed.

Dental hygiene leadership embraces the following concepts:
- Social responsibility
- Professionalism
- Ethics
- Communication

A leader in dental hygiene works within the community to develop consensus on what "oral health care for all" might look like. He or she enables others to see the problem firsthand and to implement solutions, and models public health practice by ensuring equal access to care and not tolerating discrimination against any person seeking care. The leader encourages other professionals in the community to participate in health promotion and disease prevention activities and celebrates successes.

The dental hygiene leader challenges "the way things have always been done" and seeks new ways to maximize resources and productivity while remaining mindful of ethical decision-making processes and commitment to quality oral care.[32] The leader respects the other health care providers in the community and forges collaborative relationships in providing total health care for the public.

Finally, the dental hygiene leader works within the profession to ensure continued competency, lifelong learning, and maintenance of quality standards of practice.

SUMMARY

The dental hygienist is a professional. Inherent in the role of the professional is the responsibility of making ethical decisions and choices and opportunities to practice dental hygiene in ways that will increase access to oral health services for all populations. The role requires the leadership to uphold the standards of dental hygiene practice and communication skills to promote optimal oral health for all.

Applying Your Knowledge

1. Conduct a survey of other students on campus, or dental professionals in the community, as to their beliefs of access to health care as a "privilege" or a "right." Present your findings to your class, allowing time for discussion of the various views collected.
2. Choose a dental treatment or preventive measure that is perceived by some members of society as carrying risk. Research two scientific articles in response to one of those perceived risks and share your expertise with the rest of your class.
3. Develop a one-page fact sheet for a legislator describing a particular oral health concern. Be succinct and avoid jargon. Include the following:
   a. The nature of the problem.
   b. Potential solutions to the problem.
   c. What you would like the legislator to do.
4. Survey local school districts to identify those that have signed contracts with soda companies to place vending machines in their schools as a money-making venture. Prepare an outline for a presentation you might make at a PTA meeting.

Dental Hygiene Competencies

Reading the material in this chapter and participating in the activities of Applying Your Knowledge will contribute to the student's ability to demonstrate the following competencies:

Core competencies

C.1 Apply a professional code of ethics in all endeavors.

C.6 Advance the profession through service activities and affiliations with professional organizations.

C.8 Communicate effectively with individuals and groups from diverse populations, both verbally and in writing.

Health promotion and disease prevention

HP.1 Promote the values of oral and general health and wellness to the public and organizations within and outside the profession.

Community involvement

CM.4 Facilitate client access to oral health care services by influencing individuals and organizations for the provision of oral health care.

Community Case

Jan has been volunteering in a second-grade school-based sealant project operated by the local health department at several elementary schools in the city. Volunteer dentists screen the children to ascertain which teeth are sealable and to prioritize children for urgency of restorative needs. The dental hygienists then apply sealant to the approved teeth, provide one-on-one oral hygiene instruction, and work with school nurses to provide case management and follow-up for restorative needs. One particular child, Joey, has six decayed primary teeth. He is irritable and fearful in the dental chair. Because he is not a legal citizen, Joey does not have insurance and is not eligible for Medicaid.

When preparing to place the sealants, Jan notices that teeth #3, 19, and 30 are approved for sealants. Tooth #14 is checked as needing a restoration; however, it is evident to Jan that tooth #3 needs the restoration and tooth #14 is perhaps sealable, suggesting that the teeth numbers have been switched at screening. Jan does not seal the upper molars until the tooth numbers can be clarified, and she seals the lower molars. She sends a follow-up note home to Joey's parents indicating the findings of the screening and the urgent need for dental care.

Jan returns to the school 3 months later to conduct a sealant retention check on the children who had received sealants. She discovers that (1) the status of teeth #3 and 14 for sealants has not been clarified and (2) Joey has not received the urgent dental treatment. When talking with the school nurse, Jan finds that the screening dentist has not been back to rescreen and that the nurse has been unsuccessful in convincing Joey's mother to take him to the dentist and has not found any local dental providers willing to donate the needed dental services.

1. What should Jan have done regarding the apparent switch in teeth numbers for sealants?
   a. Do as she did, do not seal either one, and wait for a rescreening by the dentist.
   b. Note the apparent switch in the child's chart, and seal tooth #14.
   c. Call the screening dentist, and explain the situation to try to get verbal approval to seal tooth #14.
   d. Indicate in the chart that tooth No. 3 is not sealable, and leave both teeth #3 and 14 for restorations.
2. What is Jan's responsibility concerning Joey's urgent need for dental care?
   a. She does not have any responsibility. It is up to the child's parents to get him into the dentist.
   b. She needs to work with the school nurse to find dental care for Joey as soon as possible.
   c. She needs to call Social Services to report a suspected case of dental neglect.
   d. She needs to talk to Joey's mother to explain the urgency of the situation.
3. What is Jan's responsibility to the dental professional community at large, in that the school nurse has not been able to find anyone to take Joey?
   a. She does not have any responsibility because dentists can decide whom they want in their practices.
   b. She should file a complaint with the state dental licensing board.
   c. She should make a presentation to local dentists regarding the oral health status of the children and their unmet dental needs.
   d. She should follow the dental professional's lead and try to convince Joey's parents that his dental needs are a priority and that they need to find the resources to pay for it.

References

1. Woolfolk MW. The social responsibility model. J Dent Educ 1993;57:346.
2. Ozar DT, Love J. Conflicting values in oral health care. J Am Coll Dent 1998;65:15.
3. Ozar DT, Sokol DJ. Dental Ethics at Chairside: Professional Principles and Practical Application. St Louis: Mosby-Year Book; 1994.
4. Gaston MA. Survey of ethical issues in dental hygiene. J Dent Hyg 1990;64:217.
5. Frankel MS. Taking ethics seriously: Building a professional community. J Dent Hyg 1992;66:386.
6. Weinstein BD. Dental Ethics. Philadelphia: Lea & Febiger; 1993.
7. Code of Ethics and Standards of Professional Conduct: American Association of Public Health Dentistry. Interim Policy adopted October 16, 1997. Springfield IL: AAPHD.
8. Christie C, Bowen D, Paarmann C. Curriculum evaluation of ethical reasoning and professional responsibility. J Dent Educ 2003;67:55.
9. Center for Ethical Leadership. Available at www.ethicalleadership.org/philosophies/ethical-leadership. Accessed January 2009.
10. Gershen JA. Response to the social responsibility model: The convergence of curriculum and health policy. J Dent Educ 1993;57:350.
11. Oral Health in America: A Report of the Surgeon General—Executive Summary. Rockville, MD: US Department of Health and Human Services, National Institute of Dental and Craniofacial Research, National Institutes of Health; 2000.
12. Children's Dental Health Project's Healthcare Reform Center. Available at www.cdhp.org/cdhp_healthcare_reform_center. Accessed January 2010.

13. Browning P, von Cube A, Leibrand H. Minimum public health standards as a basis for secure public health funding. J Public Health Manag Pract 2004;10:19.
14. Stewart GT. Health care in America: Privilege or right? Lancet 1971;2:1305.
15. Burt BA, Eklund SA. Dentistry, Dental Practice, and the Community. 4th ed. Philadelphia: WB Saunders; 1992.
16. ADEA President's Commission—Improving the oral health status of all Americans: Roles and responsibilities of academic dental institutions. J Dent Educ 2003;67:563.
17. Goldsmith MF. Health and human rights inseparable. JAMA 1993;270:553.
18. United Nations. Universal declaration of human rights. Available at www.un.org/en/udhr/index.shtml. Accessed October 2010.
19. Isman R, Isman B. Oral Health America White Paper: Access to Oral Health Services in the U.S. 1997 and Beyond. Princeton, NJ: Robert Wood Johnson Foundation; 1997.
20. Herrell IC, Mulholland CA. Reflections on health in development and human rights. World Health Stat Q 1998;51:88.
21. Medical Expenditure Panel Survey. Total Health Services—Median and Mean Expenses per Person with Expense and Distribution of Expenses by Source of Payment. U.S. 1996. Available at www.meps.ahrq.gov.
22. Valacovic R. 2010 ADEA Executive Directors Report: Meet the Future. Available at www.adea.org/about_adea/who_we_are/documents/forms/allitems.aspx. Accessed October 2010.
23. Sarll DW. Who is responsible for good oral health? Br Dent J 1996;180:164.
24. Bent JP. Health access and social responsibility. Arch Otolaryngol Head Neck Surg 1992;118:344.
25. Health Insurance Portability and Accountability Act. ADA Fact Sheet for Providers. Available at www.ada.org/prof/resources/topics/hipaa/hipaa_faqs.pdf. Accessed January 2010.
26. Bennett P, Calman K. Risk Communication and Public Health. Oxford, UK: University of Oxford Press; 1999.
27. Weinstein N, Sandman P. Some criteria for evaluating risk messages. Risk Analysis 1993;13:103.
28. Slovic P. Informing and educating the public about risk. Risk Analysis 1986;6:403.
29. Deahl ST II, Kromer ME. A taxonomy for lay risk perceptions of dentistry. J Public Health Dent 1996;56:213.
30. Jenny J. Basic social values, structural elements in oral health systems and oral health status. Int Dent J 1980;30:276.
31. American Academy of Pediatrics/American Academy of Pediatric Dentistry. Oral and dental aspects of child abuse and neglect: Joint statement. Pediatrics 1999;104:348.
32. Kouzes JM, Posner BZ. The Leadership Challenge. San Francisco: Jossey-Bass; 1995.

Additional Resources

Braveman, P. Health disparities and health equity: Concepts and measurement. Annu Rev Public Health 2006;27:167.
Garrett B, Holahan J, Doan L, et al. The Cost of Failure to Enact Health Reform: Implications for States. The Urban Institute.
www.urban.org/publications/411965.html
Sgan-Cohen, Mann J. Health, oral health, and poverty. J Am Dent Assoc 2007;138:1437.
Timeline tracing the history of attempts and successes in health care reform in the United States since 1900.
www.nytimes.com/interactive/2009/07/19/us/politics/20090717_HEALTH_TIMELINE.html

10

Cultural Competency

Magda A. de la Torre, RDH, MPH

Objectives

Upon completion of this chapter, the student will be able to:

- Describe key demographic, social, and cultural shifts and trends influencing oral health among culturally diverse groups in the United States.
- Discuss the impact of population trends in oral health and provision of oral health services to individuals and groups.
- Define the terms *cross-cultural communication, health disparities,* and *cultural diversity.*
- Define culture and cultural competence and explain why they are important.
- Identify the Oral Health Care Culturally Competent (OHCCC) Guidelines.
- Discuss the components of the Cultural Competency Continuum Ladder.
- Describe the application of strategies and approaches that enhance cross-cultural communication and education in oral health care settings.
- Apply the models described in the chapter for the provision of culturally competent health care.
- Discuss the responsibility of the dental hygienist with respect to cultural competence and the role in providing care to special populations.

Key Terms

Cultural diversity	Knowledge	Cross-cultural encounters
Health disparity	Skill	Cross-cultural communication
Culture	Cultural destructiveness	Purnell Model for Cultural
Ethnocentrism	Cultural incapacity	Competence
Cultural competency	Cultural blindness	Patient-Centered Model
Cultural Competency	Cultural precompetence	Culturally and Linguistically
Education Model	Cultural competence	Appropriate Services
Self-exploration	Cultural proficiency	(CLAS)

Opening Statements

Status and Future of Oral Health Care

- Closing the gap on health disparities and inequalities among diverse cultures will lead to better health for all Americans and is a responsibility of all health care providers.
- Race, ethnicity, gender, and socioeconomic levels are powerful factors that affect health status, access to health care services, and the quality of health care.
- We must commit ourselves to living in a world and society in which respect for human dignity and equality is valued.

- It has been said that the mark of a great community is how well it cares for its most vulnerable citizens.
- There are important variations among and within people from the same country or culture, and there may be cultural variations among generations.
- There are noticeable disparities in dental disease by income. Poor children suffer twice as many dental caries as their more affluent peers.
- *Healthy People 2020* goals are to eliminate preventable disease, disability, injury, and premature death; achieve health equity, eliminate health disparities, and improve health for all groups; create social and physical environments that promote good health for all; and promote healthy development and healthy behaviors at every stage of life.[1]
- A common goal for health professionals is to provide the best care to all patients.[2]

TODAY'S EVOLVING DIVERSE POPULATION

The United States is highly diverse, as evidenced in individual's neighborhoods, schools, and communities. Diversity extends to integral parts of our existence as human beings such as race, culture, social and economical status, language, and national origin. Diversity also extends to lifestyles, traditions, personal and family histories, ages, abilities, and other dimensions that constitute who we are and where we come from. In most communities, many languages are spoken in schools, workplaces, and homes. All of these components of our being are fundamental in interpersonal interactions and community settings. Previously, societies primarily functioned with a monocultural and monolingual perspective. People were expected to give up the values, norms, and beliefs of the society they were emigrating from in favor of new opportunities.[3] The United States has lost the image of a "melting pot" of racial and ethnic groups. **Cultural diversity** in American society is more realistically an intricate mosaic consisting of numerous racial and ethnic groups.[4,5]

The concept of diversity encompasses acceptance and respect. It means understanding that each individual is unique and recognizing our individual differences. These can be along the dimensions of race, ethnicity, gender, sexual orientation, socioeconomic status, age, physical abilities, religious beliefs, political beliefs, or other ideologies. It is the exploration of these differences in a safe, positive, and nurturing environment. It is about understanding each other and moving beyond simple tolerance to embracing and celebrating the rich dimensions of diversity contained within each individual.[6]

Today's evolving society is a multiracial, multicultural, and multilingual world (**Tables 10-1 and 10-2**).[7] The matters of race, ethnicity, and cultural differences have great significance for all who live in the United States. Society has embraced the concepts of cultural competency, cultural diversity, cultural sensitivity, cultural pluralism, and multiculturalism. These concepts are being incorporated not only into health care but also business, education, and policies. In health care, these concepts have implications on how care is provided for clients and a community that may not share the same culture and language as the provider. The clients may have different beliefs, values, attitudes, and behaviors.

Three reasons for a health care provider to be in the constant pursuit of cultural competency are the societal realities of a changing world, the influence of culture and ethnicity on human growth and development, and the challenge of providing effective and quality health care to all people.[4] These reasons indicate the need and importance of cultural competency but also the

Table 10-1   **Ethnicity in the United States (US) Population, 1990 and 2000 Census***

	ETHNICITY PERCENTAGE	
	1990	*2000*
White/Caucasian	71.3	75.1
Hispanic/Latino	8.9	12.5
Black/African-American	12.0	12.3
Asian-American/Pacific Islander	2.9	3.6
American Indian/Alaskan Native	0.7	0.9

From US Bureau of the Census, 2000.
*The 2010 Census began on April 1, 2010, and more current information can be obtained in the future at www.census.gov/.

Table 10-2   **Linguistic Diversity in the United States (US) Population***

Population	Percentage
US population (5 years old and older) speaking a language other than English at home	17.9%
Foreign-born US population	11%

From US Bureau of the Census, 2000.
*The 2010 Census began on April 1, 2010, and more current information can be obtained in the future at www.census.gov/.

emphasis of developing skills and knowledge to communicate and collaborate with persons of other cultures.

The 2000 Oral Health in America: A Report of the Surgeon General focused on oral health issues and improvements in oral health over the past century. The report reminds us that there are serious challenges for the future and that although oral health has improved in the United States over the past century, disparities in oral health still exist. Special population groups, such as infants and young children, the poor, those living in rural areas, the homeless, persons with disabilities, racial and ethnic minorities, the institutionalized, and the frail elderly, experience a greater burden of oral and craniofacial diseases. Great disparities also exist in access to oral health care and use of oral health promotion and disease prevention services, each vital to the establishment and maintenance of optimal health.[8]

CONSIDERING CULTURE

It is understood in the health, medical, and dental communities that there is a critical need to eliminate disparities in health care among the diverse populations in the United States. A **health disparity** is a population-specific difference in the presence of disease, health outcomes, or access to health care.[9] Disparities in heath status are compounded by reduced access to health care services. Although many factors affect health status, the lack of health insurance or underinsurance, and other barriers, such as transportation, rural settings, and hours of operations of facilities, are key components of reduced health care access. Underserved populations' use of medical and dental preventive services is diminished by an inability to obtain providers and services. Increased use of health services can reduce disease and contribute to improved health status (**Figure 10-1**).[10]

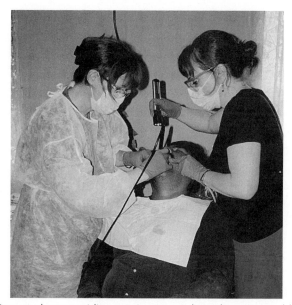

Figure 10-1 Dental hygiene students providing care in a nontraditional setting to address the needs of access by underserved populations.

Health care access problems include several components. Two important components are (1) the influences of race or ethnicity on an individual's perception of a given illness and (2) the decision to seek health care. A primary requirement in providing culturally sensitive medical care is a basic knowledge of the health status and needs of those groups being served. Health care providers traditionally have their own expectations of how health care should be delivered and how patients are supposed to respond to care. However, if they are to effectively work with a multicultural population, health care providers must alter their traditional ways of treating patients. Historically, many of the health care providers serving ethnic populations have been members of these same ethnic/racial groups themselves. It is imperative that all professionals who provide health care have the knowledge and communication skills that will make them attentive to the cultural differences of their patients.[11]

What is Culture?

Culture is an integrated pattern of human behavior that includes thoughts, communications, languages, practices, beliefs, values, customs, courtesies, rituals, manners of interacting, roles, relationships, and expected behaviors of a racial, ethnic, religious, or social group, as well as the ability to transmit these to succeeding generations.[12] Culture can also be defined as a specific set of social, educational, religious, and professional behaviors, practices, and values that individuals learn and adhere to while participating in or out of groups with whom they usually interact daily.[13a] In common terms, culture is what we live every day, our daily interactions at work, school, or in our community. It is the lens that we use to view the world and to form our opinions, thoughts, aspirations, and goals in life. Culture is both inherent and learned; it is a shared way of interpreting the world. Culture is simple yet complex, common yet unique, and constantly evolving based on our life experiences. Several factors influencing culture are listed in **Box 10-1**.

BOX 10-1 **Factors that Influence Culture**

- Age
- Socioeconomic status
- Gender
- Educational attainment
- Geography
- Family
- Place of birth
- Length of residency in the United States
- Religious beliefs
- Individual experiences
- Sexual preference
- Power relationships

Why Consider Culture?

Given the wide diversity present in modern societies, cultural competence is a necessary skill, allowing us to provide appropriate services to all individuals and communities. Given our modern technologies, it is also a skill we need for global survival. Historically, the challenges of insufficient cultural competence for cross-cultural collaboration go back to the earliest beginnings of humanity. Every human culture teaches its members to value their beliefs, morals, and views of reality as the best, as the ideal; in some cases, cultures teach that their beliefs are the ONLY acceptable way to be or think. The resulting lack of cultural interchange and adaptation could be called **ethnocentrism**—judging other cultures by your own standards consistent with your values, not theirs.[13b]

Reasons to incorporate culture in your daily activities include the following:
- To understand the values, attitudes, and behaviors of others
- To avoid stereotypes and biases that can undermine efforts
- To develop and deliver services responsive to the needs of the patients
- To focus on commonalities not differences (**Figure 10-2**)

CULTURAL COMPETENCY

Cultural competency in health care describes the ability to provide care to patients with diverse values, beliefs, and behaviors.[14] Included in cultural competency is the adaptation of oral health promotion and disease prevention and clinical dental hygiene services to meet the patient's social, cultural, and linguistic needs. Individuals who must be treated in a culturally competent manner include children, the elderly, and people with disabilities. Cultural competency is a developmental process that evolves over an extended period of time. Effective cultural competency needs to be implemented on an individual, organizational, and community level. All three entities can be at various stages of awareness, knowledge, skills, and attitudes along the cultural competence continuum (**Figure 10-3**).[15]

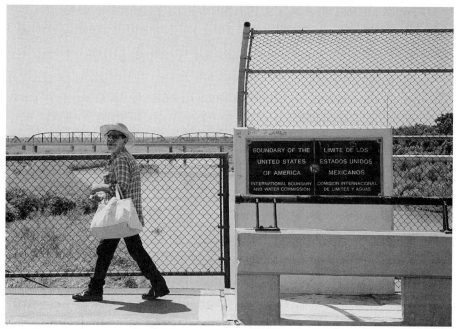

Figure 10-2 Cultural competency should be an integral part of quality oral health care to the population on the United States–Mexico border.

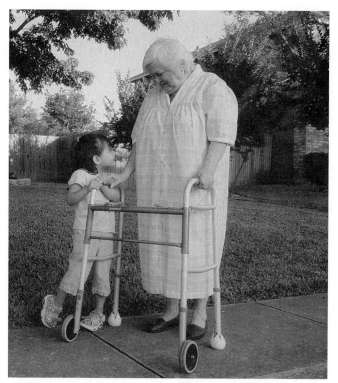

Figure 10-3 Individuals who must be treated in a culturally competent manner include children, the elderly, and the disabled.

Cultural Competency Models, Frameworks, and Strategies

Models exist that enable us to acquire the skills for self-assessment, to determine implementation of cultural competency in organizations and systems, and to evaluate effectiveness of appropriate community outreach. Following are examples of models that can be implemented in various settings and cross-cultural encounters to ensure that culturally competent attitudes, knowledge, and behaviors are implemented when providing oral health care in either a clinical or community setting. **Box 10-2** outlines the Oral Health Care Culturally Competent (OHCCC) Guidelines.[9]

Cultural Competency Education Model

The **Cultural Competency Education Model** is a conceptual model that focuses on the process of developing cultural competency in health care practices. This model is designed to foster understanding, acceptance, knowledge, and constructive relations between persons of various cultures. The model is designed as a tool for developing the knowledge and skills that health care providers need to provide quality care.[4] The model is framed on three areas of intervention: self-exploration or awareness, knowledge, and skills (**Figure 10-4**).

BOX 10-2 Oral Health Care Culturally Competent (OHCCC) Guidelines

- Develop the capacity for cultural self-assessment.
- Value diversity among peers and clients.
- Understand the dynamics of the interactions between and within cultures.
- Institutionalize and implement cultural knowledge in a nonjudgmental manner.
- Adapt preventive and clinical oral health service with an understanding, acceptance, appreciation, and respect of cultural diversity.
- Be creative in finding ways to communicate with population groups that have limited English-speaking proficiency.
- Understand cultural competency is continually evolving and a long-term developmental process.

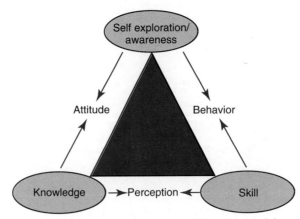

Figure 10-4 Cultural Competency Education Model.

Self-exploration: Awareness of one's own cultural heritage and increased acceptance of different values, attitudes, and beliefs.

Knowledge: To understand that one culture is not intrinsically superior to another and to recognize individual and group differences and similarities.

Skill: To master appropriate and sensitive strategies and skills in communicating and interacting with persons from different cultures and to seek information about various cultures within a society.

It is through the development of self-exploration/awareness and skill that behaviors are adapted and implemented. The development of skills and knowledge creates the perception that is formed about and by people of diverse cultures. Attitude is explored, enhanced, and broadened by the growth of an individuals' self-exploration/awareness and the gaining of knowledge about diversity and the importance of culture to our daily life.

Cultural Competency Continuum

The Cultural Competency Continuum is extensively referred to in cultural competency literature and training programs. It can serve as a guide to determine the functional competency or organizational activities and philosophies and also as a guide to personal development and expansion on becoming a culturally competent oral health care provider. The continuum has been described as a ladder in which an individual can self-assess, plan to move to another step, and then progress in the personal and professional development of cultural competence. The six stages or steps are defined here and are illustrated in **Figure 10-5**.

Cultural destructiveness: The most negative end of the continuum. It is represented by attitudes, policies, and practices that are destructive to culture, communities, and individuals. The most extreme example of cultural destructiveness is actively participating in cultural genocide, which is the purposeful destruction of a culture.

Cultural incapacity: The next step is one in which systems, agencies, or individuals do not intentionally seek to be culturally destructive but lack the capacity to help clients or communities of diverse backgrounds. The systems remain extremely biased and believe in racial superiority.

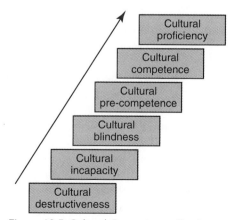

Figure 10-5 Cultural Competency Continuum.

Cultural blindness: At this level of the continuum, systems, agencies, or individuals provide services with the philosophy of being unbiased. It is believed that cultures make no difference and all people are the same. This is a well-intended philosophy; however, the consequences of such a belief are to make services ethnocentric and therefore only useful for the most assimilated. People of diverse cultures are anticipated to meet the needs and expectations of the dominant group.

Cultural precompetence: This step is on the positive end of the scale, awareness of some sensitivity but not sure what to do or "what is right." A system, agency, or individual recognizes its weaknesses in serving clients of cultural diversity and attempts to improve. Care must be taken at this level so that a false sense of accomplishment does not prevent the movement along the continuum.

Cultural competence: Culturally competent systems, agencies, or individuals are characterized by acceptance and respect for difference. There is ongoing self-assessment regarding culture, expansion of knowledge, and adaptation of service models to better meet the needs of specific populations. Cultural competence is also characterized by acknowledging similarities between diverse cultures.

Cultural proficiency: This is the most positive end of the continuum, advanced cultural competency. Culture is held in high self-esteem, and there is high regard in adding to the knowledge base of culturally competent practices, services, research, and approaches. Cultural proficiency indicates advocating for cultural competence through all systems and improves relations between cultures throughout society.[15-17]

COMMUNITY AND ORGANIZATIONAL CULTURAL COMPETENCE

Organizations must have the capacity to value diversity, conduct self-assessment, manage the dynamics of differences, acquire and institutionalize cultural knowledge, and adapt to diversity in the cultural contexts of the community they serve.[10] In addition, organizations must incorporate cultural competency principles in all aspects of policy making, administration, practice, and service delivery and systematically involve clients, stakeholders, and the communities they will serve. Training to increase cultural competence must be incorporated into our national and local infrastructures.[18] Efforts must be made with schools, the media, politicians, and administrators to emphasize the value of cultural competency. Current and future leaders need specific training to increase their cultural competence. It is important for public health agencies to include training and education to ensure that both service providers and clinical providers communicate in a culturally competent manner with every person during health care encounters and in a variety of settings with diverse communities.[19] Several models have been described in the literature that are effective in cross-cultural encounters in health settings, including the LEARN (an acronym for Listen, Explain, Acknowledge, Recommend and Negotiate) Model. The LEARN Model (**Box 10-3**) applies behaviors and attitudes during **cross-cultural encounters.** These encounters or interactions can provide opportunities for personal growth, often challenging in situations that are unfamiliar to daily living and beliefs.

The Kleinman Explanatory Model assists with the gathering of information by asking the client questions (**Box 10-4**). This model ensures appropriate individualized care when a health care provider encounters interactions with a patient and family from an unfamiliar culture. Questions of what, why, how, and who are asked to understand and implement individualized

BOX 10-3 LEARN Model of Cross-Cultural Encounter Guidelines for Health Practitioners[19]

Listen with sympathy and understanding to the patient's perception of the problem.
Explain your perceptions of the problem and your strategy for treatment.
Acknowledge and discuss the differences and similarities between these perceptions.
Recommend treatment while remembering the patient's cultural parameters.
Negotiate agreement. It is important to understand the patient's explanatory model so that the treatment fits in his or her cultural framework.

BOX 10-4 Kleinman's Explanatory Model

Kleinman's Explanatory Model to elicit health beliefs in clinical encounters provides a sensitive approach to asking about health problems.[20]
- What do you call your problem? What name does it have?
- What do you think caused your problem?
- Why do you think it started when it did?
- What does your sickness do to you? How does it work?
- How severe is it? Will it have a short or long course?
- What do you fear most about your disorder?
- What are the chief problems that your sickness has caused for you?
- What kind of treatment do you think you should receive?
- What are the most important results you hope to receive from the treatment?

health care encounters.[20] Both models are best used in clinical encounters for communication with clients in private, community, and organizational systems. These models foster our creativity when interacting with clients, families, or communities of diverse populations.

EFFECTIVE CROSS-CULTURAL COMMUNICATION

Cross-cultural communication is effectively communicating with someone of a different culture. It is important to learn all that you can about the individual, family, or the community's way of life. Two important points to remember are as follows:
1. Do not expect to ever completely understand a culture that is not your own. For example, no matter how much you study the Italian culture, you will never be Italian or share the experiences of growing up in Italy or with an Italian family rich in traditions.
2. Do not fall into the stereotyping or overgeneralization trap. Do not look at people stereotypically and then never move beyond that point. The skill of cultural competency is to learn useful general information and at the same time be aware and open to variations and individual differences.

Identifying communication strategies that positively influence basic lifestyle behaviors has become increasingly important for improving the health of millions of Americans.[21] Some skills to assist and produce effective cross-cultural communication are listed in the Guiding Principles.

GUIDING PRINCIPLES

Skills that Foster Effective Cross-Cultural Communication
- Communicate in a language that is clear and at the client's level of understanding; send clear messages.
- Define any dental terminology; avoid jargon.
- Listen well to the client's questions and stories.
- Carefully observe the client's body language.
- Look beyond the superficial.
- Be patient, persistent, and most important, flexible.
- Recognize your own cultural biases.
- Emphasize common ground; do not focus on differences, instead focus on similarities.
- Withhold judgment; accept others' differences.
- Empathize; treat each person as an individual.
- Do not assume understanding; ask for clarification.
- Always communicate in a respectful manner.
- Increase your knowledge and skills of cultural competence.

Purnell Model for Cultural Competence

The **Purnell Model for Cultural Competence** is a holistic organizing framework to guide cultural competence among multidisciplinary members of the health care team in a variety of primary, secondary, and tertiary settings. It is designed to learn about a person's own cultures and the culture of patients, families, communities, and society. The model can be utilized in an indi-

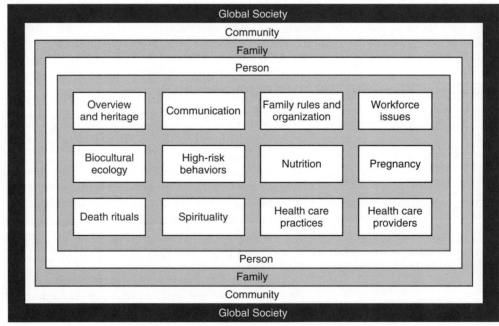

Figure 10-6 The Purnell Model for Cultural Competence.

vidual one-on-one setting, community, or organizational environment.[22] The model may guide the practice of health professionals across settings in interdisciplinary teams.

The model has an outlying rim representing global society, a second rim representing community, a third rim representing family, and an inner rim representing the person. The interior of the circle is divided into 12 sections depicting cultural domains and their concepts (**Figure 10-6**).

Health care providers can use this same process to understand their own cultural beliefs, attitudes, values, practices, and behaviors (**Table 10-3**). Health care professional societies and organizations have standards, initiatives, or statements encouraging their members to become culturally sensitive and culturally competent.

Table 10-3   **Twelve Cultural Domains in the Purnell Model for Cultural Competence**

Cultural Domain	*Related Concepts*
Overview and heritage	Country of origin; current residence; effects of the topography of country of origin on health; effects of current residence on health, economics, policies, migration, education status, occupations
Communication	Dominant language, dialects, cultural communication patterns, personal space, volume and tone, eye contact, body language, facial expressions, temporal relationships, touch, time, names, greetings
Family roles and organization	Head of household, gender roles, goals and priorities, development tasks, roles of the aged, roles of extended family members, individual and social status in the community, alternative lifestyles
Workforce issues	Autonomy, acculturation, gender roles, language barriers
Biocultural ecology	Biologic variations, skin color, body type, heredity, genetics, ecology, drug metabolism
High-risk behavior	Drug use, alcohol use, tobacco use, use of safety equipment (e.g., seat belts, helmets), high-risk behaviors, lifestyles
Nutrition	Common foods, rituals and taboos associated with food, meaning of food to the culture, how food is used in sickness and in health, limitations, deficiencies
Pregnancy and childbearing practices	Fertility practices, birthing practices, views toward pregnancy, postpartum
Death rituals	Views toward death, euthanasia, preparation for death, burial practices, bereavement practices
Spirituality	Meaning of life, religious practices, use of prayer, individual strength, spirituality and health
Health care practices	Focus on health care, magicoreligious beliefs, traditional practices, individual responsibility for health, self-medicating practices, views toward issues such as organ donations, transplantation, mental illness, rehabilitation, expression of pain, sick role, barriers to health care
Health care practitioners	Type of practitioners: Biomedical, traditional, or folk; perceptions of practitioner; gender and health care

Adapted from Purnell D, Paulanka J, editors. Guide to Culturally Competent Healthcare. Philadelphia: F.A. Davis; 2005.

Patient-Centered Model

Balint's **patient-centered model** emphasizes that each patient "has to be understood as a unique human-being." Subsequently, Levenstein and colleagues described the patient-centered clinical method as one in which the health care provider aims to gain an understanding of the patient, as well as the disease, as opposed to an approach focusing strictly on the disease.[23,24] Through patient centeredness and the patient-centered approach, health care providers place themselves in the patient's role and view the illness as the patient views the illness, health, and the health care system.[25] One major common goal between both cultural competence and patient centeredness is to improve health care quality.[23,26]

Cultural competence and patient-centeredness both began as interpersonal interaction guides for effective communication to maintain unconditional positive regard, effective rapport, and understanding of the patient's beliefs, values, and attitudes about health and illness. The role of dental professional advocates preparing to work in the community and public health settings is to encourage the implementation of culturally competent and patient-centered care in health care systems. The integration of patient-centeredness and cultural competence are initiatives to promote and improve health care quality (**Figure 10-7**).

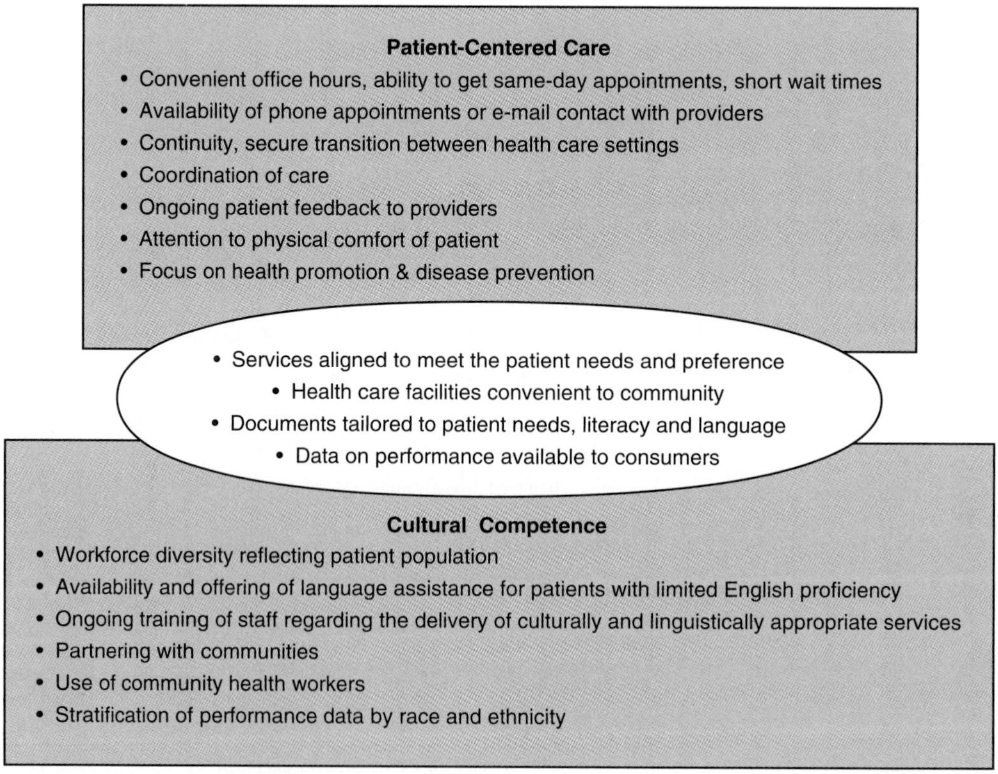

Patient-Centered Care
- Convenient office hours, ability to get same-day appointments, short wait times
- Availability of phone appointments or e-mail contact with providers
- Continuity, secure transition between health care settings
- Coordination of care
- Ongoing patient feedback to providers
- Attention to physical comfort of patient
- Focus on health promotion & disease prevention

- Services aligned to meet the patient needs and preference
- Health care facilities convenient to community
- Documents tailored to patient needs, literacy and language
- Data on performance available to consumers

Cultural Competence
- Workforce diversity reflecting patient population
- Availability and offering of language assistance for patients with limited English proficiency
- Ongoing training of staff regarding the delivery of culturally and linguistically appropriate services
- Partnering with communities
- Use of community health workers
- Stratification of performance data by race and ethnicity

Figure 10-7 Overlap between patient-centered care and cultural competence in the health system.

Culturally and Linguistically Appropriate Services

The Office of Minority Health (OMH), US Department of Health and Human Services (DHHS), published the final recommendations on National Standards for **Culturally and Linguistically Appropriate Services (CLAS)** in health care. Federal and state health agencies, policymakers, and national organizations now have a blueprint to follow for building culturally competent heath care organizations and workers.[27,28] The CLAS standards are primarily geared to health care organizations but individual providers are also incorporating the standards, especially when forming partnerships with communities. There are 14 national recommended standards to inform, guide, and facilitate implementation of CLAS (**Box 10-5**). Within this framework, there are three types of varying standards:

1. Mandates: Current Federal requirements for all recipients of federal funds (Standards 4, 5, 6, and 7).
2. Guidelines: Activities recommended by OMH for adoption as mandates by federal, state, and national accrediting agencies (Standards 1, 2, 3, 8, 9, 10, 11, 12, and 13).

BOX 10-5 Culturally and Linguistically Appropriate Services (CLAS)

Culturally Competent Care (Standards 1-3)
1. Patients and consumers receive effective, understandable, and respectful health care.
2. Recruitment, retention, and promotion of diverse staff and leadership.
3. All staff receive ongoing education and training.

Language Access Services (Standards 4-7)
4. Language assistance services, including bilingual staff and interpreters, must be offered at no cost to the patient.
5. Patients and consumers must be informed of their right to language assistance services.
6. Health organizations must ensure the competence of language assistance provided by interpreters/bilingual staff.
7. Availability of easily understood patient materials and applicable signage posted.

Organizational Support for Cultural Competence (Standards 8-14)
8. Written strategic plan with clear goals, policies, and accountability mechanisms.
9. Conduct initial and ongoing organizational self-assessments, and integrate cultural and linguistic competence measures into overall program activities.
10. Patient data collection to include race, ethnicity, and spoken and written language.
11. Maintain current demographic, cultural, and epidemiologic community profiles, and conduct needs assessment on cultural and linguistic characteristics of the service area.
12. Participatory, collaborative partnerships to facilitate community and patient/consumer involvement.
13. Ensure that conflict and grievance resolution processes are culturally and linguistically sensitive.
14. Keep the public informed about progress and successful innovations in implementing the CLAS standards.

From US Department of Health and Human Services, Office of Minority Health. Closing the Gap: National Standards for Culturally and Linguistically Appropriate Services, Rockville, MD: USDHH; 2001. Available at www.omhrc.gov/clas/.

3. Recommendations: Suggestions by OMH for voluntary adoption by health care organizations (Standard 14).

The standards are organized by three themes, as follows:

1. Culturally competent care (Standards 1-3)
2. Language access services (Standards 4-7)
3. Organizational supports for cultural competence (Standards 8-14)[29]

THE CULTURE OF HEALTH

Cultural competence integrates health beliefs and cultural values, disease prevalence and incidence, and treatment efficacy in the following statements:

- Health is culture-bound.
- Culture influences the approaches to and definitions of health and healthy living.
- The conceptions and expressions of health are culturally determined and vary both between and within cultural groups.

How an individual or community perceives health, illness, and a disability is influenced by culture. Also influenced are attitudes toward health care providers and facilities and how health information is communicated. Culture can even have an impact on health-seeking behaviors, preferences for traditional versus nontraditional approaches to heath care, and perceptions regarding the role of family in health care.[30] It is important to know that individual beliefs about health and illness affect the delivery and provision of health care. Why groups are affected differently is also important, but this is sometimes more challenging to differentiate. Some cultural factors to consider include the following:

- Self-treatment strategies
- Body image
- Social networks and social support
- Family rituals
- Crisis management
- Dietary patterns
- Child-rearing practices
- Gender roles
- Beliefs about origins of disease
- Folklore
- Traditional healing beliefs and folk medicine

Why do we need to consider these cultural factors when working with clients and communities if, as health care providers, we are taught to treat everyone the same? People want to have their differences acknowledged and respected. By incorporating individualized, patient-centered care in the context of everyone's own culture, a higher quality of care is achieved (**Figure 10-8**).[31]

A cross-cultural approach to health care and healing does not eliminate the foundation of Western medical methods. Instead, it expands and enhances the ways that assess and deliver health care services by acknowledging, appreciating, and incorporating the beliefs, values, rituals, symbols, and standards of conduct that belong to the community we work with that may also affect its health status. The cross-cultural approach combines medical science and social science for the most effective outcomes.[31]

SUMMARY

To become a culturally competent oral health care provider, it is important to pursue broad efforts at all levels of oral health promotion and disease prevention. Cultural competency needs to be incorporated into all levels: personal, family, educational, community, organizational, administra-

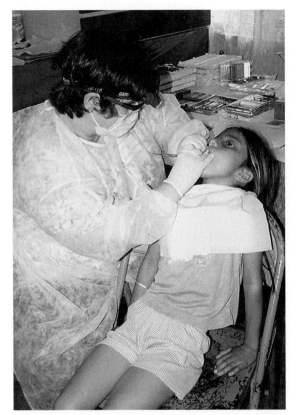

Figure 10-8 A dental hygiene student providing culturally competent oral health care to a patient at a nontraditional community setting with minimal resources.

tion, programs, and policies. It is up to the oral health care delivery system, the clinician, the health educator and wellness promoter, the consultant, the advocate, the researcher, and the administrator to value, implement, support, and foster cultural competency in every encounter made with a client. As oral health care providers, appreciating the key role culture plays in our ability to influence behavior in our clients in both one-on-one and community settings is vital. We cannot afford to let cultural barriers limit our ability to meet the oral health needs of our patients or reduce the opportunities to benefit from the services we can provide.

Community Case

You are the dental hygienist in a Community/Migrant Health Center. You have been asked by the Health Center Director to participate in applying for a grant to fund an interdisciplinary project for the elderly Asian clients of the health center. The grant will focus on health promotion and disease prevention.
1. Which of the following is not an important factor to learn about the community to enhance the cultural competency of the proposed grant?
   a. Social network and social support
   b. Tooth loss

    c. Dietary patterns

    d. Traditional healing beliefs and folk medicine

2. Select a cultural competency model that can be implemented into the grant that would meet the goals of the proposed grant, the community, and the researchers especially in six stages of personal development and expansion of becoming a culturally competent health care provider:

    a. Cultural Competency Continuum

    b. Cultural Competency Education Model

    c. LEARN Model

    d. OHCCC Guidelines

3. You are planning interdisciplinary service trainings for the health professionals that will be gathering and recording the data collected for the grant. Which of the following is not a factor that needs to be included in the training that can enhance cross-cultural communication?

    a. Be patient and flexible.

    b. Observe the client's body language.

    c. Demonstrate your professional knowledge by incorporating your discipline's terminology.

    d. Listen well to the client's questions and stories.

4. Health care providers working with a multicultural population do not need to alter their traditional ways of treating patients. It is understood in the health, medical, and dental communities that there is critical need to eliminate health disparities.

    a. The first statement is true, the second statement is false.

    b. The first statement is false, the second statement is true.

    c. Both statements are true.

    d. Both statements are false.

5. For the grant proposal, the interdisciplinary team will be developing appropriate educational materials for the clients. Utilizing the OHCCC guidelines, which is the most relevant for this task?

    a. Value diversity among peers and clients

    b. Adapt preventive and clinical oral health services with an understanding, acceptance, appreciation, and respect of cultural diversity.

    c. Be creative in finding ways to communicate with population groups that have limited English-speaking proficiency

    d. Understand the dynamics of the interactions between and within cultures

References

1. Krisber, K. Healthy People 2020 Tracking Social Determinants of Health: Input sought from Health Workforce. Nations Health 2008;38:1. American Public Health Association.
2. Cappelli, DP, Mobley, CC. Prevention in Clinical Oral Health Care. St. Louis, MO: Elsevier; 2008.
3. Parillo VN. Strangers To These Shores: Race and Ethnic Relationships in the United States. 5th ed. Boston: Allyn & Bacon; 1997.
4. Wells SA, Black RM. Cultural Competency For Health Professionals. Albany, NY: Boyd Printing; 2000.
5. Morey DP, Leung JJ. The multicultural knowledge of registered dental hygienists. J Dent Hygiene 1993;67:4.
6. University of Oregon's Summer Diversity Internships and Objectives, 1999.
7. US Bureau of the Census (2000). Available at www.census.gov/. Accessed August 2010.
8. US Department of Health and Human Services. Oral Health in America: A Report of the Surgeon General. Rockville, MD: US Department of Health and Human Services, National Institute of Dental and Craniofacial Research, National Institutes of Health; 2000.
9. Health Resources and Services Administration (HRSA). Eliminating Health Disparities: HRSA's Strategic Directions for Health Disparities. Washington, DC: US Department of Health and Human Services; 2001.

10. UCLA Center for Health Policy Research and Henry J. Kaiser Family Foundation. Racial and Ethnic Disparities in Access to Health Insurance and Health Care. Report #1525, April 2000, 800-656-4533. Los Angeles: UCLA; www.healthpolicy.ucla.edu. Accessed August 2010.

11. Mutha S, Allen C, Welch M. Toward Culturally Competent Care: A Toolbox for Teaching Communication Strategies. Center for the Health Professions, UCSF. Available at www.11.georgetown.edu/research/gucchd/ncc/. Accessed August 2010.

12. National Center for Cultural Competence of Georgetown University Center for Child and Human Development. Conceptual Frameworks, Models, Guiding Values and Principles. 2004. Available at www.11.georgetown.edu/research/gucchd/ncc/. Accessed August 2010.

13a. Diversity Rx Website. Supported by the National Conference of State Legislatures (NCSL), Resources for Cross Cultural Health Care (RCCHC). Washington, DC: Henry J. Kaiser Family Foundation. Available at www.diversityrx.org/HTML/ ESGLOS.htm. Accessed August 2010.

13b. US Department of Health and Human Services. Health Care Rx: Access For All Chartbook. Washington, DC: US Department of Health and Human Services; 1998.

14. Bentacourt, JR, Green AR, Carillo JE. Cultural Competence in Health Care: Emerging Frameworks and Practical Approaches. Washington, DC: Commonwealth Fund; October 2002.

15. Cross TL, Bazron BJ, Dennis KW, et al. Towards a Culturally Competent System of Care: Vol 1. Washington, DC: National Technical Assistance Center for Children's Mental Health, Georgetown University Child Development Center; 1989.

16. Pursuing Organizational and Individual Cultural Competency: An Epistemology of the Journey Toward Cultural Competency. Austin, TX: Texas Department of Health; 1998.

17. National Alliance of Hispanic Health. Quality Health Services for Hispanics: The Cultural Competency Component. DHHS Publication No. 99-21, 2001. Available at www.hispanichealth.org. Accessed August 2010.

18. Cohen E, Goode TD. Policy Brief 1: Rationale for Cultural Competence in Primary Health Care. Washington, DC: National Center for Cultural Competence; 1999. Available at www.dml.georgetown.edu/depts/pediatrics/gucdc/nccc6.html. Accessed August 2010.

19. US Department of Health and Human Services, Office of Minority Health. Closing the Gap: Moving Toward Consensus on Cultural Competency in Health Care. Rockville, MD: US Department of Health and Human Services; January 2000. Available at www.omhrc.gov/clas/. Accessed August 2010.

20. Kleinman A. Patients and Healers in the Context of Culture. Oakland, CA: The Regents of the University of California; 1981. Available at www.diversityrx.org/HTML/MOCPT3.htm. Accessed August 2010.

21. Institute of Medicine (IOM), Committee on Communication for Behavior. Change in the 21st Century: Improving the Health of Diverse Populations: Speaking of Health: Assessing Health Communication Strategies for Diverse Populations. Washington, DC: National Academies Press; 2003.

22. Purnell L. The Purnell model for cultural competence. J Transcult Nurs 2002;13:193.

23. Saha S, Beach MC, Cooper LA. Patient centeredness, cultural competence and healthcare quality. J Natl Med Assoc 2008;100:1275.

24. Levenstein JH, McCracken EC, McWhinney IR, et al. The patient-centered clinical method. 1. A model for the doctor-patient interaction in family medicine. Fam Pract 1986;3:24.

25. Stewart M, Brown J, Weston W, et al. Patient-Centered Medicine: Transforming the Clinical Method. London: Sage; 1995.

26. Stewart M, Brown JB, Weston WW, et al. Transforming the clinical method: patient-centered medicine. Abingdon, UK: Radcliffe Medical Press; 2003.

27. US Department of Health and Human Services, Office of Minority Health: Closing the Gap: Office of Minority Health Publishes Final Standards for Cultural and Linguistic Competence. Rockville, MD: February/March 2001. Available at www.omhrc.gov/clas/. Accessed August 2010.

28. US Department of Health and Human Services, Office of Minority Health. Closing the Gap: National Standards for Culturally and Linguistically Appropriate Services. Rockville, MD: March 2001. Available at www.omhrc.gov/clas/. Accessed August 2010.

29. US Department of Health and Human Services, Office of Minority Health. National Standards for Culturally and Linguistically Appropriate Services (CLAS). Rockville, MD: April 12, 2007. Available at www.omhrc.gov/clas. Accessed August 2010.

30. Denoba DL, Bragdon JL, Epstein LG, et al. Reducing health disparities through cultural competence. J Health Educ 1998;29(suppl):5.

31. Kaiser Permanente. Multicultural Caring: A Guide to Cultural Competence for Kaiser Permanente Health Professionals, 2000.

Additional Resources

Cotton CE, Tolman EE, Cardona Mack J. A Su Salud! New Haven, CT: Yale University Press; 2004.
www.yale.edu/yup/salud/

Addressing Cultural and Linguistic Competence in the HCH Setting. A Brief Guide.
www.nhchc.org/culturalcompetence0406.pdf

Bonder B, Martin L, Mireicle A. Culture in Clinical Care. Thorofare, NJ: Slack; 2002.

Bureau of Health Professions Division of Interdisciplinary Community-Based Programs
http://bhpr.hrsa.gov/interdisciplinary/

Bureau of Primary Health Care
http://bphc.hrsa.gov/

Centers for Disease Control and Prevention (CDC)
www.cdc.gov/

Centers for Medicare & Medicaid Services
www.cms.gov/

Cross-Cultural Health Care
www.xculture.org/

Cultural Competence Resources for Health Care Providers
www.hrsa.gov/culturalcompetence/

DHHS Initiative to Eliminate Racial and Ethnic Disparities in Health
www.raceandhealth.hhs.gov/

Diller JV, Moule J. Cultural Competence: A Primer for Educators. Belmont, CA: Thomas Wadsworth; 2005.

Diversity Rx
www.diversityrx.org/

Gropper RC. Culture and the Clinical Encounter: An Intellectual Sensitizer for the Health Professions. Yarmouth, MA: Intercultural Press; 1996.

Hogg Foundation for Mental Health
www.hogg.utexas.edu/PDF/Saldana.pdf

Health Resources and Services Administration
www.hrsa.gov/

Indian Health Service
www.ihs.gov/

Jeffreys MR. Teaching Cultural Competence in Nursing and Health Care. New York: Springer; 2006.

Lynch EW, Hanson MJ. Developing Cross-Cultural Competence: A Guide to Working with Children and their Families. Baltimore: Paul H. Brookes Publishing; 1998.

National Center for Cultural Competence (1-800-788-2066)
http://nccc.georgetown.edu/index.html

National Clearinghouse for Alcohol and Drug Information (1-800-729-6686)
http://ncadi.samhsa.gov/

National Education Association
www.nea.org/tools/30402.htm

National Institutes of Health (NIH)
www.nih.gov/

Office for Civil Rights
www2.ed.gov/about/offices/list/ocr/index.html

Office of Minority Health Resource Center (1-800-444-6472).

Pengra LM. Your Values, My Values: Multicultural Services in Developmentally Disabled. Baltimore: Paul H. Brookes Publishing; 2000.

Purnell LD, Paulanka BJ. Transcultural health care—a culturally competent approach. Philadelphia: F.A. Davis; 1998.

Rundle A, Carvalho M, Robinson M. Cultural Competence in Health Care: A Practical Guide. Hoboken, NJ: Jossey-Bass; 2002.

Srivastava R. The Healthcare Professional's Guide to Clinical Cultural Competence. St. Louis: Elsevier; 2007.

Substance Abuse and Mental Health Services Administration
www.samhsa.gov/

Service-Learning

Sheranita Hemphill, RDH, MPH, MS

Objectives

Upon completion of this chapter, the student will be able to:
- Discuss traditional outreach efforts.
- Discuss experiential learning methods and their unique purposes.
- Define service-learning and list distinguishing characteristics.
- List benefits of service-learning
- List the challenges of service learning.
- Use resources to plan and implement service-learning.

Key Terms

Experiential learning	Collaboration	Clinical rotation
Service-Learning (SL)	Orientation	Internship
Service objectives (SO)	Preparation	Practicum
Learning objectives (LO)	Reflection	Volunteerism
Service-Learning objectives (SLO)	Evaluation	Risk management
	Community service	

Opening Statements

Findings of Service-Learning Research in Higher Education Include the Following
- Service-Learning has a positive effect on student personal development such as a sense of personal efficacy, personal identity, spiritual growth, and moral development.
- Service-Learning has a positive effect on interpersonal development and the ability to work well with others, leadership skills, and communication skills.
- Service-Learning has a positive effect on reducing stereotypes and facilitating cultural and racial understanding.
- Service-Learning has a positive effect on social responsibility and citizenship skills.
- Service-Learning has a positive effect on commitment to service.
- Service-Learning contributes to career development.
- Students and faculty report that service-learning improves students' ability to apply what they have learned in the "real world."

From Eyler JS, Giles DE Jr, Stenson CM, et al. At a glance: What we know about the effects of service-learning on college students, faculty, institutions and communities, 1993–2000. 3rd ed. Boston: Learn and Serve America National Clearinghouse; 2001. Available at www.servicelearning.org/filemanager/download/aag.pdf.

Recent national health initiatives emphasized the need for community-based strategies to address oral health disparities. Consequentially, the national attention has caused a significant interest in the nation's oral health. Oral health conversations at the national, regional, and local sectors have increased and have led to extensive research, comprehensive publications, numerous conferences, and targeted programs focused on treatment and health promotion. The entire dental community has become involved in advancing the public's interest. The increasing national momentum has served to advance "dental" concerns to authentic public health issues and has presented an opportunity for dental hygiene education programs to contribute to the improvement of the oral health of the nation starting right in our neighborhoods.[1-7]

The oral health recommendations found in *Healthy People 2020* (see Chapter 4) and *Oral Health in America: A Report of the Surgeon General* (OHARSG) are a road map for change to the current method of teaching community dental health by dental hygiene education programs. If integrated into the dental hygiene curriculum, the recommendations will positively influence community dental hygiene instruction for students and community outreach dental hygienists. Preparing students for the public health workforce is arguably one of the most important outcomes for today's dental hygiene programs. Use of dental hygienists in community health programming requires that students acquire the knowledge and skills of the public health worker as this will contribute to advancing students' career options. These public health initiatives have made it clear that the dental community must respond to broader community issues, and the community dental health curriculum must be positioned to prepare students to work in this changing public health environment.[2,3,6-8,9]

This chapter focuses on a learning technique through which the existing community-based dental hygiene curriculum can be enhanced to better meet the oral public health needs of the community. In addition, it provides guidance and suggestions designed to prepare dental hygiene students to address oral health disparities in their communities. It challenges students to use their dental hygiene education as the foundation for future public health career opportunities. Integrating the objectives of the nation's health agenda, as outlined in national public health initiatives, into the dental hygiene curriculum positions the dental hygiene profession into the public health arena more decisively and affects the public's oral health positively.

DENTAL HYGIENE COMMUNITY SERVICE OUTREACH EFFORTS

Traditional Outreach Efforts

Historically, dental hygiene students have provided community dental health outreach for diverse populations. Educational methods used to prepare dental hygiene students to instruct these populations include health education lectures with a focus on lesson plan development and implementation. The benefits of these methods are excellent in preparing dental hygiene students to deliver effective oral health messages but fall short of preparing students to anticipate or meet the needs of the public's oral health challenges.[10-13] Further assessment reveals that the primary benefit of traditional outreach instruction and methodology is the acquisition of technical skills in a short time frame.[14-17] Though these methods provide practical experience in organizing a presentation, and they assist dental hygiene students in perfecting their presentation techniques, they are prone to be one-shot, short-term projects, rendering the aim to favorably affect oral health behavior as insufficient.

Long-term strategies are needed to improve the oral health behavior of populations for lifelong benefits. Behavioral change is an integral component of effective oral health promotion strategies (see Chapter 8). Students often complain that their patients do not follow their oral health instructions. Practicing dental hygienists are all too familiar with this sentiment. However, once the experienced hygienist realizes that oral health "instructions," delivered in one appointment, do not translate into better oral health behaviors, they eventually start treating their patients as individuals.

They design oral health education messages that are spread out over time, and they ensure that the messages are individually tailored to the language, reading level, and cultural perspective. They stop assuming that everyone values oral health as much as they do; instead, they ask the patients what is important to them. Experienced hygienists begin to incorporate the assistance of the patients' significant others for support, and they integrate cultural specific information so that the patients can perceive benefits for themselves (see Chapter 10). In effect, they use theories of health education to motivate, educate, and empower their patients. To positively affect health behavior, dental hygiene students must acquire knowledge of health education theories and the basic principles of health promotion and they must design and implement ongoing projects using them.[8,15,16]

Dental hygiene students can contribute to the national oral health agenda. Imagine the oral health benefits if the dental hygiene programs in the United States adopted a standard approach of instructing students in community dental health outreach efforts. What would be the impact if all the programs used *Healthy People 2020* Objectives in developing durable community dental health projects? Likewise, envision the possibilities of comparing oral health outcomes across the country.

Adopting a standard teaching method for implementing community dental health outreach would prepare the dental and dental hygiene programs to answer such questions as asked by Indiana University School of Dentistry professor, Dr. Karen Yoder: "Do dental graduates internalize an appropriate vision of their role as a health professional in the context of community?"[17] Programs would be able to consistently evaluate and measure the impact of their collective public health efforts. The oral health promotional efforts and results of dental hygiene students could then move beyond the anecdotal; their efforts could have a lasting impact on the nation's oral health.

Short-term community outreach provides little opportunity for community members to become empowered with the skills and knowledge they need to sustain the intended goals of the program. Likewise, short-term community dental health outreach provides inadequate opportunity for dental hygiene students to become proficient in applying theoretic concepts and for investigating public health career options in depth. Finally, short-term community dental health outreach efforts inhibit the development of a collective national oral health agenda for the dental hygiene programs in the country.[3,4,8,18-19]

Experiential Outreach Efforts

Experiential learning, commonly referred to as "practical learning" or "real-world learning," originated from the grassroots research of such theorists as John Dewey, Kurt Lewin, Jean Piaget, and Carl Rogers. Experiential learning is an umbrella term that references various models of learning in which experience governs the learning process.

A specific example of experiential learning is first-year dental hygiene students who enrolled in a didactic dental radiology course are learning how to interpret radiographic findings. Thus far, the instructor and the dental hygiene students are not pleased with the retention and comprehension of the content. The dental radiology course instructor and a secondary education teacher decide to collaborate for mutual benefit by providing an environment in which experience is

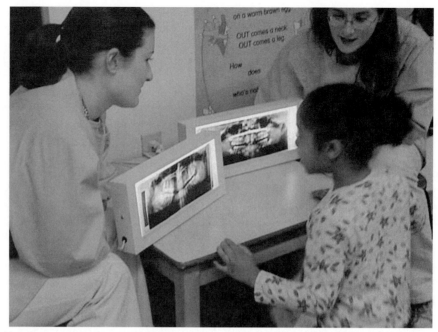

Figure 11-1 First-year students reinforcing their acquired radiographic interpretation skills through teaching.

dominant in the learning process. The dental hygiene students can connect their didactic learning with the real need of the high school teacher's objectives for his or her students through experiential learning. The dental hygiene students have to design age-appropriate activities and present on radiographic findings to the group of high school students. The traditional methods of lectures, textbook reading, and even radiographic interpretation exercises are enhanced because of the practical application of those methods. Active learning becomes experienced learning just as experience learning becomes active learning.

Experiential learning changes the focus of learning, shifting it from the confines of the classroom to the community. Classroom learning is supplemented with purposeful work-based learning opportunities within the community, and to ensure that the course objectives are being met, the students apply their program planning skills with guidance from their faculty and from the community partner. Experiential outreach efforts should place emphasis on tasks that contribute to the students' knowledge base (**Figure 11-1**).

Experiential Learning Theory is Different from Cognitive Learning Theory

In the cognitive approach, theorists see learning as primarily a mental process in which the learner is able to recall acquired facts and figures. Unlike cognitive learning, experiential learning incorporates personal experiences (a known concept) with the application of new skills. For example, here is a case in which personal experience is incorporated in the learning. A service-learning team of dental hygiene students meets to plan oral health activities for a youth group. Only one of the dental hygiene students has previous experience working with this population and quickly mobilizes the dental hygiene team into action. Experiential learning benefits students through growth opportunities resulting from civic participation.

Cognitive knowledge is very important in experiential learning, but it should be used in conjunction with experiential methods for increased proficiency in interpreting situations and acting appropriately. If, for example, a dental hygiene student finds that the caregivers in a long-term facility are reluctant to provide frequent oral health care to the patients, the student's efforts may be better spent by having the group of caregivers brainstorm for a decision regarding what is reasonable in their circumstances. In this example, although the student is fully aware of what the literature says regarding the removal of prostheses during the night, they are also able to interpret the fact that the habits of the staff are not going to be changed quickly but gradually.

GUIDING PRINCIPLES

Outcomes of Experiential Learning
- Connects classroom learning with authentic situations
- Continuously reinforces learned knowledge and skills through practical experience
- Challenges the student to think critically in addressing real needs
- Increases aptitude for teaching various populations
- Enhances the skills of the dental hygiene workforce

Experiential learning takes place in authentic situations. A Women, Infant, and Children's (WIC) facility is a good example of a service-learning setting in which a broader understanding of oral health is necessary to effect change for a lifetime. In the community health course, students are learning about the social determinants of oral health. They are shown an image of a woman standing in line at a local WIC facility. They are asked to document their thoughts about this woman, and this is followed by small group discussions that explore the social determinants of oral health. Without actually interacting with the woman, how can they really know what her visits to the WIC facility signify? Perhaps she is seeking nutritional provisions for her child, but is that all? In assisting this woman, the students will have to use their learned skills to "see" beyond the obvious. The dental hygiene students need to apply cognitive skills, such as the recall of facts regarding the mission of the public health facility, but they will also need to construe other oral health needs that the mother and her family may have; the reality is bigger than the image. In this case, the dental hygiene students will learn more because they construct the strategies that they will use to assist this family. They are brainstorming, sharing, and reminding each other to be thoughtful and use evidence-based discussions rather than anecdotal opinionated fragments of thought. In essence, they are learning through experience. Experiential learning links genuine learning opportunities to the classroom and the textbook material.[20-22]

THE ARRAY OF EXPERIENTIAL LEARNING METHODS

The spectrum of experiential learning methods in health professions education is broad, and the decision regarding which method to use should be determined by the intended goal. As such, care must be taken in choosing methods that are reflective of the goal. It is not unusual for multiple experiential methods to be used in health professions education. **Box 11-1** is a list of common experiential methods and their unique purposes.

BOX 11-1 **Experiential Learning Methods**

Community Service

Students provide a service to the community, and the primary focus is on the community's needs. This activity may or may not have a curriculum connection. The student may provide the service for reasons other than a classroom assignment (e.g., club requirement, religious obligation).

Clinical Rotation

Clinical rotation is a curriculum-based activity not necessarily associated with a service outcome and is designed primarily to benefit the student learning. Students are assigned rotation through clinical experiences so that their skills, knowledge, and expertise are enhanced.

Practicum/Internship

A practicum/internship is typically longer than a clinical rotation and is designed to benefit the student. In this instance, the student may be assigned to work in a particular specialty area for an entire academic quarter or semester. An example of practicum/internship is when a dental hygiene bachelor's completion program assigns senior students to various public health agencies, higher education institutions, and governmental agencies for the practical experience of on-the-job exposure and training.

Volunteerism

Students provide a service to the community, and the major benefit is for the community. This activity is not necessarily associated with an academic course. Examples include assisting at the concession stands at an athletic event and/or participating in a secondary tutoring program.

SERVICE-LEARNING AND ITS DISTINGUISHING CHARACTERISTICS

Service-Learning Defined

Service-Learning (SL) is one of the many techniques of experiential learning. Definitions of SL may vary, but they all imply equality between the service as received by the community partner and the learning for the dental hygiene students. Essentially, SL is a jointly structured learning experience between the community partner and the academic course of instruction. The definition of SL by the Community Campus Partnership for Health (CCPH), a nationally recognized organization whose mission includes the improvement of the health of the public, has remained relevant and consistent in its description. CCPH executive director, Sarena Seifer, MD, has defined SL in the following manner[23]:

> Service-Learning is a structured learning experience that combines community service with preparation and reflection. Students engaged in service-learning provide community service in response to community-identified concerns and learn about the context in which service is provided, the connection between their service and their academic coursework, and their roles as citizens.

This definition promotes collaboration between communities and health professions educational institutions, and the planning and implementation of SL clearly illustrates the collaboration. The community partner's objectives are called **service objectives (SO)**—a service is desired. The academic course objectives are called **learning objectives (LO)**—academic course desired learn-

BOX 11-2 **Service-Objectives Defined**

Service Objectives (SO)	Learning Objectives (LO)	Service-Learning Objectives (SLO)
The SO is a written statement of need provided by the agency. Through this process, dental hygiene students are positioned to provide a needed service as opposed to what they think is needed.	This is the course LO. Note that not all LO are appropriate for SL programs. LOs that require higher-level thinking (e.g., exploring barriers to oral health access) are best for SL experiences.	The SLO is the result of combining the LO with the SO. Ideally, the community partner should work with the students to combine the objectives. If this is not possible, the partner should be given the chance to modify the SLO.

ing. Through intentional thoughtfulness, the SO and the LO are combined, forming **service-learning objectives (SLO)**. **Box 11-2** summarizes each of the three objectives.

The equal weighing of the SO and the LO is a classic feature of SL. Note that even the configuration of the words "service-learning" illustrates that both the service and the learning are equivalent. The "S" in service and the "L" in learning are always written in identical fashion, either capitalized or in lower-case letters.[19,23,24] Also note that, in this chapter, a hyphen is used to emphasize that the service and the learning are "connected." The service is a community task, and the learning is the academic goal.[19,24,25]

The end-product of SL is not a one-way directional process. In other words, both the community and the academic institution's students are learning from the experience. What about the service aspect of SL; do both parties contribute to the service side of SL? If service is thought of as something received, both sides are beneficiaries. The community partner is a recipient of the skills, knowledge, and expertise of the dental hygiene program, and the dental hygiene student is the recipient of the outcomes of the exposure afforded by way of the community partner.[25]

GUIDING PRINCIPLES

Ideas that Can Be Integrated into Service-Learning Projects
- Develop a brochure listing dental public health resources, including Safety Net facilities.
- Plan and conduct a Basic Screening Survey (BSS) and issue oral health "report cards."
- Identify public and private dental facilities that are currently accepting public health insurance (Medicaid) and assist families in finding dental homes.
- Assist the school nurse in following up with dental referrals.
- Collaborate with local law enforcement/students to promote child safety by performing bite impressions for use in identification of children.
- Assist the community in assessing the adequacy of their community water fluoridation.
- Develop and implement oral health lesson plans for allied health students and/or other health professionals (e.g., medical doctors, nurses).

SL is not a substitute for traditional classroom instruction nor does it assist in the learning pursuit. For example, when students are learning about the socioeconomic status of the population, the textbook may be used to convey background information about the subject. In addition to specific textbook readings, students may also read a journal article and additional details may be gathered from the Internet, other media, and classroom lectures. Each of these assignments may add to the knowledge base; however, all require little active involvement, hence retention and comprehension are compromised.[26] An active learning approach requires multiple levels of consideration and can contribute to a deeper understanding of the subject. With SL, students are expected to integrate the SO of the community partner and incorporate previous and concurrent learning into the assignment. In this way, students are assisting in the construction of their own learning and fulfilling the course objectives while fulfilling the desires of a community partner.

GUIDING PRINCIPLES

Service-Learning Contributions to Classroom Learning
- Students become active learners as they construct much of the learning experience.
- Exposure to oral public health becomes a reality as SL projects require action such as the utilization of national and local public health resources.
- Course content is relevant and timely as the national and local oral public health issues are firmly linked to the curriculum.
- Students see the big picture; their professional roles are clearly linked to the national health issues identified in *Healthy People 2020* (the nation's health objectives).

The following is an example of how the SO and the LO may be combined. A community organization, which educates children with social learning disabilities such as Asperger syndrome and attention deficit disorder, wants the children to recognize the social context of the smell of breath and its relationship to oral hygiene behaviors. The organization's SO is for the dental hygiene students to teach the children how and why they should keep their mouths clean. The two most fitting academic course LOs for the dental hygiene students are (1) to discuss the current literature regarding the oral microbial flora and its relationship to halitosis and (2) to deliver educational content in an appropriate approach. Combining the community partner's objectives and the academic course objects may result in a SL objective such as "the dental hygiene students will use imagery of a pollution overcast caused by the varied automotive fumes as an analogy to relate halitosis as the result of the crowded collection of bacteria on the tongue."

In this case, as in all SL experiences, the dental hygiene students will have provided a community service in response to community-identified needs. In the process, the dental hygiene students are provided an opportunity to learn about oral bacteria in a different way, they learn about the circumstances of the group, they work synergistically to generate creative and appropriate learning opportunities, and they contribute a public health service. Learning is optimized. What about the needs of the community partner—the children? What could the possible outcomes be? How could those outcomes be assessed? The next section provides some answers by elaborating on the unique features and requirements of a true SL experience.

Distinguished Characteristics of Service Learning

Service-Learning is distinguished from other experiential methods by distinct features. Characterized as principles of SL, these features are universally understood as ideals that must be present for an experiential learning experience to truly be a SL experience. Through comparison of other types of experiential learning experiences and teaching and learning methods, it should

BOX 11-3   Yoder's Framework for Service-Learning in Dental Education

Scholarship	Partnerships	Programs	Growth
Academic link Community-engaged scholarship	Sustained community partnerships Service-Learning objectives Broad preparation	Sustained service Reciprocal learning	Guided reflection Community engagement Evaluation and improvement

be noted that the collective use of these principles is not typical in educating dental hygiene students.

The literature on SL spans many disciplines in higher education. The terms used to define and discuss SL are assorted; however, the mixed terminology used to discuss SL is often no more than a collection of mere synonyms. SL models serve to protect the integrity of SL as a teaching method by acting as blueprints for the construction of SL experiences. The SL Protocol for Health Professions Schools (SLPHPS) consists of seven guidelines used as a model for SL in any health profession. Collectively, these are referred to as the essential components of SL (see Guiding Principles). Developed by the Center for Healthy Communities (CHC), a nationally known academic-community partnership in Ohio, SLPHPS is one of the most-often used models. Yoder's framework of SL in dental education consists of ten essential components, with a clear-cut emphasis on dental professions education (**Box 11-3**). Both models provide a structure to discuss, plan, implement, and evaluate SL experiences, and both emphasize the necessity of integrating the community partner in all aspects of the experience, from conceptionalization to the ongoing evaluation phase. SL models promote the essential characteristics and serve as a solid foundation, without which SL is ill defined.*

Community Partner Collaboration

Collaboration means working together to accomplish a goal. Other words that may come to mind when thinking about collaboration include "joint effort," "teamwork," or "partnership." In SL projects, the program is jointly planned by the course instructor, the community partner, and the students. The parties collaborate to ensure that the needs of all are met. The faculty is interested in making sure that student LOs are attended to, the community partner is interested in ensuring that its organization's needs are met, and the dental hygiene students are interested in applying their health education knowledge and skills.

In traditional community projects, dental hygiene faculty typically initiated the communications leading to a community service experience for the dental hygiene students. The faculty would contact an agency representative and inform them that they wanted to place dental hygiene students in their organization to gain community experience. With SL, either the faculty, community partner, or the student can initiate the conversation. The community agency can contact the faculty to request the services of the dental hygiene students, and likewise, the student can initiate the discussion by contacting an agency to discuss the possibility of developing a mutually beneficial project. In this instance, the students must identify the appropriate LO from the course syllabus,

*References 8, 17, 19, 23-25, 28.

work with the agency representative to identify their needs or SO, and must also receive consent from the faculty.

Mutual Objective Formation

The needs of the community partner are referred to as the SOs, and they are developed from their mission statement. Student course objectives are referred to as LOs, and they originate from the guidelines of the Commission on Dental Accreditation (CODA) Standards for Dental Hygiene Education Programs and the dental hygiene competencies developed by the Section on Dental Hygiene Education of the American Dental Education Association (ADEA). The collective standards serve as the model for all dental hygiene programs.[29,30]

The SO and the LO are deliberately combined for mutual benefit to form the SLO, and this is not completed in isolation. It is important for the students, the agency, and the faculty to become acquainted with each other's missions, populations, objectives, operations, and facilities. Clear communication and face-to-face meetings are good approaches to gaining insight to the different perspectives, after which they can jointly determine how their objectives may be combined for mutual benefit.

In an example of mutual objective formation, an elementary district's school nurse contacts the dental hygiene faculty for assistance in securing dental homes for children needing immediate care. The faculty meets with the school nurse, preferably face-to-face, and they discuss a possible collaboration. The faculty then presents the project of finding "dental homes" for low socioeconomic status (SES) public elementary school children. The school teacher is satisfied because this meets the needs of the school district's curriculum; the summarized SO is to keep children healthy for classroom learning. The LO of the dental hygiene faculty are met in that the project will actively engage their students in demonstrating proficiency in advocating for populations with no or inadequate dental insurance. The dental hygiene students are equally satisfied because they finally get the opportunity to apply their program planning skills.

After considering the SO, the students decide which of the course's LOs will work best with the school's need. They may choose one or multiple LOs. After informing the school nurse of their LO, the students and the school nurse jointly combine their respective objectives, which are then presented to the faculty for assessment. The planning for the SL program can now proceed.

Exercise. In the space below, combine the LO and SO from the scenario above into at least one SLO.

_____

_____

Orientation

A formal **orientation** provides an opportunity for all parties to get acquainted, to become familiar with each other's facilities, and to plan the SL experience. A formal orientation provides a forum for the agency representative to become more familiar with the level of student expertise, the course objectives, and the history of the students' community service exposure. Similarly, students become familiar with the agency, its staff, and the population. The smallest of details is addressed.

The agenda for the orientation should include a community partner presentation, which will provide an overview of the organization and its needs. The overview is often accomplished through an oral presentation supplemented with informational pamphlets and followed by a question and answer session. Ideally, the orientation should occur in two steps; one should take place at the dental hygiene program's site, and the other should occur at the community agency's site. Orientations serve several purposes, including increasing the familiarity of all stakeholders with each location. A few of the purposes of orientation are listed below, and many more can be found by searching through the Internet resources at the end of this chapter.

- Risk management and relevant policy and procedures guidelines can be discussed.
- The Health Insurance Portability and Accountability Act (HIPAA) regulations can be reviewed.
- Appropriate attire, including protective wear, can be determined.
- The expectations of the community partner and those of the students can be discussed.
- Issues of transportation, directions, and parking can be assessed.
- Work space for student workers may not be available, yet may be needed.
- The availability of lockers for students' personal belongings can be assessed.

A formal orientation minimizes disruptions to the SL program. It ensures the appropriateness of the facilities, and it provides an occasion for all parties to discuss concerns and resolve issues for the success of the SL program.

Preparation

Preparation involves program planning skills that have been presented in another chapter in this textbook. With the use of previously learned team-building skills, activities are brainstormed, roles are identified, action plans and contingency plans are developed, and timelines are set. Student leadership skills evolve as each student takes responsibility for the success of the program outcomes.

In a scenario illustrating preparation, an urban child-development program partnered with a dental hygiene program to expand oral health access for the children in three of the public elementary schools. Ms. Kane, the director of a local children's program, and the three principals participated in the orientation phase. Ms. Kane presented background information using oral presentation and multimedia resources that depicted captivating scenes from each of the schools.

The principals introduced themselves and provided an overview of their school's history, demographics, and the economic status of the families. The dental hygiene students were divided into three teams, and each team was assigned to one of the three schools. The students then met with the respective principal and began the process of team building.

Eventually, each team developed an overall goal for their SL project, uniquely tailored for the particular school's needs. Using relative course objectives from the syllabus and the service objective articulated by the principals, the teams developed SLO and evaluation measures. Everyone took an active role in the program planning, and this contributed to the overall success of the SL plan.

This is but one example of the process. Alternate planning strategies could include having the dental hygiene students select a school rather than being assigned, or they could also be assigned randomly. The dental hygiene students could have also visited each school for observational purposes before deciding on a choice. The LO could have been taken directly from the public school district's curriculum, or the elementary children could have generated their own "wish list" of desired learning. Regardless of the process, LO could have also been distributed to the dental hygiene students for further consideration.

Service-Learning Experience

At this point, the program is ready to be implemented. Previously developed SL lesson plans and evaluation tools are used in this phase of the SL project. **Figure 11-2** is a SL lesson plan template.

Reflection

Reflection involves critical thinking and critical expressions about the SL experience and the specific encounters. The aim of reflection is to draw meaning from the experience. The aim is not to develop skills of criticizing for the sake of being critical. Empathy, public health advocacy, and solutions are necessary. Reflection involves self and societal appraisal. A desired outcome is for the dental hygiene student to intellectually discuss the surrounding social, cultural, and economic events that have contributed to the shape of the situation.

Reflection is not intended to be a condemning session aimed at the "system"; its purpose is to assist in the formation of informed knowledge by permitting the dental hygiene students to consider course content in relation to the multiple sociologic factors affecting the situation.[8,25,31] Essentially, theoretic content has been applied in the community, and reflective activities permit the students to process the experiences encountered and place them in the context of the course objectives.

Some researchers liken the hyphen in SL to the idea of reflection. In this instance the hyphen forces the dental hygiene student to pause and consider the implications of the SL project. Students should entertain critical questions regarding the experience. The hyphen symbolizes the importance of processing the SL experience. One could question whether an experience without reflection was really an experience. Ideally, students should first consider the SL experience introspectively and then dialog with the other students, the instructor, and the community partner.

Deliberate reflection that is connected to the LO and the SO helps to illuminate the SL project in its entirety. Reflection helps to clarify the thinking process. Questions are carefully considered and posed with the objectives in mind. Thinking skills are challenged in the process of helping students see the connection between course content, dental public health issues, and the sociocultural environment from which they exist.

Review **Box 11-4** for further reflection ideas. Specific formats for conducting reflective sessions offer additional guidance and can be located by researching the Internet resources located at the end of this chapter. Questions, poster presentations, roundtable discussions, audiovisual presentations, and keeping journals all offer reflective opportunities to help students consider the quality of the process and the outcome.

Evaluation

Implementation of the **evaluation** phase actually begins with the initial program planning conversations, at the orientation when all stakeholders are present. In order to evaluate any program the criteria for measuring the project's objectives must be determined first. Establishing a way to measure the degree of satisfaction with a particular objective outcome must be made explicitly at the onset.

Take a look at the following SLO. At the end of this module, the dental hygiene student will explain three characteristics of manual dexterity of a specific population of children 3 to 6 years old and present at least one strategy to assist in daily oral hygiene care.

SERVICE-LEARNING LESSON PLAN

Student Hygienist's Name _____

Date _____

Agency _____

Contact Person _____

Address _____ Phone _____ FAX _____

Email _____

Audience _____ Age _____

Service Objective	Learner Objective	Service-Learning Objective

Concepts	Strategies	Time
1	1	1
2	2	2

Materials Needed	Resources Used

EVALUATION

Basic Questions: What went well? What will I change in the future? What additional materials or resources were needed?

Formative Measures:

Summative Measures:

Figure 11-2 Service-learning lesson plan template.

BOX 11-4 Reflection Methods

- Have the community partners facilitate prepared and impromptu discussion sessions
- Present a poster session and invite the entire college and community
- Organize roundtable discussions where the senior students present their findings to the junior students
- Incorporate audiovisual into any reflection method
- Perform guided journaling that addresses the connection, challenges, context, and continuity of the service-learning (SL) experience
- Create a website that highlights the continuous nature of the SL efforts of your school
- Develop an evaluation instrument to be implemented in future SL programs
- Publish an article in a dental hygiene newsletter or journal

This is the point from which the evaluation discussions should start. The dental hygiene students may draft the initial evaluation procedure, but the community partner must provide input into the shaping of the evaluation procedure. Collaboration is an integral component of the SL process. Remember, including the community partner is not a courtesy, it is an obligation in SL.

A main point of evaluation is to strengthen programs. If there is no standard way of assessing satisfaction, there is no objective way for all of the stakeholders to continuously assess and improve the SL program. The evaluation phase presents an opportunity to increase the sustainability of the program, to keep it going, to fortify the program and make it stand on its own. The task of developing standards to judge program outcomes is a very important joint process and should involve all patients.[5,18,24-26]

Evaluation: Work Smarter Not Harder

Evaluation is both a formative (continuous) and summative (end) process. If your team knows that program evaluation is continuous, they may be able to work smarter. For example, one group of students wrote in their journal, "We were prepared for a much larger crowd, so the presentation had to become much more informal. The program became more personal due to the small size of the group." In this example, the dental hygiene students were able to assess the situation while executing the program and they made changes based upon their collective knowledge of the SL components. Because it is a dynamic process it is very constructive in increasing the potential for program success.

Evaluation that occurs at the end of the program is known as summative evaluation. It can be thought of as an end-report which summarizes the degree of success of each objective. It compares the actual outcomes against standards of measurement previously developed. A well written report summarizes the program, objectively informs all parties regarding the impact of the program, and can go a long way in determining the future of other programs. **Table 11-1** provides formative and summative evaluation measures.

USING NATIONAL DATA SOURCES IN EVALUATING SERVICE-LEARNING

Program objectives and evaluation measures do not have to be created from scratch. National agendas, such as *Healthy People,* provide a perfect platform for program planning for smaller

Table 11-1 **Formative And Summative Evaluation Measures**

Category of Evaluation	*Service-Learning Objective*	*Example Measures*
Summative	At the end of this program, the dental hygiene students will be able to conduct an oral health family assessment to determine and incorporate the resources, priorities, and concerns of the family.	Increase in skill development (interviewing skill), awareness (cultural awareness), knowledge (knowledge of resources), and outlook (socioeconomic perspective).
Formative	At the end of this program, the dental hygiene students will be able to use national data sources to compile appropriate oral health information from different ethnic and racial populations.	Number of resources used, adequacy of materials, scope of resources, and accuracy of measurement.

communities. State, regional, and local oral health advocacy organizations work smarter when they realize that their goals are not necessarily unique and that many resources are available to assist in their goals.

One example is *Healthy People 2020.* The oral health chapter in the *Healthy People 2020* publication provides criteria that could serve as common standards for meeting the oral health objectives of the nation. Specific oral health objectives, baseline data, and targets for improvement of oral health diseases for a variety of populations are included. These standards can be modified for use in dental hygiene programs across the country. Use of the *Healthy People 2020* baseline and targets as the evaluation norm adds a dimension of consistency to community dental health programs, and it assists everyone in assessing the success of the community dental health program objectives.[3-5]

BENEFITS OF SERVICE-LEARNING

Student Benefits

Service-Learning can foster leadership, cultural competency, lifelong learning, and a commitment to caring for the underserved. SL involvement may ultimately contribute to increased civic responsibility. SL projects can increase students' awareness of the social and political topics and processes, and it may encourage students to become actively involved in civic responsibilities.[1,24,28]

In SL projects, dental hygiene students are exposed to multiple aspects of diversity, which can foster a healthy appreciation for the differences they experience and thereby reduce stereotypical ideas and behaviors. These opportunities include exposure to different populations, different religions, various neighborhoods, different levels of wellness, and mental and physical abilities. When students reflect about the social determinants of health that are known factors in health and wellness conditions, they are challenged to view the community's endurance in a nonstereotypical manner, perhaps even as an asset. They are able to explore sensitive issues in the secure environment of the classroom, before they encounter such instances in the world of work.

Personal contact with community members that are different from "you" encourages personal growth, broadens horizons, decreases the tendency to stereotype, and increases interpersonal skills.

Many health profession students have never cared for or spoken to someone of a different culture or race, and understandably the first time may be uncomfortable. But when placed into perspective, it is much simpler to gain this exposure in the comfort of an SL experience. In this instance faculty guidance, community partnering mentoring, and multiple opportunities for reflection can make a great difference in personal and professional growth.[10,18,22,27,28]

As dental hygiene students become acquainted with the local resources in their communities, the practical implications become clearer. Students can apply this knowledge to the patients that they care for in the clinical dental hygiene settings. SL turns the theoretic into the practical when concepts that were once considered complex and ambiguous become clearer to students who put them into practice. In summary, students engaged in SL are more likely to make the connection between their service and their academic coursework. They provide community service in response to community-identified concerns, and they learn in the context of the service provided.

Community Partner Benefits

A major benefit to the community partner is the opportunity to create long-term community-campus relationships. Activities to foster retention of the community partners are essential, and they are specific to the needs of the community partner. The dental hygiene faculty can invite a particularly supportive community partner to serve on the dental hygiene department's advisory committee. Or, the dental hygiene faculty could provide the agency's staff with an oral health continuing education session during an academic term in which the dental hygiene students are not available to participate in an SL project. Thus the continued contact with the community partner serves to minimize the disruption of the established SL program, and the continuity of the SL project is maintained. Additional community partner benefits are listed below. See if you can add one more benefit to the list. Add your selection as number 5, and see what your peers developed.

Additional Community Partner Benefits

1. Increased access to expertise from the academy
2. Affirmation of the agency's mission
3. Contribution to health professions education through mentoring
4. Extended service delivery through student contributions
5. _____

Benefits for the Nation's Oral Health Agenda

Oral Health in America: A Report of the Surgeon General clearly articulated the public health benefit of expanding the services provided by dental hygienists. SL, while rapidly evolving as a teaching and learning development, has also shown promise in its ability to assist health profession students meet the health objectives that are outlined in the nation's health agenda. In addition to placing dental hygiene students in the customary sites for dental health education, students can also be placed in long-term community-based settings. Long-term SL projects provide for expanded access, continuity of care, curriculum integration, outcomes assessment, and evaluation.[6,7,23-25]

Issues of access to health care are challenging, and nationally health profession schools are moving towards sustained community-based partnerships. As such, the dental health professions need to actively investigate effective means to instruct students to participate fully in these part-

BOX 11-5 Summary of Service-Learning Benefits

Students	Agency	Faculty
Exposure to multiple aspects of diversity	Partnering in educating future health professions students	Increases the training sites
Practical application of team skills and didactic content	Lasting community-campus relationships	Course enrichment
Secure environment for discussing sensitive issues	Real needs addressed	Increased awareness of community needs, resources, and strengths
Enhance self-confidence, interpersonal and leadership skills	Continuous community-campus relationships	Support the mission of the institution
Preparation for leadership role in dental hygiene organizations	Increased visibility of agency and its mission	Enhancement of scholarship and professional growth
Potential for interdisciplinary learning and collaboration	Increased networking opportunity	Meets core educational requirements
Cross-cultural skill development	Continuing education	Work experience with experts in the field
Explore career options	Use of academic resources such as Institutional Planning and Research	Meeting of academic goals of service, scholarship, and teaching

nerships. Service-Learning has tremendous potential to reduce the unmet dental needs of the underinsured, uninsured, underserved, and underrepresented. **Box 11-5** presents a summary of the SL benefits for the various stakeholders.

CHALLENGES OF SERVICE-LEARNING

Service-Learning challenges are encountered by all of the stakeholders: students, faculty, and academic partners. However, the approaches to managing the issues encountered with SL are unique in that they vary depending upon the SL project. However, SL challenges are embraced as a valuable element in experiential learning. **Table 11-2** is a partial listing of the challenges facing students, faculty, and the community partner.

Program planning for SL does not occur in a space devoid of situational challenges. **Risk management** is a phrase that suggests that such exposures might be managed with organizational influence. Academic institutions and community organizations are likely to have their very own risk management departments. The function of such offices may serve as an institutional clearinghouse whose primary responsibility is guidance in formulating risk management procedures for the purpose of implementing SL experiences. The academic institution may have an affiliation agreement that it requires the community partner to sign, and likewise, the community partner may have a similar agreement for the faculty and a policy document for the students to sign. Management of challenges and resources to assist with sustaining SL provide essential quality control.

Table 11-2   Challenges Facing Students, Faculty, And The Community Partner

Student Challenges	Suggestions
Indifference	Provide service-learning (SL) training
	Link the experience to future employment options
	Include students in the planning
Optional status in curriculum	Integrate SL into the curriculum
	Course credit should be awarded
Dilemmas	Develop contingency plans for unexpected occurrences
	Develop the objectives with the agency partner

Community Agency Challenges	Suggestions
Previous negative experience with faculty and/or students	Get to know each other's programs, services, and needs
	Develop a mutual mission statement
	Plan the SL experience together
	Emphasize team planning, shared responsibility, and individual accountability
	Provide SL training session
Lack of continuity of service	Provide agency staff with professional development sessions in the nonacademic quarters
Lack of real authority	Reference the partner as "community faculty"
	Partner participation in reflection and evaluation
Time	Advance planning is critical
	Heavy workload initially, but diminishes with time

Faculty Challenges	Suggestions
Hidden agendas	Conduct research jointly with the agency
Time	Advance planning is critical
	Heavy workload initially, but diminishes with time
	Secure grants to support your service outreach
	Get a faculty mentor
Promotion	Document your work using portfolios, publications, and presentations
	Examine the institution's mission for service statements. Serve on the promotion and tenure committees to ensure a voice at the table
Colleagues' acceptance	Advocate for the inclusion of SL as a topic at conferences
Assumptions	What is obvious to faculty is not the case for students
	Do the work required to get students to perceive the obvious

Leaders in the field of experiential learning suggest that all stakeholders involved in the planning and implementing of SL projects should also be involved in planning for risk management. The issue of risks involving the students, the faculty, the academic institution, the community agency, and the community members should be discussed openly, and strategies should be developed and distributed to all parties. Contingency planning, documentation, and review are prudent components of experiential learning opportunities.[14,23] A few of the issues that will need to be considered for inclusion in risk management discussions include those found in **Box 11-6**.

BOX 11-6 **Risk Management Considerations**

- Service-Learning (SL) agreement
- Special insurance policies
- Policies/procedures
- Contact information
- Emergency procedures
- HIPAA compliance
- Background checks
- Student misconduct
- Travel and transportation
- Record of SL placements
- Approved lesson plan
- Storage of personal items
- Orientation checklist
- Evaluation documentation
- Scope of practice
- Attendance policies

SUMMARY

Traditional methods of familiarizing dental hygiene students with community-based outreach methods such as community service, volunteerism, clinical rotations, and/or field experiences, though limited in scope, are useful in the dental hygiene curriculum. The dental hygiene community outreach efforts can be enhanced with SL, an underused instructional method.

Service-Learning has the potential to enhance the students' educational experiences and to affect the oral health of the public in a positive fashion. SL emphasizes partnership stability. This, in turn, results in continuity of services, which contributes to the success of SL programs. SL challenges students and compels them to become more active in their learning. In addition to listening to lectures, participating in classroom discussions, and completing other assignments, students can tailor their own learning opportunities so that they improve in areas that are important to them. SL transforms the learning experiences for dental hygiene students and the oral health of the community.[23-25]

Applying Your Knowledge

Service-Learning Objectives Writing Exercise

The ideal time to combine objectives is during the orientation phase. The community partner's needs are more likely to be met when they take an active role in forming the SLO. **Table 11-3** provides examples of SO, LO, and SLO to facilitate skill development in writing objectives. A few of the examples have been intentionally left blank for you to practice the objectives. Your job is to complete the SLOs for the blank examples and compare your results with those of your classmates.

Table 11-3 Service-Learning Grid Exercise

Example	Service Objective (SO)	Learning Objective (LO)	Service-Learning Objective (SLO)
1	Dental hygiene students will support the school nurse with follow-up and referral dental services, including the identification of resources.	Dental hygiene students will demonstrate knowledge of health and non-health barriers to dental hygiene services.	Dental hygiene students will learn about the health and non-health barriers to dental hygiene services by assisting the school nurse with follow-up and dental referrals.
2	Children and parents will receive age-appropriate and culturally sensitive dental health education.	Dental hygiene students will prepare dental health education lessons for children in inner-city public schools.	Dental hygiene students will prepare and present age-appropriate and culturally sensitive dental health education to families.
3	Adolescents will be able to list the oral health consequences of a diet high in sugar.	Dental hygiene students will demonstrate skills in communicating effectively with adolescents.	
4	Adolescent minority youth at the Jefferson House will be encouraged to consider careers in dental hygiene.	First- and second-year dental hygiene students will demonstrate an understanding of basic principles of adolescent learning, including behavior management.	
5	Schoolteachers will learn basic pediatric oral health information that will assist them to recognize the need for urgent dental treatment.	Dental hygiene students will be able to demonstrate effective skills and knowledge when communicating with schoolteachers.	
6	The adults will receive a confirmation of oral findings.	Dental hygiene students will demonstrate knowledge and skills in collecting and analyzing the results of an adult Basic Screening Survey.	
7	The participants will receive a dental health report card that illustrates the results of a screening.	Dental hygiene students will develop a reporting instrument for a longitudinal study that will convey the results of an oral screening.	

Dental Hygiene Competencies

At the end of this chapter the student should be able to demonstrate success in the following competencies:

Health promotion and disease prevention
HP.1 Promote the values of oral and general health and wellness to the public and organizations within and outside the profession.
HP.4 Identify individual and population risk factors and develop strategies that promote health-related quality of life.

Community involvement
CM.1 Assess the oral health needs of the community and the quality and availability of resources and services.
CM.3 Provide community oral health services in a variety of settings.
CM.4 Facilitate client access to oral health services by influencing individuals and organization for the provision of oral health care.
CM.6 Evaluate the outcomes of community-based programs, and plan for future activities.

Professional growth and development
PGD.1 Identify alternative career options within health care, industry, education, and research, and evaluate the feasibility of pursing dental hygiene opportunities.
PGD.3 Access professional and social networks and resources to assist entrepreneurial initiatives.

Community Case

The local dental society and the local dental hygiene program collaborated on the Give Kids a Smile Day (GKSD) national event. The dental hygiene department at Your Community College (YCC) and volunteers from the dental society conducted a massive oral screening on area under-served children. The results revealed that 60% of the 250 children aged 7 to 13 years had an urgent need for dental treatment, and 75% had never visited the dentist.

The dental hygiene faculty, community dentists, and dental hygiene students want to provide dental services for this group of children. You are a student in the dental hygiene program, and you have agreed to serve as a member of the planning committee. The committee members consist of community members, agency members, dental hygiene faculty, dental hygiene advisory board members, and dentists from the local dental society.

1. Which national data source can be used as a model for the formation of program objectives?
   a. *Healthy People 2020*
   b. *Oral Health in America: Report of the Surgeon General*
   c. Association of State & Territorial Dental Directors
   d. Basic Screening Survey
2. Which of the following teaching methods provides concentrated benefit to the recipients of service and to the learner?
   a. Community service
   b. Volunteering
   c. Service-Learning
   d. Clinical rotations

3. In the development of this community dental program, which category of evaluation is it that allows the planners to assess the program while it is in progress so that modifications, if necessary, can be instituted?
   a. Summative evaluation
   b. Formative evaluation
   c. Normative evaluation
4. Which of the following core functions is addressed in the screening phase?
   a. Assessment
   b. Policy development
   c. Assurance
5. What type of objective is the following? "Dental hygiene students will be able to identify five major sources of public health financing for oral health services."
   a. Service objective
   b. Learning objective
   c. Service-Learning objective

References

1. Haden NK, Catalanotto FA, Alexander CJ, et al. Improving the oral health status of all Americans: Roles and responsibilities of academic dental institutions. J Dent Educ 2003;67:563.
2. Hemphill SL. Curriculum as intervention: Transforming a dental hygiene community dental health course into a service-learning course [Newsletter]. Washington, DC: American Public Health Association Oral Health Section; 2003.
3. Hemphill SL. Public health advocacy and access through education [Newsletter]. Washington, DC: American Public Health Association Oral Health Section Newsletter; 2003.
4. Rice A. Interdisciplinary collaboration in health care: Education, practice and research. National Academies of Practice Forum 2000;2:59.
5. US Department of Health and Human Services. Proposed Healthy People 2020 Objectives. www.healthypeople.gov/hp2020/Objectives/TopicAreas.aspx. Accessed October 2010.
6. US Department of Health and Human Services, Public Health Service. National Call to Action to Promote Oral Health. Rockville, MD: National Institutes of Health, National Institute of Dental and Craniofacial Research; NIH Publication No. 03-5303, 2003.
7. US Department of Health and Human Services. Oral Health in America. A Report of the Surgeon General, Executive Summary. Rockville, MD: National Institutes of Health, National Institute of Dental and Craniofacial Research; 2000.
8. Kolb DA, Boyatzis RE, Mainemelis C. Experiential learning theory: Previous research and new directions. In: Sternberg RJ, Zhang LF, editors. Perspectives on Cognitive, Learning, and Thinking Styles. Mahwah, NJ: Lawrence Erlbaum; 2000.
9. American Dental Hygienist's Association. Public Health ADHA. Available at http://adha.org/publichealth/index.html. Accessed January 2010.
10. Canfield A, Clasen C, Dobbins J, et al. Service-Learning in Health Professions: Education: A Multiprofessional Example. Academic Exchange, Winter, 2000; 102.
11. DePaola DP, Slavkin HC. Reforming dental health professions education: A white paper. J Dent Educ 2004;68:1139.
12. Hood JG. Service-learning in dental education: Meeting needs and challenges. J Dent Educ 2009;73:454.
13. Aston-Brown RE, Branson B, Gadbury-Amyot CC, et al. Utilizing public health for service-learning rotations in dental hygiene: A four-year retrospective study. J Dent Educ 2009;73:358.
14. Bailey TR, Hughes KL, Moore DT. Working Knowledge: Work-Based Learning and Education Reform. New York: RoutledgeFalmer; 2004.
15. Bensley LB. Using theory and ethics to guide method selection and application. In: Bensley RJ, Brookins-Fisher J, editors. Community Health Education Methods. 2nd ed. Sudbury, MA: Jones & Bartlett; 2003. p. 1-130.
16. Bringle RG, Hatcher JA. Institutionalization of service-learning in higher education. J Higher Educ 2000;71: 273.
17. Yoder KM. A framework for service-learning in dental education. J Dent Educ 2006;70:115.

18. McKenzie JF, Pinger RR, Kotecki JE. An Introduction to Community Health, 4th ed. Boston: Jones & Bartlett; 2002.

19. Rice C, Brown JR. Transforming educational curriculum and service-learning. J Experiential Educ 1998;12:140.

20. Cashman SB, Seifer SD. Service-learning an integral part of undergraduate public health. Am J Pre Med 2008;35:273.

21. Forrest JL, Miller SA, Overman PR, et al. Evidence-based decision making. A translational guide for dental professionals. Philadelphia, PA: Lippincott Williams & Wilkins; 2009.

22. Farley CL. Service Learning: Applications in midwifery education. J Midwifery Women's Health 2003;48:444.

23. Seifer SD. Service-learning: Community-campus partnerships for health professions education. Acad Med 1998;73:273.

24. Furco A. Service-learning: A balanced approach to experiential learning. In: Expanding Boundaries: Service and Learning. Columbia, MD: Cooperative Education Association; 1996.

25. Eyler J, Giles DE. Where's the Learning in Service-Learning? San Francisco: Jossey-Bass; 1999.

26. Angelo TA, Cross KP. Classroom Assessment Techniques: A Handbook for College Teachers. 2nd ed. San Francisco: Jossey-Bass; 1993.

27. Mofidi M, Gambrell A. Community-based dental partnerships: Improving access to dental care for persons living with HIV/AIDS. J Dent Educ 2009;73:1247.

28. Cauley K, Canfield A, Clasen C, et al. Service-learning: Integrating student learning and community service. Educ Health 2001;14:173.

29. Commission on Dental Accreditation. Accreditation Standards for Dental Hygiene Education Programs. Chicago: American Dental Association; 2010. [Electronic version]. Available at www.ada.org/sections/educationandcareers/pdfs/dh.pdf. Accessed October 2010.

30. American Association of Dental Schools (AADS). Competencies for Entry into the Profession of Dental Hygiene. Washington, DC: AADS Section on Dental Hygiene Education; approved March 1999.

31. Strass R, Mofidi M, Sandler ES, et al. Reflective learning in community-based dental education. J Dent Educ 2003;67:1234.

Additional Resources

Community-Campus Partnership for Health
http://depts.washington.edu/ccph/

Learn and Serve America: Corporation for National Service
www.learnandserve.org/

National Oral Health Surveillance System
www.cdc.gov/nohss/

Learn and Serve America's National Service-Learning Clearinghouse
www.servicelearning.org/

Risk Management and Liability in Higher Education Service-Learning
www.servicelearning.org/instant_info/fact_sheets/he_facts/risk_mgmt/index.php

12

Planning a Student Community Project with Head Start

Robin Brocato, MHS
Kathy Voigt Geurink, RDH, MA

Objectives

Upon completion of this chapter, the student will be able to:
- Define the purpose of a student community project.
- Define needs assessment as it applies to selecting a target population.
- Prepare planning forms, including selection of the target population, assessment visit, and written agreement of project goals and objectives.
- Define the goals and mission of Head Start.
- Describe the oral health component of Head Start.
- Apply the knowledge of planning, implementation, and evaluation to set up a community project.

Key Terms

Community projects	Evaluation	Early Head Start
Planning	Target population	Head Start Program
Implementation	Head Start	Performance Standards

Opening Statements

Goals of Student Community Projects
- To improve the oral health of Head Start children and families in a local Head Start Program
- To improve the oral health of children residing in a state-supported home
- To improve the oral health of mentally and physically challenged adults and children at a group home
- To improve the oral health of pregnant teens attending health classes in a public school setting
- To improve the oral health of senior citizens living in an assisted living center
- To improve the oral health of hearing impaired children attending a community school for the deaf

THE COMMUNITY ORAL HEALTH PROJECT

Community Oral Health Project Description

The community oral health project is an opportunity for dental hygiene students to take what they have learned in the Community Oral Health course and apply it in a setting of their choice. **Community projects** allow students to interact in the community at a level that will produce positive behavioral change and impact the oral health of the population being served. Because of the constraints of time within a dental hygiene curriculum, the project impact may be limited. Therefore it is important to include follow-up plans for sustainability of the project activities once the initial project is complete. The student community project varies from the traditional one-time presentations since it includes assessing the needs of the population, **planning** for and **implementation** of disease prevention and health promotion activities, and **evaluation** of the project. The project can be a service-learning project if it contains service-learning components, including learning objectives and service objectives that will equally benefit both the student and the population being served (see Chapter 11). The goal of the community project is to improve the oral health of the selected population, although the project does provide a learning experience for the student.

Selecting a Target Population

In the previous chapters, it has been documented that despite improvements in oral health, profound disparities remain in specific population groups in the United States. People who are at highest risk for poor oral health are children from low-income families, children and adults with special health care needs, and vulnerable elderly citizens. If 80% of dental disease is found in 25% of the citizens, as stated in *Oral Health in America: A Report of the Surgeon General*, it makes sense to plan community projects that will target the 25% who are at most risk.[1] Students can use community resources, the Internet, and organizations such as the United Way to select a facility that serves the population they want to work with. The needs of at-risk populations have been documented and described in various journals and publications. Students should do a literature search (see Chapter 7) and review two to three recent articles describing the oral health status for the population they target for their community project. *Healthy People 2010* and *Healthy People 2020* provide data on oral health status and trends, as well as goals for improving the oral health of the nation (see Chapter 5). Students should also review the *Healthy People* national health objectives (see Chapters 4 and 5) that relate to the selected **target population.** This connection will allow the students to see how their project not only makes a difference in the health of persons in one local site but also persons in the nation.

Next Steps in the Planning Process

Once the target population has been selected and a form is turned in to the instructor (Form A can be accessed on the Evolve website), the following steps should be taken (see also Guiding Principles). The first step would be to contact the intended site through a phone call to explain interest in setting up a community project to improve the oral health of the population served by this organization. If there is interest by the site, a visit is set up to discuss the project, which would include a tour of the facility and time to discuss the needs of the target population. If necessary, a letter of introduction for the students, written by the community instructor, can be obtained and brought to this first meeting. A first-visit form (Form B can be accessed on the Evolve website) is filled out listing attendees at the meeting, describing the target population, and their oral health needs. The student group (usually two to four students) needs to gather enough information at this meeting to prepare a written agreement of the project goal, objectives, activities, and evaluation methods. Dates for conducting the project should also be discussed with a minimum of two visits: to conduct pretesting and begin project activities. A third visit will be needed to complete activities and conduct final evaluation or posttesting. The length of time is important to the impact on the population. Once the agreement is written and signed, the project can begin as planned. (Form C can be accessed on the Evolve website.) Evidenced-based practices should be employed as the interventions that will make a difference in the oral health of the target population. For an example, see the Head Start Project in the section on Head Start Oral Health Project.

GUIDING PRINCIPLES

Steps in Planning the Project (see forms on Evolve website)
- Contact the site
- Visit the site
- Write a project agreement

Evaluation

Evaluation measures are to be designed during the planning of the project. Evaluation measures should be connected to the project objectives and are the means of determining if the project accomplished what it was designed to do. Evaluation can include information from questionnaires, pretests, and posttests of knowledge, focus groups, numbers of participants, and student reflections (see Chapters 6 and 11). The student community project can be considered a "mini" project compared with a state level intervention or a government-organized program; however, many of the same steps and efforts can be applied (see Chapter 6). For example, short-term measurement of knowledge and attitude change can be determined as evaluation within the target population and possibly some short-term behavioral changes might be measured if time allows. The long-term changes, however, such as disease rates or health changes, take more time than the student project can determine. With the student project, long-term health outcomes cannot be guaranteed. The student community project provides a taste of public health and how to plan, implement, and evaluate a project to improve oral health. It is a valuable tool in getting students involved in their communities with the hope that they will continue to be involved as professionals in future interventions and educational programs in their communities.

The next section describes the Head Start population as a possible target population for conducting student community oral health projects, as well as a population needing the continued support and involvement of oral health professionals to improve the oral health of Head Start children and families.

HEAD START

Head Start Program Description

The **Head Start** program was founded in 1965 as part of President Johnson's War on Poverty. It began as a summer program that was designed to break the cycle of poverty by providing comprehensive services to low-income preschool children and their families. The overall mission of Head Start is to prepare children for school. Head Start programs promote school readiness by enhancing the social and cognitive development of children through the provision of educational, health, nutritional, social, and other services to enrolled children and families. They engage parents in their children's learning and help them make progress toward their educational, literacy, and employment goals. Significant emphasis is placed on the involvement of parents in the governance

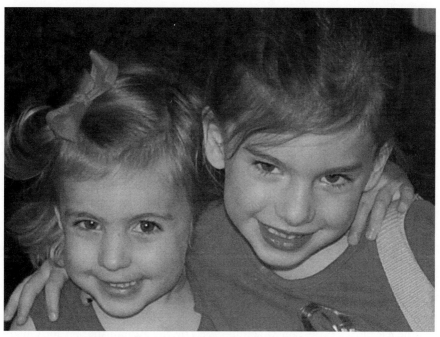

Figure 12-1 Happy children, healthy smiles.

of local Head Start programs. Parents are an integral part of the program and are seen as the child's primary and first teacher (**Figure 12-1**).

In terms of socioeconomic status, the Head Start program serves our nation's most vulnerable children. From 1965 until the most recent Head Start Reauthorization in December 2007, eligibility for Head Start services was at or below 100% of the federal poverty level (FPL). The 2010 FPL for a family of four is $22,050.00.[2] The 2007 Reauthorization of Head Start allows Head Start programs to serve up to 35% of children whose family income is up to 130% of the FPL. For a family of four, this is $28,665.00. In contrast, eligibility for Medicaid is 133% of the FPL (states have the option to expand eligibility beyond federal guidelines); eligibility for the Children's Health Insurance Program (CHIP) has been set by the states as up to or above 200% of the FPL. In 2009, eligibility for the Special Supplemental Nutrition Program for Women, Infants and Children (WIC) was increased to 185% of the FPL.

Head Start primarily serves 4-year-old children. The racial/ethnic composition of children in Head Start is presented in **Table 12-1**.

More than 140 languages are spoken by Head Start children and families, and 31% speak a language other than English. Head Start also serves migrant and seasonal farm workers' children and families, as well as American Indian/Alaska natives.

In recognition of the mounting evidence that the earliest years matter a great deal to a child's growth and development, the **Early Head Start** program was established in fiscal year 1995 to serve children from birth to age 3. Funds were awarded to Early Head Start programs in 1995. According to the 2006–2007 Program Information Report data compiled by the Office of Head Start (OHS), the number of Early Head Start grantees has since risen to 734. In 2009, the American Recovery and Reinvestment Act increased funding for Early Head Start by $1.1 billion,

Table 12-1   **Fiscal Year 2007 Program Statistics**

Enrollment	*908,412*
Ages	
Number of 5-year-olds and older	3%
Number of 4-year-olds	51%
Number of 3-year-olds	36%
Number younger than 3 years of age	10%
Racial/Ethnic Composition	
American Indian/Alaska Native	4.0%
Black/African American	30.1%
White	39.7%
Asian	1.7%
Hawaiian/Pacific Islander	0.8%
Bi-Racial/Multi-Racial	4.9%
Unspecified/Other	18.8%
Hispanic/Latino	34.7%

From *Head Start Fact Sheet,* fiscal year 2008.

which will result in Early Head Start being able to serve 55,000 more pregnant women, infants, and toddlers and their families.

The Head Start program is administered by the Administration for Children and Families (ACF) within the US Department of Health and Human Services (DHHS). Head Start agencies receive grant funding directly from ACF (rather than the state) and may either directly operate Head Start programs (72%) or delegate operations (23%), or may either directly operate the program and delegate service delivery (4%) or maintain central staff only and operate no program directly (1%).

Agencies receiving Head Start funding include community action agencies (32%), public/private schools (17%), private/public nonprofit agencies (37%), government agencies (7%), and tribal governments or consortiums (American Indian/Alaska native) (7%).

All Head Start and Early Head Start programs must follow a set of federal program performance standards in each of these service areas: Child development and health, family and community partnerships, and program design and management. As mandated by Congress, Head Start and Early Head Start programs are monitored every 3 years to ensure compliance with these performance standards.

Health Services in Head Start

Head Start health services focus on prevention and early intervention and encompass medical, nutrition, oral health, and mental health services. The **Head Start Program Performance Standards** require that when a child enters the program, Head Start staff must work in partnership with parents to ensure the child has a medical home and health insurance and is up-to-date on a schedule of primary and preventive health care (including dental) and fully immunized. Early in the program year, Head Start children also receive sensory, behavioral, and developmental screenings. In the event a potential health concern is identified during the well-child visit or when the child is screened, Head Start works with the parents in making referrals for further diagnosis, evaluation, and treatment. Head Start can provide transportation to medical or dental appointments and also provide child care as needed. Programs are required to have procedures in place

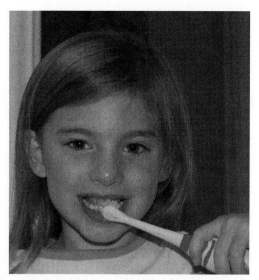

Figure 12-2 Head Start teaches children healthy lifestyle behaviors, such as tooth brushing.

to make sure that children receive needed services and that parents understand any procedures that their child may receive.

Head Start programs are required to participate in the US Department of Agriculture (USDA) Child Nutrition Programs: the School Breakfast Program, the School Lunch Program, or the Child and Adult Care Food Program. Meals are either prepared on-site or prepared by an outside vendor and delivered to the program and must be high in nutrients and low in sugar, fat, and salt.

Head Start programs are required to establish and maintain a Health Services Advisory Committee (HSAC) comprised of local health care professionals, Head Start staff, and parents. Typically, health professionals serving on the HSAC include pediatricians, nurses, nurse practitioners, dentists, dental hygienists, nutritionists, and mental health providers (therapists, social workers). Other HSAC members can include representatives for the local education agency, fire and police departments, and first responders.

The HSAC can be instrumental in identifying community resources, assisting programs in developing and implementing policies and procedures, keeping the program informed of emerging research and practice guidelines, as well as providing education to program staff and parents.

Health education for both children and parents is an important requirement of Head Start. Children are taught healthy behaviors, such as handwashing and toothbrushing, and can learn about injury prevention, physical activity, and making healthy food choices (**Figure 12-2**). Parents participate in health education workshops or receive health education services in the home.

Oral Health Services

The oral health status of Head Start children has long been a concern of the OHS. In 1972, the OHS published a series of training and technical assistance educational materials known as "The Rainbow Series." The guide on Dental Services discusses the importance of dental care for the preschool child and states: "Dental decay is the single most common health defect in Head Start children."[3] In the early days of Head Start, basic dental services were often provided by dentists who volunteered their services and included an oral examination and treatment planning;

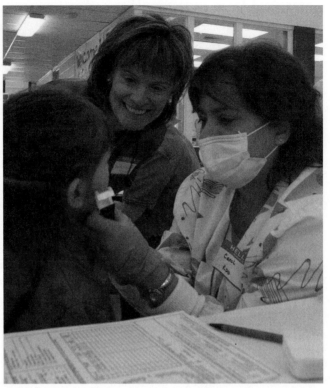

Figure 12-3 Dental hygienists provide fluoride varnish to Head Start child.

dental prophylaxis, direct application of fluoride in communities that lacked adequate fluoride levels in the public water supply, restoration of decayed primary and permanent teeth, pulp therapy for primary and permanent teeth, extraction of nonrestorable teeth, and services required for the relief of pain or infection (**Figure 12-3**).

Over the years, Head Start programs have faced many challenges in meeting the oral health performance standard requirements. During much of the 1990s, poor access to oral health services was the number one health issue affecting Head Start programs nationwide as reported by Head Start directors, training and technical assistance providers, and Administration for Children and Families Regional Office Head Start Program Specialists.[4] The main challenges Head Start programs and parents face when it comes to receiving oral health services include a limited number of dentists who accept Medicaid, lack of transportation (or long travel time to see the dentist), inability to take time off work to keep dental appointments, lack of child care, and language/cultural barriers. In addition, some Head Start parents are reluctant to take their child to the dentist because of their own negative experiences with the dentist, or they do not understand the important role of oral health for young children because baby teeth "just fall out."

OHS has employed a variety of strategies to support Head Start programs in meeting the performance standards, including establishing partnerships with federal agencies with oral health expertise, such as the Maternal and Child Health Bureau within the Health Resources and Services Administration (HRSA) or DHHS, and by providing training and technical assistance through a national network of training and technical assistance providers. In 1999, the Head Start and Partners Forum on Oral Health was held in Washington, DC. Head Start staff and parents; training and technical assistance providers; pediatric dentists; representatives from local and

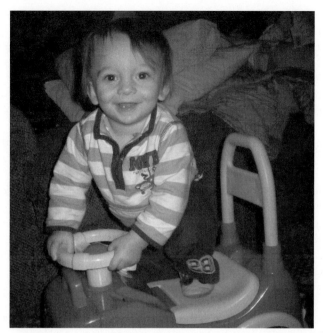

Figure 12-4 Early Intervention through Head Start—Oral Health Programs will put children on the road to healthy teeth and gums starting with "the first tooth."

state WIC programs, Medicaid, maternal and child health, child care, and the Centers for Medicare & Medicaid Services; and regional ACF staff met to discuss oral health issues impacting Head Start children families. The Forum provided an opportunity for Head Start participants to hear first-hand the latest research on caries prevention, nutrition, and oral health and access to care. The proceedings of the Forum were published in the 2000 *Journal of Public Health Dentistry.*[5,6] In 2006, the OHS invested $2 million in grants to 52 Head Start, Early Head Start, and American Indian/Alaska native and Migrant/Seasonal Head Start programs to design and implement oral health models that met the needs of communities and populations they serve.

The goals of the Oral Health Initiative (OHI) were to do the following:

1. Improve oral health care delivery systems for children from birth to age 5 and for pregnant women in Head Start programs.
2. Learn about the influences of culture on the oral health practices of Head Start families.
3. Develop high-quality service delivery models that promote oral health as integral to physical health, as well as oral health prevention principles supported by evidence-based curricula that include use of promising practices, oral health education, and counseling for parents and staff.
4. Develop models of oral health care that are sustainable in communities through the development of collaborative partnerships with community and state agencies, as well as with other providers such as local dentists, dental and dental hygiene schools, local and state health and dental associations, WIC clinics, pediatricians, dieticians, and other dental-related groups.
5. Solicit buy-in from key stakeholders and demonstrate strategies for future funding and related support after federal grant support ends.
6. Develop models of care that integrate oral health into existing local public or private health systems to improve access to care for young children and pregnant women, including the

development of referral systems to access pediatric dental services, referral systems for pregnant women, and oral health education.

7. Identify models of care that are replicable and develop strategies to share models of care and to disseminate information and lessons learned about the OHI.

8. Respond to issues addressed in regional and state/jurisdiction oral health strategic plans developed through Head Start Oral Health Forums.

OHI grantees employed a variety of strategies to address the goals of the OHI, including the following:

- Having children act as role models to reduce classmate fear of the dentist
- Involving all staff (e.g., center directors, family service workers, and teachers) in oral health education efforts
- Establishing personal relationships with local dentists in an effort to recruit more dentists to serve Head Start children
- Hiring dental hygienists to provide oral health education, screenings, and apply fluoride varnish
- Building on existing community resources to develop and strengthen community partnerships
- Building on existing local/state oral health efforts to maximize resources and to coordinate efforts
- Analyzing program information report data to assess the success of oral health efforts
- Focusing on oral health of pregnant women
- Developing training materials including videos and/or public services announcements
- Recruiting dentists to serve on the HSAC
- Developing and disseminating parent newsletters, oral health fact sheets, and/or brochures
- Conducting oral health screenings to assess children's oral health needs
- Conducting parent surveys to assess attitudes toward oral health
- Developing strategies to support parents who were ready to address their fear of the dentist

Opportunities for Dental Hygiene Students

The Head Start setting provides myriad opportunities for dental hygiene students to support Head Start programs in achieving the Head Start Program Performance Standards. As mentioned previously, many of the OHI grantees hired hygienists to provide oral health education to children, parents and staff, provide fluoride varnish, and to conduct oral health screenings. Hygiene students can also assist local Head Start programs in identifying local oral health resources or in establishing partnerships with local providers and programs. In addition, students may serve on the local program's HSAC.

Students interested in working with their local Head Start program may visit the Head Start website at http://eclkc.ohs.acf.hhs.gov/hslc/HeadStartOffices.

HEAD START ORAL HEALTH PROJECT

Community Project Goal

Initiating a community oral health project with Head Start is a rewarding experience and contributes to the improvement of oral health for children, especially those from minority, racial and ethnic backgrounds and children from socioeconomic disadvantaged families. America's youngest and poorest children, aged 2 to 4 years old and living below poverty level, have nearly three times the dental caries as children of higher income families.[7] A comprehensive goal of a Head Start community oral health project would be to improve the oral health of Head Start children and families through oral health education, disease prevention, and referrals to dental homes for treatment. Students conducting oral health education projects in Head Start are often also involved with conducting fluoride varnish projects, including screenings and referrals for dental care.

Example: Community Oral Health Project with Head Start

Dental hygiene students conducted the Head Start Community Project as described in the following:

Community Project

Goal: To improve the oral health of Head Start children through an educational program for Head Start parents, staff and children who attend a program at a local Head Start Center.

Objectives: On completion of three educational sessions at the Head Start Center, the parents and staff will be able to do the following:
1. Answer a posttest with 90% accuracy on the following topics:
   • The importance of primary teeth
   • Early childhood caries (a transmissible infectious disease)
   • Feeding practices and nutrition
   • Fluoride modalities, including fluoride varnish
   • Daily oral hygiene care for mom and child
2. Demonstrate correct brushing techniques for themselves and the children. The Head Start children will be able to do the following:
   • Participate willingly in the classroom brushing.
   • Repeat through song three reasons why we brush our teeth: To smile, eat, and chew.
   • Fill out a weekly coloring chart of the days they brushed their teeth at home with help from a parent.

Activities

Session One:
Pretest
Educational presentation for parents /staff
Song for children
Question and answer

Session Two:
Educational presentation continued
Practice brushing session by children and parents
Practice singing the children's song
Practice brushing on a large model/brush
Parents practice brushing a child's teeth

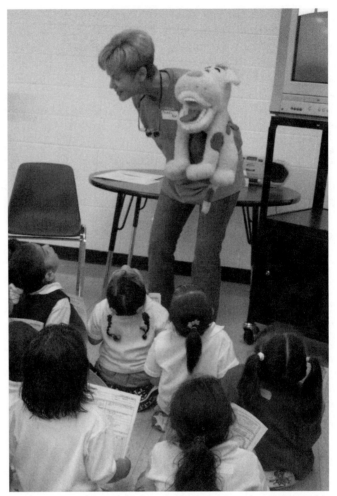

Figure 12-5 Dental hygienist provides education to Head Start children.

Session Three:
Educational presentation and review of material
Posttest
Question and answer
Healthy snacks shared at the last session

Resources

PowerPoint presentations on the selected topics
AAPD Educational flipchart on the selected topics (www.aapd.org)
Head Start Early Childhood Learning and Knowledge Center (www.eclkc.ohs.acf.gov)
Fact sheets on Head Start children's oral health from the Maternal and Child Oral Health Resource Center (www.mchoralhealth.org)

Toothbrushes for adults and children
Large puppet/typodont and brush for demonstrating toothbrushing to the children

Sustainability

The dental hygiene students provided educational materials that can be used by staff in continuing oral health education for parents and children. Dental hygiene students worked with volunteer dental hygienists from the local dental hygiene component to start a fluoride varnish project, including two applications of fluoride varnish during the school year, as well as a basic screening survey (BSS) and referral as needed for dental care. Dental hygiene students suggested the next class will continue the educational program and work with dental hygienists from the community to provide services needed by Head Start children, families, and staff.

DENTAL HYGIENISTS WORKING WITH HEAD START

Dental Hygienists: A Valuable Resource

As licensed professionals, dental hygienists are a valuable resource in the process of establishing dental homes for Head Start children.[8] Their services include screenings, prevention and education, referral for treatment and assistance in the coordination of follow-up care. They are facilitators for finding and establishing dental homes that will allow the Head Start child an opportunity to receive comprehensive oral health care. Dental hygienists working with Head Start are enabling the Head Start grantee to meet the oral health–related performance standards and to bring improved oral health to every Head Start child.

Examples of programs where dental hygienists are involved with finding dental homes for Head Start children are seen nationwide. Many states have adopted less restrictive practice acts to allow dental hygienists to work in public health settings, including Head Start. Promoting expanded practice settings and removing restrictive supervision barriers are essential to the success of improving the oral health of underserved populations.[9]

The National Maternal and Child Oral Health Resource Center

The National Maternal and Child Oral Health Resource Center's Head Start activities are supported by the intraagency agreement between the OHS and the Maternal and Child Health Bureau with the goal of enhancing the quality of oral health services for pregnant women, infants, and children enrolled in Head Start. The resource center has developed a wealth of educational materials, such as brochures for pregnant women and parents of infants and young children; tip sheets for Head Start staff and parents; and fact sheets, including "What Dental Hygienists Need to Know About Head Start" and an electronic newsletter titled "Oral Health Alert: Focus on Head Start" that can assist dental hygienists and dental hygiene students learn about and become involved in Head Start programs.

Call to Action

Dental hygienists and dental hygiene students interested in working with Head Start should contact their state dental hygienists' association and their component dental hygiene organization to determine the level of services presently being offered and how best to organize efforts and get involved. Review of state Head Start Oral Health Action plans online at www.astdd.org will provide valuable background information.[10] Dental hygienists can also locate a Head Start center directly by visiting the website (www.adha.org/public health/index.html) and following the link titled "Find a Head Start Center near you." Dental hygienists can contact Head Start centers and offer assistance with parent and staff education, as well as participation on the health services advisory board. The common goal of the dental profession and Head Start is to see that the children obtain the dental care essential to their health and school readiness. There will be various paths and collaborative opportunities for accomplishing this task.

References

1. US Department of Health and Human Services. Oral Health in America: A Report of the Surgeon General. Rockville, MD: US Department of Health and Human Services; 2000.
2. US Department of Health and Human Services. The 2010 HHS Poverty Guidelines. Available at: http://aspe.hhs.gov/poverty/. Accessed April 2, 2010.
3. Project Head Start, Dental Services, US Department of Health, Education and Welfare. Washington, DC; 1972.
4. Head Start Bulletin on Oral Health. Issue No. 71, May 2001.
5. Brocato R. Head Start and Partners Forum on Oral Health. Washington, DC: Head Start Bulletin 2001;71:1.
6. Proceedings from the Head Start and Partners Forum on Oral Health. J Public Health Dent 2000;60: summer issue.
7. Vargas CM, Crall JJ, Schneider DA. Sociodemographic distribution of pediatric dental caries: NHANES III, 1988–1994. J Am Dent Assoc 1998;129:1229.
8. Geurink KV. Dental Hygienists' Role in Establishing Dental Homes for Head Start Children. Access 2008.
9. American Dental Hygienists' Association (ADHA). Supervision by States. Available at www.adha.org/governmental_affairs/index.html. Accessed April 2010.
10. State Head Start Oral Health Forum Action Plans. Association of State & Territorial Dental Directors web site. Available at www.astdd.org/head-start-oral-health-project/. Accessed October 2010.

Additional Resources

Head Start Early Childhood Learning and Knowledge Center
    http://ecklc.ohs.acf.hhs.gov/hsl
Maternal and Child Oral Health Resource Center
    www.mchoralhealth.org/HeadStart
Regional, State and Professional Head Start Oral Health Forum reports
    www.mchoralhealth//hsforums.htm
Association of State & Territorial Dental Directors Head Start Oral Health Project Evaluation Report 2001-2008
    www.astdd.org/index.php?template=head_start.html
Office of Head Start Oral Health Webinars. Partnerships to Improve Oral Health in Head Start. 2007
    www.mchoralhealth.org/HeadStart/presentations.html
Association of State & Territorial Dental Directors Basic Screening Survey (BSS)
    www.astdd.org/index.php?template=surveybss.html
American Academy of Pediatrics. Dental Home Initiative
    www.aapd.org/headstart/

Test-Taking Strategies and Community Cases

13

Kathy Voigt Geurink, RDH, MA

Objectives

Upon completion of this chapter, the student will be able to:
- Develop an overview of the National Board Dental Hygiene Examination.
- Develop guidelines for answering multiple-choice test items and community testlets.
- Identify tips for examination preparation.
- Take a practice examination on community cases.
- Increase his or her confidence level in preparing for the examination.

Key Terms

Community health activities   Multiple-choice questions   Critical thinking
Community cases

OVERVIEW OF THE EXAMINATION

The National Board Dental Hygiene Examination (NBDHE) is written and administered by the Joint Commission on National Dental Examinations of the American Dental Association (ADA). The purpose of the examination is to determine professional competency in the various subject areas that are taught in the schools of dental hygiene.

According to the NBDHE Candidate Guide, the examination consists of 350 multiple-choice questions and is administered during 1 full day consisting of two 4-hour periods. Component A (4 hours in the morning) contains approximately 200 multiple-choice questions; Component B (4 hours in the afternoon) contains 150 questions based on 12 to 15 dental hygiene cases. Component A is composed of the following three major areas:
- Scientific basis for dental hygiene practice
- Provision of clinical dental hygiene services
- **Community health activities**

In the community health activities area, approximately four **community cases** are presented with a series of **multiple-choice questions** related to the situation described. The community cases are simulated situations that might occur in the community. They usually involve the dental hygienist's participation in a community oral health activity. Multiple-choice questions after the community cases require that the dental hygiene student apply information, such as that within this textbook, to select the correct answer. The community cases and the related questions are referred to as *testlets* within the examination.

MULTIPLE-CHOICE QUESTIONS

Multiple-choice questions are used to test the student's knowledge and understanding of content. A multiple-choice test item consists of a stem, which poses a problem that is followed by a list of answers. The stem is presented either as a question or as an incomplete statement. A choice of four or five answers is given per question. Only one of the answers is correct or best. The other answers are called distracters. Some suggestions are as follows:

1. When answering multiple test questions, use your time wisely. Look over the test initially to determine how many questions are presented, and calculate approximately how much time you will need to answer them.
2. Read directions and questions carefully.
3. Attempt to answer every question; if you are unsure of an answer, mark or flag that question to enable you to return to it later if time permits.
4. Actively reason through each question, and read all answers before making your choice.

Here are some tips that may help you answer the questions. Look for the following within the questions and answers:

- Logical clues that help you select the correct answer
- A repeated word or concept in both the question and answer
- Length of the correct response; often the longest answer is correct
- A similarity in or a direct opposite of responses; you can eliminate contradictory answers or complete opposites to the question

Examples of Multiple-Choice Questions

The following multiple-choice test questions relate to information in Chapter 8 and demonstrate how to answer multiple-choice questions using the clues already presented. Answer the following questions using your knowledge and these clues.

1. Which choice describes the Stages of Change Theory?
   a. It is an example of ways to effect changes in public policy.
   b. It assesses a person's readiness to change and adopt behaviors that lead to a healthy lifestyle.
   c. It includes key concepts such as reciprocal determination, observational learning, and reinforcement.
   d. It directly assesses how susceptible to paridontitis a patient perceives oneself to be.
2. An example of the tailoring technique that is used in formulating an individual's oral health plan is:
   a. Highlighting one or two messages that might apply to your patient.
   b. Using photographs of American Indian women for posters in the Indian Health Service clinic.
   c. Providing three individualized recommendations based on risk factors identified during a personal risk assessment.
   d. Asking a group whether they prefer a video, slides, or a demonstration.
3. You have developed a new program to promote oral health to teenage mothers. You would like to discuss your ideas with other health professionals at an upcoming public health conference. Which of the following formats would be best for presenting your information?
   a. Roundtable discussion
   b. Oral presentation
   c. Research poster presentation
   d. Table clinic

4. Which of the following formats would you use to ensure the highest retention of information about oral cancer in a group of adults?
   a. Reading a booklet about oral cancer
   b. Using a multimedia presentation
   c. Demonstrating an oral examination, followed by a discussion and a return demonstration of how to perform the oral cancer examination
   d. Watching a video

The answers to these questions are provided here using clues versus a knowledge rationale. See Chapter 8 for a knowledge review.

1. b. This is the logical answer because Chapter 8 is on health promotion and behavioral change. Although a. has the word *changes,* the topic is not relevant. Answers c. and d. have no wording similar to that of the question.
2. c. This answer uses a similar idea—the concept of individualization—even if one does not connect risk with tailoring. Answers b. and d. can be eliminated because they are opposites of the question, referring to groups rather than an individual. Answer a. uses the vague term *might,* which makes it a less viable answer than c.
3. a. This answer uses repetition of the term *discuss,* which gives the clue to the best answer. The other three answers are ways to present the information, but a. is the best answer.
4. c. This answer has length, and it is logical that you will retain information better when you involve more of your senses.

ANSWERING COMMUNITY CASE QUESTIONS (TESTLETS)

When answering the community cases, you must change your train of thought from thinking about private practice to thinking about community. Recall the definitions from within this text and the comparisons of private practice and community oral health practice. Your selection of the correct answer must be in relation to what is best for the community as a whole. You will be applying the information you have learned in your community course to a simulated situation in the community.

In most dental hygiene schools, students have an opportunity to apply the information that they have learned in the community course by conducting projects in the community. These projects require **critical thinking** skills to determine the best way to achieve maximum oral health for the target population the student chooses to work with. Studying the "Applying Your Knowledge" features at the end of each chapter in this textbook is a good way for students to practice their critical thinking skills. Testing with cases requires students not only to retrieve knowledge, as in the stand-alone multiple-choice questions, but also to use their knowledge and critical thinking skills to make choices. Your critical thinking skills are just that—thinking about what you know. The NBDHE measures your ability to solve problems and to make decisions based on the knowledge you have acquired in your coursework.

Once you are in a community frame of mind, read carefully through the community situation. Then start on the multiple-choice questions; remember that the questions refer to the case presented. Some of the questions can probably be answered on a stand-alone basis, but they are intended to relate only to the case presented. The best answer is the one related to the information in the case.

If time permits, rereading through the case one more time after answering the questions allows you to catch any incorrect answer you may have selected without recalling important information from within the case. The community cases are located in the test in the latter half of the morning.

If you do better with case-type questions early in a 4-hour period, consider answering the cases first and then the other multiple-choice questions in this section.

In your general preparation for the examination, try to identify your weak areas and concentrate your review on them. Do not cram for an examination of this magnitude. Set aside scheduled time for review, possibly using a calendar to set aside hours weekly to use for study. Some people study well in groups. Group studying can be beneficial because you learn other students' ideas and ways to recall information. Other students do better alone. It is your choice, but perhaps you can try a little of both.

Previous examination questions give you practice in test taking and often cover material that never changes. Alternate your review periods with practice examinations. Staying calm is important to your psyche. Remember, you will not know everything. A positive attitude always helps!

Examples of Critical Thinking: Community Oral Health Practice Testlets

The following four testlets and community cases are compiled as a practice test in community oral health. The number and type of questions are similar to what you will encounter on the NBDHE in this area. You should complete these questions in less than 40 minutes so that you will still have about 1 minute per question on the other multiple-choice questions in the morning section. There are four testlets with five questions each.

Testlet No. 1

You practice dental hygiene in a low-socioeconomic-level, multicultural city with a population of 1.5 million. The office you work in, however, serves a relatively higher socioeconomic population of the city. The city water supply is not fluoridated; consequently, dental decay is prevalent in the mouths of children residing in the poorer sections of the city. Most families in the city are of Hispanic descent. You recently assisted the public health dental hygienist in conducting a screening on the children in a local elementary school to document their oral health status. Fluoridation was defeated 10 years ago because of a strong antifluoridation campaign. Fluoridation will be on the ballot again in 8 months. The following questions relate to this situation:

1. What would be the best thing for you, as a private practice dental hygienist, to do to help get the fluoride referendum passed?
   a. Continue educating your patients on the benefits of fluoride as you have been doing.
   b. Start calling community leaders.
   c. Make a financial contribution to the cause.
   d. Check with your local dental hygiene component to determine whether a unified plan of action has been developed and how you might help.
2. The following political tactics will be beneficial in ensuring that the fluoridation referendum will pass except one:
   a. Public debate with the antifluoridationists
   b. Analysis of the referendum of 10 years ago
   c. Endorsements by community leaders
   d. Distribution of literature in Spanish and English throughout the community
3. The best index to use to determine the decay rate in the elementary school-aged children would be:
   a. DMFT
   b. CPI
   c. OHI
   d. PDI

4. To make sure that your data will be reliable before you conduct the screening, you should:
   a. Contact the parents of the children.
   b. Inform the children about oral hygiene.
   c. Calibrate the examiners.
   d. Plan how many children will be included.
5. If the fluoridation referendum fails to pass once again, which alternative plan would be the most effective?
   a. Sending letters to parents requesting them to take their children to the dentist for treatment and fluoride
   b. Giving oral hygiene lessons in the classrooms
   c. Initiating a school fluoride mouth rinse program
   d. Getting the children to participate in a sealant program

Testlet No. 2

You have recently been employed as a public health dental hygienist in a local health department. You have been asked to plan, implement, and evaluate a school-based educational and preventive program for selected elementary schools located in your school district. The program is to be based on the *Healthy People 2020* oral health objectives. Your plan includes classroom education and the use of a mobile dental van to provide cleanings, sealants, and fluorides. The following questions relate to the formation of this program.

1. All of the following are *Healthy People 2020* objectives that will be affected by your program except:
   a. Increasing the proportion of health departments that have an oral health component
   b. Increasing the proportion of children who receive preventive dental services
   c. Increasing the proportion of children who are provided with topical fluoride
   d. Reducing the incidence of periodontitis and gingivitis in children
2. Your planning includes collecting data using the DMFT Index. This tool of measurement will be helpful in assessing which of the following?
   a. The demand for services from your oral health program
   b. The amount of gingivitis and periodontitis in children's teeth
   c. The need for services from your oral health program
   d. The children's risk of contracting other health diseases
3. In the evaluation phase of your program, you plan to measure the children's performance skills in the area of oral hygiene. Which method would be best to accomplish this?
   a. A written pretest and posttest
   b. A demonstration of the procedures by the children
   c. An oral survey of the children's attitudes on oral health
   d. A surprise index at the school after lunch
4. On the dental van, you want to assess the needs of the children and make appropriate referrals for treatment. Which of the following methods would be best to relay to the parents the overall needs of their children after the screening?
   a. Sending the DMFT Index numbers home with the children
   b. Mailing literature on the importance of oral health to the parents
   c. Phoning the parents and reporting on the finding
   d. Using the Basic Screening Survey (BSS) and sending the results home with a list of local community clinics
5. All of these programs would be resources for payment in treating the children's teeth at the dentists' offices except:
   a. Medicare
   b. Medicaid

    c. State Children's Health Insurance Program (CHIP)
    d. Private insurance

Testlet No. 3

One of your private practice patients is a nursing home administrator. She requests your assistance in providing an oral health care program for the patients with Alzheimer's disease who reside at the Manor Care. The program is to include education, screening, and referral. The residents are from a lower socioeconomic group and have complex health histories. The social worker has consents for dental treatment, if needed, and a vehicle for transportation.

1. What would the first step be in planning this program?
    a. Arranging a time for an in-service for the nursing home staff
    b. Assessing survey attitudes of the residents to determine what is needed
    c. Arranging a meeting of the people to be involved to assess the needs and to determine goals and objectives for the program
    d. Planning an educational session for the residents
2. Which activity would be most beneficial to the goal of improving the residents' oral hygiene?
    a. Providing toothbrushes for the staff
    b. Purchasing electric toothbrushes for the residents
    c. Educating the staff on the importance of good oral hygiene self-care
    d. Educating the residents on oral disease
3. The screening indicates that there is a need for better oral hygiene and dental restorative work. All of the following are possibilities for dental care for the patients who are mobile except:
    a. Taking the elderly residents to a private practice dentist who accepts Medicare patients, since Medicare pays for dental treatment
    b. Checking with the nearby dental school for arranging to transport residents to their clinic for care on a reduced-fee or no-cost basis
    c. Taking the residents to a community clinic that bases its fees on a sliding scale
    d. Asking the dentist and hygienist in your community who use portable equipment to include Manor Care on their list of nursing homes to visit
4. The Gingival Index (GI) was performed on the residents with natural teeth. The following scores were recorded: 2.5, 2.7, 2.8, 3.0, 2.5, 2.4, and 2.9. Which score represents the mean GI score of the residents?
    a. 2.50
    b. 2.55
    c. 2.61
    d. 2.69
5. In analyzing the assessment data, the dental hygienist found the correlation between age and oral cancer to be +.80. This relationship could be described as:
    a. Weak
    b. Negative
    c. Strong
    d. Moderate

Testlet No. 4

You reside in a small town and work in a community clinic. The regional public heath dental hygienist asks for your assistance in assessing, planning, and implementing oral health programs in your town. She is especially concerned about the elderly population and about developing a tobacco awareness program in the middle school.

1. You perform an assessment of the community's needs, including a description by age, gender, and socioeconomic status. This assessment is referred to as the:
   a. Design of your plan
   b. Community profile
   c. List of priorities
   d. Needs assessment
2. You decide to collect some baseline data to document the needs of the adults in the community and, possibly, to secure funds for program development. You want to measure healthy gingiva, presence or absence of bleeding, supragingival or subgingival calculus, and periodontal pockets. Which index would you use to screen the adults who visit your clinic?
   a. OHI
   b. DMFT
   c. PDI
   d. CPI
3. You intend to survey the middle school students to assess their perception of how susceptible they are to addiction and cancer caused by tobacco products. In your prevention program, you will present the benefits of not smoking or chewing and will discuss the results of their decisions. Which model of health promotion are you using?
   a. Stages of Change Theory
   b. Social Learning Theory
   c. Community Organization Theory
   d. Health Belief Model
4. Upon completion of your tobacco awareness program, you intend to present the results to other health care professionals at a health promotions meeting. Which strategy would you choose if you wish to reach a large number of people, have time for interaction, and do not intend to use audiovisual equipment?
   a. Poster presentation
   b. Roundtable discussion
   c. Oral paper
   d. Table clinic
5. You bring your tobacco awareness program to the state public health dental hygienist. In attempting to follow the essential services of the public health core functions, the state dental hygienist wants to support and implement programs at all levels of prevention. At which level of prevention is your tobacco program?
   a. Primary
   b. Secondary
   c. Tertiary
   d. Planning

Answers and rationales to the questions are presented next. Also, see the chapters in which the information can be retrieved from within the text.

Answers And Rationales

The answers, rationales for each answer, and chapter cross-references are presented next.

Testlet No. 1

1.   d.   A unified plan of action is the best defense against a strong antifluoridation group. Answers a., b., and c. are also possibilities of things you can do, but d. is best and foremost (see Chapter 6).

2.	a.	A public debate with antifluoridationists only provides them with an opportunity to reach more people with their scare tactics (see Chapter 6).
3.	a.	The DMFT Index is used to determine the decay rate in children (see Chapter 4).
4.	c.	Calibration of examiners is the best way to make sure that the data that you are collecting are reproducible or reliable (see Chapter 7).
5.	c.	A school fluoride mouth rinse program would be the next choice because it is inexpensive and would benefit all the children in reducing dental decay. Sealants are more expensive, and education does not guarantee a reduction in decay. These programs should be used in conjunction with fluoride (see Chapter 6).

Testlet No. 2

1.	d.	Reducing the incidence of periodontitis and gingivitis in children is not an objective of *Healthy People 2020;* all the other choices are objectives (see Chapter 5).
2.	c.	An assessment such as that conducted using the DMFT Index determines the need for oral health services. Answers b. and d. would not be appropriate because the DMFT Index is an assessment tool for determining decay. (see Chapters 4 and 9).
3.	b.	Evaluation of performance is best conducted with an activity or demonstration by the person being evaluated (see Chapters 6 and 8).
4.	d.	The Basic Screening Survey (BSS) is an easy tool to let parents know whether the child needs emergency care, whether treatment is necessary, or whether routine care is recommended. Local community clinics provide the best fee for service for low-income patients. It is difficult to reach people by phone, and the follow-up list for referral is very important to the screening process (see Chapters 2 and 4).
5.	a.	Medicare is a program for elderly people, and it does not cover dental services. All of the other programs offer oral health treatment for children (see Chapter 6).

Testlet No. 3

1.	c.	Assessment of needs is always the first step in program planning (see Chapters 3 and 8).
2.	c.	The residents in nursing homes rely on the staff or caregivers to assist them with oral hygiene. Therefore the staff must be educated on the importance of their own oral health first (see Chapters 2, 6, and 8).
3.	a.	All of these ideas would work except a., since Medicare does not offer dental benefits (see Chapter 6).
4.	d.	To find the mean, add the scores and divide by the total number of scores (see Chapter 7).
5.	c.	In comparing two variables, if the correlation is .70 or higher, the relationship is strong (see Chapter 7).

Testlet No. 4

1.	b.	"Community profile" is the term used to describe the community, including gender, age, and socioeconomic status (see Chapter 3).
2.	d.	The Community Periodontal Index (CPI) entails gathering data in all the areas described. It is a modification of the Community Periodontal Index of Treatment Needs (CPITN) and is more readily used. The other indexes are too specific and not as inclusive. The PDI is not widely used anymore (see Chapter 4).

3. d. The Health Belief Model is the only one listed that includes information on the people's perceptions or beliefs about oral health (see Chapter 8).
4. a. The poster presentation allows for the most interaction with the largest number of people. This is a popular presentation method at health promotion meetings. Audiovisual equipment is not used, and personal interaction is foremost (see Chapter 8).
5. a. Preventive services, such as a tobacco awareness program, are at the primary prevention level; they prevent the disease before it occurs. Secondary prevention reduces or eliminates disease in the early stages. Tertiary prevention limits disability from disease in later stages. Planning and implementing are phases of program development (see Chapters 1, 2, and 6).

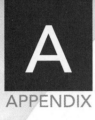
Academy of General Dentistry
www.agd.org
American Academy of Pediatric Dentistry (AAPD)
www.aapd.org
American Association of Endodontists (AAE)
www.aae.org
American Association of Orthodontists
www.aaortho.org
American Association of Public Health Dentistry (AAPHD)
www.aaphd.org
American Dental Assistants Association (ADAA)
www.dentalassistant.org
American Dental Association (ADA)
www.ada.org
American Dental Hygienists' Association (ADHA)
www.adha.org; www.adha.org/governmental_affairs
American Medical Association (AMA)
www.ama-assn.org
American Public Health Association (APHA)
www.apha.org
Association of State & Territorial Dental Directors (ASTDD)
www.astd.org
Centers for Disease Control and Prevention (CDC), Oral Health Resources
www.cdc.gov/oralhealth/index.htm
Centers for Medicare & Medicaid Services (CMS)
www.cms.hhs.gov
Colgate Company
www.colgate.com
Federation Dentaire Internationale (FDI) World Dental Federation
www.fdiworldental.org
Government Grants
www.grants.gov

*Updated URLs for these resources and more can be found on this book's Evolve site.

Health Resources and Services Administration (HRSA)
www.hrsa.gov
International and American Associations for Dental Research (IAADR)
www.iadr.com
National Institute of Dental and Craniofacial Research (NIDCR)
www.nidcr.nih.gov
National Maternal and Child Oral Health Resource Center
www.ncemch.org/oralhealth
National Oral Health Information Clearinghouse
www.nidcr.nih.gov
Occupational Safety and Health Administration (OSHA)
www.osha.gov
Oral Health America
www.oralhealthamerica.org
Procter & Gamble
www.dentalcare.com
Synopsis of State Dental Public Health Programs
www.astdd.org/docs/StateSynopsisReport2010Summary.pdf
The American Academy of Periodontology
www.perio.org
The American College of Prosthodontists
www.prosthodontics.org/acpros/index.html
US Department of Health and Human Services (DHHS)
www.dhhs.gov
World Health Organization (WHO)
www.who.ch

Dental Hygiene Competencies*

According to the "Competencies for Entry into the Profession of Dental Hygiene" approved and adopted by the American Dental Education Association (ADEA) House of Delegates in 2003, the dental hygienist must exhibit competencies in the five following domains:

1. The dental hygienist must possess, first, the Core Competencies (C): the ethics, values, skills, and knowledge integral to all aspects of the profession. These core competencies are foundational to all of the roles of the dental hygienist.
2. Second, inasmuch as Health Promotion (HP) and Disease Prevention is a key component of health care, changes within the health care environment require the dental hygienist to have a general knowledge of wellness, health determinants, and characteristics of various patient/client communities. The hygienist needs to emphasize both prevention of disease and effective health care delivery.
3. Third is the dental hygienist's complex role in the Community (CM). Dental hygienists must appreciate their role as health professionals at the local, state, and national levels. This role requires the graduate dental hygienist to assess, plan, and implement programs and activities to benefit the general population. In this role, the dental hygienist must be prepared to influence others to facilitate access to care and services.
4. Fourth is Patient/Client Care (PC), requiring competencies described here in ADPIE format. Because the dental hygienist's role in patient/client care is ever changing, yet central to the maintenance of health, dental hygiene graduates must use their skills to assess, diagnose, plan, implement, and evaluate treatment.
5. Fifth, like other health professionals, dental hygienists must be aware of a variety of opportunities for Professional Growth and Development (PGD). Some opportunities may increase clients' access to dental hygiene; others may offer ways to influence the profession and the changing health care environment. A dental hygienist must possess transferable skills (e.g., in communication, problem solving, and critical thinking) to take advantage of these opportunities.

Core Competencies

C.1 Apply a professional code of ethics in all endeavors.

C.2 Adhere to state and federal laws, recommendations, and regulations in the provision of dental hygiene care.

C.3 Provide dental hygiene care to promote patient/client health and wellness using critical thinking and problem solving in the provision of evidenced-based practice.

---

*Also available on this book's Evolve website.

C.4 Assume responsibility for dental hygiene actions and care based on accepted scientific theories and research as well as the accepted standard of care.

C.5 Continuously perform self-assessment for lifelong learning and professional growth.

C.6 Advance the profession through service activities and affiliations with professional organizations.

C.7 Provide quality assurance mechanisms for health services.

C.8 Communicate effectively with individuals and groups from diverse populations both verbally and in writing.

C.9 Provide accurate, consistent, and complete documentation for assessment, diagnosis, planning, implementation, and evaluation of dental hygiene services.

C.10 Provide care to all clients using an individualized approach that is humane, empathetic, and caring.

Health promotion and disease prevention

HP.1 Promote the values of oral and general health and wellness to the public and organizations within and outside the profession.

HP.2 Respect the goals, values, beliefs, and preferences of the patient or client while promoting optimal oral and general health.

HP.3 Refer patients or clients who may have a physiologic, psychologic, or social problem for comprehensive patient and client evaluation.

HP.4 Identify individual and population risk factors and develop strategies that promote health-related quality of life.

HP.5 Evaluate factors that can be used to promote patient or client adherence to disease prevention or health maintenance strategies.

HP.6 Evaluate and use methods to ensure the health and safety of the patient or client and the dental hygienist in the delivery of dental hygiene.

Community involvement

CM.1 Assess the oral health needs of the community and the quality and availability of resources and services.

CM.2 Provide screening, referral, and educational services that allow clients to access the resources of the health care system.

CM.3 Provide community oral health services in a variety of settings.

CM.4 Facilitate client access to oral health services by influencing individuals and organizations for the provision of oral health care.

CM.5 Evaluate reimbursement mechanisms and their impact on the patient or client's access to oral health care.

CM.6 Evaluate the outcomes of community-based programs and plan for future activities.

Patient and Client Care

Assessment

PC.1 Systematically collect, analyze, and record data on the general, oral, and psychosocial health status of a variety of patients or clients using methods consistent with medicolegal principles. This competency includes the following steps:
   a. Select, obtain, and interpret diagnostic information, recognizing its advantages and limitations.
   b. Recognize predisposing and etiologic risk factors that require intervention to prevent disease.
   c. Obtain, review, and update a complete medical, family, social, and dental history.

   d. Recognize health conditions and medications that affect overall patient or client care.

   e. Identify patients or clients at risk for a medical emergency, and manage the patient or client care in a manner that prevents an emergency.

   f. Perform a comprehensive examination using clinical, radiographic, periodontal, dental charting, and other data collection procedures to assess the patient's or client's needs.

Diagnosis

PC.2 Use critical decision-making skills to reach conclusions about the patient's or client's dental hygiene needs based on all available assessment data. This competency includes the following steps:

   a. Use assessment findings, etiologic factors, and clinical data in determining a dental hygiene diagnosis.

   b. Identify patient or client needs and significant findings that affect the delivery of dental hygiene services.

   c. Obtain consultations as indicated.

Planning

PC.3 Collaborate with the patient or client or other health professionals to formulate a comprehensive dental hygiene care plan that is patient-centered or client-centered and based on current scientific evidence. This competency includes the following steps:

   a. Prioritize the care plan based on the health status and the actual and potential problems of the individual to facilitate optimal oral health.

   b. Establish a planned sequence of care (educational, clinical, and evaluation) based on the dental hygiene diagnosis; identified oral conditions; potential problems; etiologic and risk factors; and available treatment modalities.

   c. Establish a collaborative relationship with the patient or client in the planned care to include etiology, prognosis, and treatment alternatives.

   d. Make referrals to other health care professionals.

   e. Obtain the patient's or client's informed consent based on a thorough case presentation.

Implementation

PC.4 Provide specialized treatment that includes preventive and therapeutic services designed to achieve and maintain oral health. Assist in achieving oral health goals formulated in collaboration with the patient/client. This competency includes the following steps:

   a. Perform dental hygiene interventions to eliminate or control local etiologic factors to prevent and control caries, periodontal disease, and other oral conditions.

   b. Control pain and anxiety during treatment through the use of accepted clinical and behavioral techniques.

   c. Provide life support measures to manage medical emergencies in the patient or client care environment.

Evaluation

PC.5 Evaluate the effectiveness of the implemented clinical, preventive, and educational services, and modify as needed. This competency includes the following steps:

   a. Determine the outcomes of dental hygiene interventions using indexes, instruments, examination techniques, and the patient or client self-report.

   b. Evaluate the patient's or client's satisfaction with the oral health care received and the oral health status achieved.

   c. Provide subsequent treatment or referrals based on evaluation findings.

   d. Develop and maintain a health maintenance program.

Professional growth and development

PGD.1 Identify alternative career options within health care, industry, education, and research and evaluate the feasibility of pursuing dental hygiene opportunities.

PGD.2 Develop management and marketing strategies to be used in nontraditional health care settings.

PGD.3 Access professional and social networks and resources to assist entrepreneurial initiatives.

The American Association of Dental Schools (AADS; now called the *American Dental Education Association [ADEA]*) drafted these competency statements. Representation was provided from both baccalaureate and associate degree dental hygiene programs. It also included representation from dental hygiene, clinical, social, and basic sciences and the American Dental Hygienists' Association (ADHA). A separate committee, the Dental Hygiene Education Competency Draft Review Committee, further reviewed and provided feedback on the document. The competency statements were presented for public comment at the 1998 AADS Annual Session, the 1998 Dental Hygiene Directors conference, and the Section on Dental Hygiene Education home page on the Internet and went into effect in January 2000.

Bibliography

American Dental Education Association (ADEA). *Competencies for entry into the profession of dental hygiene: ADEA Section on Dental Hygiene Education* (approved March 2003 House of Delegates).

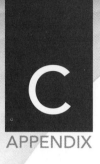

Community Partnerships for Oral Health

APPENDIX C-1 POTENTIAL COMMUNITY PARTNERS

Patients, Clients and Consumers of Services

- Patients and clients
- Parents and family representatives
- Advocacy groups for patients, clients, and consumers of services
- Advocacy groups for parents and family representatives
- Consumers of services
- Public representatives
- Support groups for patients, clients, and consumers of services
- Support groups for parents and family representatives

Government Agencies and Programs

- State, territorial, and tribal departments of health (e.g., administrators and staff for oral health, maternal and child health, WIC, primary health care, family planning, rural health, health disparities, minority health, HIV, chronic diseases, tobacco control, etc.)
- State, territorial, and tribal human service agency staff and administrators (e.g., programs for individuals with mental illness and mental retardation, developmental and acquired disabilities, government hospitals, clinics, and institutions, programs for individuals with special health care needs [e.g., blind, deaf, etc.], state units on elder affairs and aging, department of corrections)
- Regional council of governments
- Area agencies on aging in local areas
- County extension agencies
- Local health departments (e.g., county and city health officials and staff)
- Local human service agency administrators and staff (e.g., programs for individuals with mental illness and mental retardation, developmental and acquired disabilities, government hospitals, clinics, and institutions, programs for individuals with special health care needs [e.g., blind, deaf, etc.], elder affairs and aging, department of corrections)
- Representatives such as county and city officials working with child care, youth services, literacy, libraries, elderly and disabled services, public transportation, public housing, workforce development, etc.
- Environmental health: community water supervisors or managers related to community water fluoridation

Policymakers and Organizations

- US Congress: Senators and Representatives
- Legislators: State Senators and State Representatives
- Local government elected officials: county judges, mayors, city councilors and county commissioners, etc.
- Policy advocates (e.g., Legal Aid, League of United Latin American Citizens [LULAC], National Association for the Advancement of Colored Person [NAACP], etc.)
- Policy institutes

Community Organizations

- Advocacy organizations for clients and consumers of services
- Advocacy organizations for children and adults with disabilities, HIV, cancer, homeless children and adults, etc.)
- United Way, American Cancer Society, Diabetes Association, March of Dimes, Easter Seals, Mental Health Association, Success by 6, Healthy Mothers/Healthy Babies Coalition, League of Women Voters, Association for Retarded Citizens (ARC), United Cerebral Palsy, American Red Cross, Urban League, American Association of Retired Persons (AARP), etc.
- Community action agencies
- Senior nutrition services and sites
- Early childhood intervention organizations
- National, state, and local information and resource (I&R) networks (community information and resource centers such as organizations coordinating non-emergency 3-1-1 telephone number call centers for government services; organizations coordinating 2-1-1 telephone number help lines with United Ways and information and referral agencies in states and local communities; organizations coordinating toll-free hotline (e.g., state Maternal and Child Health (MCH) Agency Title V toll-free hotline; aging and disability information and referral support centers)
- Representatives of consumer and regional advisory groups
- Religious organizations
- Faith-based organizations (e.g., Catholic Charities, Salvation Army, etc.)
- Local representatives active in collaborative service programs with health and human service agencies that specifically address key issues (e.g., community planning)
- Service organization for vulnerable population groups (e.g., literacy, elderly and disabled services, youth services, veterans, women, public transportation, public housing, workforce development, child care, food banks, homeless shelters, migrant and seasonal farm workers, etc.)
- Administrators and staff for programs and supportive services, including Alzheimer's facilities and care, assisted living, programs for assistive technology and disability aids, eldercare agencies, geriatric and professional care manager, home care services, home maintenance and chore services, hospice care, programs for long-term care insurance, medicaid, and medicare supplement, advantage and drug planning, medical equipment and medical alert programs, nursing homes, retirement communities with care, senior health care and house call doctors, and veterans' benefits consultants
- Corporation for National and Community Service, AmeriCorps, Senior Corps, Learn and Serve America, Volunteers in Service to America (VISTA), Youth Service Corps, and City Year
- Business leaders and Chamber of Commerce (e.g., Women Chamber of Commerce, Hispanic Chamber of Commerce)

- Community centers and neighborhood associations
- State and local coalitions, collaborations, initiatives, outreach staff, community-based organizations and advocacy organizations for oral health, public health issues, access to health care (e.g., insuring children, adults, uninsured, vulnerable groups, etc.)
- Foundations and corporate giving programs: international, national, state, and local community grant makers and philanthropy sector administrators and staff
- Unions and organized labor
- Civic organizations: Junior League, Rotary International, Kiwanis, Lions Club, Elks
- Youth Groups: Boys and Girls Clubs, YMCA, YWCA, Big Brothers/Big Sisters, Special Olympics
- Media: international, national, state, and local media, including newspapers, television, radio, magazines/journals, internet, websites, blogs, social media, social networking pages, Facebook, Twitter, Flickr, YouTube, etc.

Education-Related Organizations and Groups

- Regional education service centers
- Local school districts and boards: superintendents, principals, teachers, school nurses, school social workers, parent liaisons
- Local child development and child care grantees and Head Start grantees and delegate agencies (e.g., Head Start executive directors, Head Start health coordinators, etc.)
- Parent-Teacher Associations/ Organizations
- Parenting education programs
- Adult education and literacy programs
- Home school programs
- Employment and vocational education
- Education-related unions
- Fraternities and sororities

Health and Human Service Providers, Groups, Organizations, and Associations

- Health systems, hospitals and clinics (e.g., rural and community, public, nonprofit, private, children's hospitals, Department of Veterans Affairs hospitals and clinics, county hospital districts, etc.)
- Community health centers
- Safety-net health and oral health programs— community dental clinics, nonprofit dental clinics
- Maternal and Child Health Programs
- State and local health professional associations
- Dentists, dental hygienists, and dental assistants
- Physicians, pediatricians, family physicians, physician assistants, etc.
- Nurses, nurse practitioners, nurse midwives, etc.
- Speech pathologists
- Dieticians
- Nursing home administrators
- Early childhood early intervention providers
- Social workers, care coordinators, and case managers
- Health educators, community health workers, community health advisors, lay health advocates, promotores/promotoras, outreach educators, community health representatives, peer health promoters, peer health educators, and patient navigators

Third-Party Payers

- Health plans
- Dental insurers
- Managed care organizations
- Health maintenance organizations (HMOs)
- Employers providing dental insurance coverage
- Employers not providing dental insurance coverage
- Medicaid, Children's Health Insurance Program (CHIP)
- Health insurance coverage high-risk pools, preexisting condition insurance plans, and health insurance exchanges
- Program established by the 2010 Patient Protection and Affordable Care Act
- Health insurance programs and special initiatives reaching out to people with disabilities, veterans and military personnel, families, children, young adults, seniors, early retirees, individuals living in rural areas, Hispanics/Latinos, African Americans, Asian Americans and Pacific Islanders, American Indian and Alaska Natives, women, lesbian, bisexual, gay, and transgender (LBGT) communities, small businesses, and employers

Higher and Professional Education

- Universities and colleges
- Dental, dental hygiene, dental therapist, dental assisting schools
- Nursing schools
- Medical schools
- Allied health schools
- Schools of public health
- Schools of social work
- Schools of public policy and health administration
- Schools for speech pathology
- Schools for dietetics

Business Organizations and Retail Outlets

- Airlines
- Banks
- Beauty and barber shops
- Chambers of commerce
- Computer companies and stores
- Grocery stores
- Delicatessens, specialty, and ethnic food stores
- Health clubs
- Insurance companies
- Shopping malls
- Maternity stores
- Movie theaters

NOTE: Territorial agencies and organizations include the following territories and jurisdictions: District of Columbia; Pacific-Basin territories and jurisdictions: Territory of American Samoa, Territory of Guam, Republic of the Marshall Islands, Federated States of Micronesia, Commonwealth of the Northern Mariana Islands, and Republic of Palau; and Eastern territories and jurisdictions: Commonwealth of Puerto Rico and US Virgin Islands. Tribal agencies and organizations include the following: American Indian/Alaska Native tribally designated organizations; Alaska Native Health Corporations; Urban Indian Health Organizations.

Bibliography

American Dental Association. Community organization for water fluoridation manual. Chicago: American Dental Association, Council on Access, Prevention and Interprofessional Relations; 1997.

Association of State & Territorial Dental Directors. Best practice approaches for state and community oral health programs: state oral health coalitions and collaborative partnerships. New Bern, NC: ASTDD; 2008.

Association of State & Territorial Dental Directors. Best practice approaches for state and community oral health programs: state oral health plans and collaborative planning. New Bern, NC: ASTDD; 2008.

Centers for Disease Control and Prevention, Division of Oral Health. Infrastructure development tools, updated. Atlanta: CDC; 2009.

Centers for Disease Control and Prevention, Division of Oral Health. Building capacity to fluoridate, literature review. Atlanta: CDC; 2003.

Centers for Disease Control and Prevention, Division of Oral Health. Infrastructure development tools: oral health coalition framework. Atlanta: CDC; 2002.

DentaQuest Foundation: An electronic compendium of resources for building oral health coalitions. Westborough, MA: DentaQuest Foundation; 2010.

Seven Days of Immunizations. National Infant Immunization Week. Atlanta: U.S. Department of Health and Human Services, Public Health Service, Centers for Disease Control and Prevention; 1995.

Steffensen JEM. Guide for oral health listening sessions: activation of a collaborative oral health plan in Texas. San Antonio: Department of Community Dentistry, University of Texas Health Science Center at San Antonio, Dental School; 2004.

Washington State Oral Health Coalition. Community roots for oral health: guidelines for successful coalitions. Olympia, WA: Washington State Department of Health, Community and Family Health; 2000.

APPENDIX C-2   ORAL HEALTH COALITION FRAMEWORK

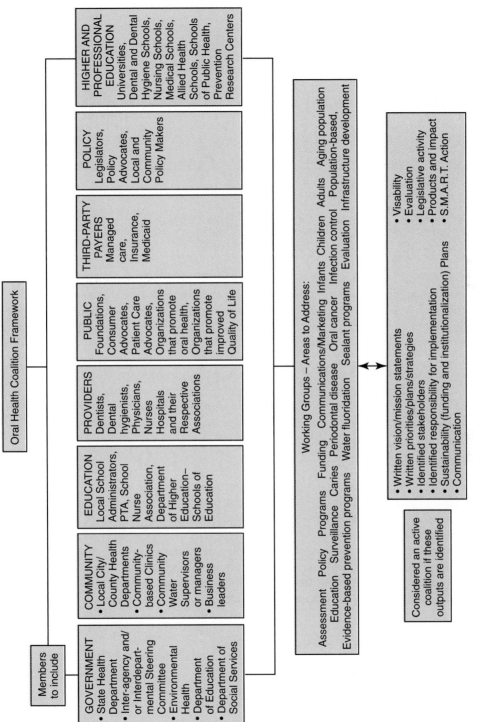

Adapted from: CDC, Division of Oral Health. Oral Health Infrastructure Development Tools, 2002.

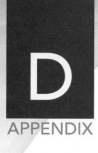

D

Resources for Community Health Assessment

APPENDIX D-1   EXAMPLES OF INFORMATION FOR A COMMUNITY PROFILE

Physical and Spatial Characteristics

Geopolitical boundaries, community-designated boundaries, geographic size, community location description, population size, population density, community type, general physical environment, geographic isolation, physical conditions of neighborhoods, community assets, people-made environment, layout of the community, residential neighborhoods, business districts, buildings, greenspace, parks, transportation routes, roads, traffic, congestion, environmental conditions, air quality, water supply, water quality, community infrastructure, education resources and facilities, location and characteristics of local institutions, landmarks, art, media, playgrounds, recreation facilities and resources, libraries, public commons and informal gathering places, number of places of worship, religious denominations, local economy and types of industry, signs of development or decay in community areas, and patterns of daily activities and everyday human interactions.

Community Inventory

History of community, community traditions, dominant values, significant beliefs, events that have occurred in the community with a short- or long-term effect on the health of the community, political system, local government structure, political structure, dominant political affiliation, number of registered voters, power structure, formal and informal community leadership, formal community support systems, informal helping networks/mutual support and trusted community members, gatekeepers, opinion leaders, community historians, communication channels, inventories of citizen's associations and community organizations, inventory of capacities of individual community members, and groups of individuals.

SOCIODEMOGRAPHIC CHARACTERISTICS

Community Demographic Data

Population distribution by age, gender, race and ethnicity composition, social class, economic status, education levels, occupations, marital status, gender ratios, socioeconomic data, employment status, neighborhood living conditions, value of housing, household living conditions, household crowding, indices of deprivation, levels of education, religions, nationality, and cultural characteristics, generational information, in-migration and out-migration, immigration status, trends of change in size and composition.

Social Demographic Data

Social attributes, social structure, community stability, social cohesiveness, civic engagement and pride, social networks, family and household characteristics, family values, family living patterns, community norms, customs and lifestyles, health-enhancing behaviors, risk and protective factors, values, attitudes, beliefs, opinions, social and cultural forces, religious beliefs, enrollment in government programs (including Temporary Assistance for Needy Families [TANF]), public assistance, food stamps, Supplemental Food Program for Women, Infants, and Children (WIC), Head Start, child care support, Medicaid, Children's Health Insurance Program (CHIP), vulnerable populations groups in community, quality of life, crime, and security.

Vital Events

Natality (births), fertility rates, life expectancy, mortality (deaths), marriages, divorces, population mobility.

APPENDIX D-2   EXAMPLES OF GOVERNMENT RESOURCES FOR HEALTH DATA

Resources for health and oral health information are available from many organizations and governmental agencies. These sources include: clearinghouses and resource centers, federal, state, and local government agencies, foundations, policy and research centers, professional, programs and initiatives, and voluntary organizations. This section will concentrate on resources available through government entities. The National Maternal and Child Oral Health Resource Center has a listing of internet links to many organizations and agencies that provide oral health information.
www.mchoralhealth.org/Links/index.html

Below are websites for some of the government resources for health data. For additional resources and definitions of the services they provide visit the Elsevier website.

National Maternal and Child Oral Health Resource Center (OHRC), Georgetown University
www.mchoralhealth.org/
National Maternal and Child Oral Health Policy Center
http://nmcohpc.net/
National Oral Health Information Clearinghouse (NOHIC)
www.nidcr.nih.gov/OralHealth/
National Oral Health Surveillance System (NOHSS)
www.cdc.gov/nohss/index.htm
Synopses of State & Territorial Dental Public Health Programs (State Synopses)
http://apps.nccd.cdc.gov/synopses/index.asp
Water Fluoridation Reporting System (WFRS)
www.cdc.gov/fluoridation/fact_sheets/engineering/wfrs_factsheet.htm

Agency for Healthcare Research and Quality (AHRQ)
www.ahrq.gov/
Administration on Aging (AOA)
www.aoa.gov
Administration for Children and Families (ACF)
www.acf.hhs.gov/
Centers for Medicare and Medicaid Services (CMS)
www.cms.gov/
Centers for Disease Control and Prevention (CDC)
www.cdc.gov/
CDC, National Center for Health Statistics (NCHS)
www.cdc.gov/nchs/index.htm
Health Resources and Services Administration (HRSA)
www.hrsa.gov/
Indian Health Service, Division of Oral Health
www.ihs.gov/MedicalPrograms/Dental/index.cfm
National Institutes of Health (NIH)
www.nih.gov/
National Institute of Dental and Craniofacial Research (NIDCR) Oral Health Data and Statistics
www.nidcr.nih.gov/
Healthy People 2020
http://healthypeople.gov/HP2020/
World Health Organization, Oral Health Databases
www.who.int/oral_health/databases/en/index.html

APPENDIX D-3   SUMMARY OF DATA COLLECTION METHODS

Method	Instrument	Cost and Time*	Advantage
Document Study Review and evaluate existing documents or records describing past events or occurrences	Information abstracted from archival sources (raw data, datasets of summary data, printed reports); qualitative or quantitative data from public legislative bodies, governmental officials and agencies, private businesses, professional and community organizations, nonprofit foundations	$-$$ ⏱–⏱⏱	Data often readily available.
Observational Field Study Assessment of actual events, objects, or people in "natural" setting	Assessors use checklists, evaluation forms, camera, tape recorder, rating scales, observation field notes. Qualitative approach with content or situational analysis	$$ ⏱⏱	First-hand information.
Windshield or Walking Tour Within community-designated boundaries, observers and recorders drive or walk in community areas at varying times of days and days of week to assess community activities, interactions and events through observation, informal conversations, and interactions with community members	Observers and recorders document community characteristics and record information using observational guides, checklists, survey tools, notes, photos, audiotapes, videotapes; qualitative approach with content or situational analysis; results summarized and displayed through written narratives, tables, diagrams, slide and video shows, maps, collages	$-$$ ⏱–⏱⏱	First-hand information.
Mailed Survey Assessment (surveys, polls, evaluations, etc.) conducted by direct mail; adaptations include questionnaire sent home with children from school, telefax survey, magazine or newsletter survey, or electronic survey (using networked computers, e-mail, Internet, websites, blogs, social media, social networking pages, Facebook, Twitter, Flickr, etc.).	Self-administered standardized, structured questionnaire with closed- and open-ended questions completed by respondent; quantitative approach with statistical analysis of responses	$$ ⏱⏱	Data can be collected from a large sample.

Continued

APPENDIX D-3   SUMMARY OF DATA COLLECTION METHODS—cont'd

Method	Instrument	Cost and Time*	Advantage
Telephone Interview Survey interview conducted by telephone.	Interviewer reads structured interview schedule (standardized, questionnaire) with closed- and open-ended questions to respondent; quantitative approach with statistical analysis of responses	$$ 🕐🕐	Data can be collected from a large sample.
Person-to-Person Interview Survey interview conducted face to face between a respondent and an interviewer.	Structured interview schedule (standardized, questionnaire) with closed- and open-ended questions read to respondent by an interviewer; quantitative approach with statistical analysis of responses	$$-$$$ 🕐🕐– 🕐🕐🕐	Face-to-face communication allows for more in-depth information.
In-Depth Personal Interview Survey conducted face-to-face to learn about life history, events, and experiences.	Interviewer uses open-ended, flexible, unstructured nondirective questions; transcriptions of tape recordings used for thematic analysis of content	$$-$$$ 🕐🕐– 🕐🕐🕐	Smaller sample with expanded perspectives
Screening Survey Rapid assessment using screening procedures.	Standardized written criteria and measurements, measuring instruments, and protocols; cursory inspection provides crude estimates; quantitative approach with statistical analysis of results	$$ 🕐🕐	Practical and uniform information in a short time period.
Epidemiologic Survey Extensive assessment using examination procedures, clinical samples, and clinical tests.	Standardized written criteria and measurements, measuring instruments, and protocols; detailed planning of examination conditions, indices, criteria, sampling approach, personnel training, data collection, data management, and analysis; quantitative approach with statistical analysis of results	$$-$$$ 🕐🕐– 🕐🕐🕐	More detailed information.

APPENDIX D-3 SUMMARY OF DATA COLLECTION METHODS—cont'd

Method	Instrument	Cost and Time*	Advantage
Asset Maps Geographic study and mapping that can identify patterns of community characteristics, physical assets, or settings of human activity and interactions.	Input and display of data from existing sources or new data onto geographic map using simple materials (land use map and adhesives or pushpins) or detailed community planning and evaluation computer software (e.g., Geographic Information System [GIS] computer software) and other powerful tools for organizing location, distribution, and mapping of spatial data	$-$$-$$ ⊕–⊕⊕	Good overview and visualization of information
Inventories or Directories Documenting and cataloging of assets and capacities of individual community members or community resources such as institutions, organizations, and associations.	Identify, evaluate, and organize assets and capacities in a community and develop adequate mechanisms for linkages that can produce opportunities for action; such capacities may include assets owned or skills processed by individual community members; may also include sources of mutual aid, connections, and resources among institutions, organizations, and associations in a community	$-$$ ⊕–⊕⊕	Data often collected previously
Focus Group Guided group discussion provides information on a specific topic from a certain population group.	Moderator leads guided group discussions among 5 to 12 individuals over ½ to 1½ hours by using a series of open-ended questions on a preestablished discussion guide; transcriptions from tape recordings and written field notes of discussions used for thematic analysis of content	$$-$$$ ⊕⊕– ⊕⊕⊕	Varied and ample information
Public Forum or Community Dialogue Event Individuals or groups provide verbal input or feedback on specific issues.	Moderator solicits, collects, and summarizes written comments or oral testimony; oral testimony recorded by tape recorder or court reporter to generate official record for analysis	$$ ⊕⊕	First-hand and ample information

Continued

APPENDIX D-3   SUMMARY OF DATA COLLECTION METHODS—cont'd

Method	Instrument	Cost and Time*	Advantage
Community Visioning Process			
Groups of community stakeholders collectively develop shared vision of their community in the future.	Through an interactive approach (retreat or workshop format), a skilled facilitator brings individuals together over one or more days and guides participants through vision process by posing questions and assisting participants to visualize the future community and possibilities for forward advancement; small groups discuss visions and images; creation of document to reflect visions; follow-up meeting held to refine visions and to develop plan for incorporation of visions into community planning process	$$-$$$ ☺☺– ☺☺☺	Broad with ample and varied input
Creative Assessment			
Community members document perceptions of community through creative means.	Creative techniques and forums for expression (photography, film, theater, music, dance, murals, puppet shows, storytelling, drawings) used to convey wide range of perceptions of a community	$$-$$$ ☺☺– ☺☺☺	Interesting and innovative

$, Inexpensive; $$, moderate cost; $$$, expensive; ☺, less time-consuming; ☺☺, moderately time-consuming; ☺☺☺, very time-consuming.

APPENDIX D-4   EXAMPLES OF INFORMATION FOR A COMMUNITY HEALTH ASSESSMENT

Community Health Measures	Examples
Health Status (measurements of natality [births], morbidity [illness], and mortality [deaths])	***Birth statistics:*** Age, parity of mother, duration of pregnancy, types of births (single, twin), complications of pregnancy, complications of birth, birth defects, birth weight (e.g., low), premature births, and births to adolescent, older, or unmarried females ***Morbidity statistics:*** Incidence and prevalence of diseases, conditions, disabilities, injuries (distribution, intensity, and duration) such as unintentional and intentional injuries, homicide, suicide, cancer, heart disease, diabetes, stroke, infectious diseases (communicable) HIV/AIDS, tuberculosis, STD, mental illness, alcohol and drug abuse problems, occupational diseases, disability and decreased independence, developmental disabilities (e.g., cleft lip and/or palate, craniofacial anomalies), oral diseases or conditions (e.g., dental caries, periodontal diseases, or oral injuries) ***Mortality statistics:*** Distribution of death rates by age, race/ethnicity, sex, cause, geographic location, leading causes of deaths such as cancer (breast, colon, lung, or oral), heart disease, stroke, homicide, motor vehicle injuries, suicide, unintentional injury, and infant, neonatal, and postneonatal mortality
Health risks and protective factors (identification of patterns of behavioral and nonbehavioral factors)	***Self-rated (self-reported) general and oral health status***, recent poor health, days of work lost, days of school lost (e.g., caused by dental problems or care), average number of unhealthy days in past month, and satisfaction with quality of life and public health, health care, and social service system ***Occupational risks and work disability*** ***Stress indicators and resources*** (drunk driving, robberies, or assaults), access to drugs, recent drug use, alcoholic beverage outlets, gang problems, family violence (child abuse and neglect, spouse and elder abuse), major depression, self-esteem, alienation, discrimination, feelings of hope and despair, feelings of anger, social and family support, social and family resources (adaptation and cohesion), life events, or stress (personal, family, or job stress). ***Levels of health knowledge, beliefs, attitudes, behaviors, practices, and skills*** about self-care (toothbrushing with fluoride toothpaste and flossing) and health interventions; lifestyle, including diet (low in sugar), physical activity, health-related substance use (tobacco and alcohol), and safety practices (seat belts, mouthguards); and knowledge about location, availability, and appropriate use of local health resources, services, programs, family health care expenditures. ***Use of child and adult preventive health services,*** including dental sealants, fluoride treatments, prenatal care in first trimester, immunizations for children and adults, Pap smear, mammogram, and sigmoidoscopy for colon cancer screening.

Continued

APPENDIX D-4   EXAMPLES OF INFORMATION FOR A COMMUNITY HEALTH ASSESSMENT—cont'd

Community Health Measures	Examples
Access to public health, health care and social service system (scope, adequacy, accessibility, and availability of services in a coordinated, integrated system)	**Access to community preventive services (community water fluoridation) and public health services:** Scope and adequacy of local health department covering essential public health services (including infrastructure and capacity measures, local voluntary health programs, operational health promotion and education programs in work sites, schools, and community) by health providers, numbers, types, locations, and adequacy. **Access to facilities for personal health care:** Assessment of numbers, types, location, and adequacy of hospitals; emergency facilities; outpatient primary care; oral health; hearing; vision care; speech, physical, and occupational therapy; urgent care; mental health; alcohol and drug treatment programs; nursing homes; community health centers **Access to health professionals:** Adequacy and numbers of educated public health professionals and personal health service professionals with expertise and competence, levels of knowledge, attitudes, and behaviors, as well as practices and skills of public health professionals and personal health service professionals **Access to health insurance and usual sources of health care:** Comprehensive benefits with dental insurance and per capita spending (Medicare, Medicaid, Children's Health Insurance Program [CHIP], private insurance, Supplementary Security Income [SSI]) **Scope and adequacy of local social service programs** in addressing basic human, family, and community needs

HIV/AIDS, Human immunodeficiency virus/acquired immunodeficiency disease; *STD,* sexually transmitted disease.

APPENDIX D-5　EXAMPLES OF PRIMARY DATA COLLECTION TASKS

Planning
- Determine scope and objectives.
- Prepare protocols describing assessment plan.
- Select data collection methods.
- Establish criteria.
- Determine sampling methods and processes.
- Obtain approval of authorities.
- Plan for personnel and physical arrangements.
- Plan for data analysis phase (recording, managing, and analyzing data).
- Plan for data reporting phase.
- Prepare budget.
- Develop timetable of main activities and responsible staff.
- Plan for referral process (for clinical findings detected in health survey).
- Plan and develop consent form.
- Translate consent form.
- Gain approval of consent form from Institutional Review Board.
- Plan and develop data collection instruments.
- Develop data collection protocols.
- Plan data entry processes.
- Plan quality assurance processes for data collection.
- Plan and develop training materials for field team.

Implementing
- Contact and recruit participants.
- Gain consent of participants.
- Record data.
- Manage data.

- Plan and develop data collection and entry process (manual collection or direct data entry into personal computer or a mobile device also known as handheld device, handheld computer, palmtop computer, or personal digital assistant [PDA]).
- Translate data collection instruments.
- Gain approval of data collection instruments from Institutional Review Board.
- Pilot test consent form and data collection instruments.
- Revise consent form and data collection instruments.
- Obtain approval of revised consent form and data collection instruments from Institutional Review Board.
- Draw sample.
- Plan fieldwork and scheduling.
- Purchase and organize supplies.
- Initiate contact with data collection sites (work through established community networks or organizational structures).
- Organize logistics for data collection, including travel and site requirements.
- Train field team.
- Calibrate field team.
- Implement pilot test of assessment.

- Analyze data.
- Maintain quality assurance processes.
- Summarize findings.
- Report findings.

APPENDIX D-6   HEALTHY PEOPLE: MEASURES TO MONITOR OBJECTIVES AND DATA SOURCES

National Oral Health Objectives

Healthy People 2010 Oral Health Goal: To prevent and control oral and craniofacial diseases, conditions, and injuries and improve access to related services.

Healthy People 2010 National Health Objective Number* (Healthy People 2020 Proposed National Health Objective Number)†: Objective Topic Summary	Proposed National Oral Health Objective (Healthy People 2020)‡	Measure to Monitor Objective (Healthy People 2010) and Data Source (Healthy People 2020)
HP2010-21-1 (OH HP2020-6): Reduce dental caries experience.	Reduce the proportion of children and adolescents who have dental caries experience in their primary or permanent teeth. a. Reduce the proportion of young children with dental caries experience in their primary teeth (aged 3 to5 years). b. Reduce the proportion of children with dental caries experience in their primary and permanent teeth (aged 6 to 9 years). c. Reduce the proportion of adolescents with dental caries experience in their permanent teeth (aged 13 to 15 years).	% of persons with ≥1 dft or DMFT National Health and Nutrition Examination Survey (NHANES); Centers for Disease Control (CDC); National Center for Health Statistics (NCHS); Oral Health Survey of Native Americans, Indian Health Service (IHS), Division of Oral Health
HP2010-21-2 (OH HP2020-7): Reduce untreated dental decay	Reduce the proportion of children, adolescents, and adults with untreated dental decay. a. Reduce the proportion of young children with untreated dental decay in primary and permanent teeth (aged 3 to 5 years). b. Reduce the proportion of children with untreated dental decay in primary and permanent teeth (aged 6 to 9 years). c. Reduce the proportion of adolescents with untreated dental decay in primary and permanent teeth (aged 13 to 15 years). d. Reduce the proportion of adults with untreated dental decay (aged 35 to 44 years). e. Reduce the proportion of adults with untreated coronal caries (aged 65 to 74 years). f. Reduce the proportion of adults with untreated root surface caries (aged 75 years and older).	% of persons with ≥1 dt or DT NHANES, CDC, NCHS

APPENDIX D-6   HEALTHY PEOPLE: MEASURES TO MONITOR OBJECTIVES AND DATA SOURCES—cont'd

Healthy People 2010 National Health Objective Number* (Healthy People 2020 Proposed National Health Objective Number)†: Objective Topic Summary	Proposed National Oral Health Objective (Healthy People 2020)‡	Measure to Monitor Objective (Healthy People 2010) and Data Source (Healthy People 2020)
HP2010-21-3 and 21-4 (OH HP2020-8): Reduce permanent tooth loss and complete tooth loss	Increase the proportion of adults who have never had a permanent tooth extracted because of dental caries or periodontal disease. a. Increase the proportion of adults who have never had a permanent tooth extracted because of dental caries or periodontitis (aged 45 to 64 years). b. Decrease the proportion of older adults who have lost all of their natural teeth (aged 65 to 74 years).	% of persons with 28 teeth, no teeth extracted % of persons with all teeth extracted, edentulous NHANES, CDC, NCHS; Oral Health Survey of Native Americans, IHS, Division of Oral Health
HP2010-21-5a (OH HP2020-9): Reduce periodontal disease: destructive periodontal disease	Reduce periodontitis (aged 45 to 74 years).	% of persons with ≥4 mm LOA in at least 1 site NHANES, CDC, NCHS
HP2010-21-5b: Reduce periodontal disease: gingivitis	Reduce gingivitis. (HP2010 objective archived; proposed to not be included in Healthy People 2020. Archived because of lack of adequate data source.)	% of persons with ≥1 bleeding site NHANES, CDC, NCHS; Oral Health Survey of Native Americans, 1999, IHS, Division of Oral Health (Healthy People 2010 Data Sources)
HP2010-21-6 (OH HP 2020-1): Early detection of oral and pharyngeal cancers	Early detection of oral and pharyngeal cancers Increase the proportion of oral and pharyngeal cancers detected at the earliest stage.	% of individuals with oral and pharyngeal cancer diagnosed at earliest stage Surveillance, Epidemiology, and End Results (SEER); National Institutes of Health (NIH); National Cancer Institute (NCI)

Continued

APPENDIX D-6 HEALTHY PEOPLE: MEASURES TO MONITOR OBJECTIVES AND DATA SOURCES—cont'd

Healthy People 2010 National Health Objective Number* (Healthy People 2020 Proposed National Health Objective Number)†: Objective Topic Summary	Proposed National Oral Health Objective (Healthy People 2020)‡	Measure to Monitor Objective (Healthy People 2010) and Data Source (Healthy People 2020)
HP2010-21-7 (OH HP2020-16): Increase annual examinations for oral and pharyngeal cancer	Increase the proportion of adults who receive preventive screening and counseling from dental professionals (developmental). a. Increase the proportion of adults who received information from a dentist or dental hygienist focusing on reducing tobacco usage or smoking cessation. b. Increase the proportion of adults who received an annual cancer screening from a dentist or dental hygienist. c. Increase the proportion of adults who are tested or referred for glycemic control from a dentist or dental hygienist.	% of individuals with recent oral and pharyngeal examination past year NHANES, CDC, NCHS (potential data source)
HP2010-21-8 (OH HP2020-10): Increase dental sealants	Increase the proportion of children who have received dental sealants on their molar teeth. a. Children aged 3 to 5 years b. Children aged 6 to 9 years c. Adolescents aged 13 to 15 years	% of persons with ≥1 sealant on permanent molars NHANES, CDC, NCHS; Oral Health Survey of Native Americans, 1999, IHS, Division of Oral Health
HP2010-21-9 (OH HP2020-2): Increase community water fluoridation	Increase the proportion of the U.S. population served by community water systems with optimally fluoridated water.	% of people served by community water systems with optimal levels of fluoride Fluoridation Census, CDC, National Center for Chronic Disease Prevention and Health Promotion (NCCDPHP)
HP2010-21-10 (OH HP2020-3): Increase use of oral health care system	Increase the proportion of children and adults who use the oral health care system each year.	% of individuals with annual dental visit Medical Expenditure Panel Survey (MEPS), Agency for Healthcare Research and Quality (AHRQ)

APPENDIX D-6   HEALTHY PEOPLE: MEASURES TO MONITOR OBJECTIVES AND DATA SOURCES—cont'd

Healthy People 2010 National Health Objective Number* (Healthy People 2020 Proposed National Health Objective Number)†: Objective Topic Summary	Proposed National Oral Health Objective (Healthy People 2020)‡	Measure to Monitor Objective (Healthy People 2010) and Data Source (Healthy People 2020)
HP2010-21-11 (OH HP2020-11): Increase use of oral health care system by residents in long-term care facilities	Increase the proportion of long-term care residents who use the oral health care system each year. (Developmental)	% of nursing home residents with dental service within past year National Nursing Home Survey (NNHS), CDC, NCHS (potential data source)
HP2010-21-12 (OH HP2020-4): Increase dental services for low-income children	Increase the proportion of low-income children and adolescents who received any preventive dental service during the past year.	% of low-income children and adolescents with preventive dental service within past year MEPS, AHRQ
HP2010-21-13 (OH HP2020-12): Increase school-based health centers with oral health component	Increase the proportion of school-based health centers with an oral health component. a. Dental sealants b. Dental care c. Topical fluoride	% of school-based health centers with an oral health component National Assembly on School-Based Health Care (NASBHC)
HP2010-21-14 (OH HP2020-13): Increase local health departments and health centers with an oral health component	Increase the proportion of local health departments and Federally Qualified Health Centers (FQHCs) that have an oral health component. a. Increase the proportion of FQHCs that have an oral health care program. b. Increase the proportion of local health departments that have oral health prevention and/or care programs.	% of local health departments and community health centers with oral health component Health Resources and Services Administration (HRSA), Bureau of Primary Health Care (BPHC); Association of State & Territorial Dental Directors (ASTDD); Association of Community Dental Programs

Continued

APPENDIX D-6   HEALTHY PEOPLE: MEASURES TO MONITOR OBJECTIVES AND DATA SOURCES—cont'd

Healthy People 2010 National Health Objective Number* (Healthy People 2020 Proposed National Health Objective Number)†: Objective Topic Summary	Proposed National Oral Health Objective (Healthy People 2020)‡	Measure to Monitor Objective (Healthy People 2010) and Data Source (Healthy People 2020)
HP2010-21-15 (OH HP2020-14): Increase number of states with a system for recording and referring infants and children with cleft lips and cleft palates	Increase the number of states and the District of Columbia that have a system for recording and referring infants and children with cleft lips and cleft palates to craniofacial anomaly rehabilitative teams. a. System for recording cleft lip/palate. b. System for referral for cleft lip/palate to rehabilitative teams.	Number of states with system for recording and referring orofacial clefts ASTDD
HP2010-21-16 (OH HP2020-5): Increase number of states with an oral health surveillance system	Increase the number of states and the District of Columbia that have an oral and craniofacial health surveillance system.	Number of states with an oral health surveillance system ASTDD
HP2010-21-17 (OH HP2020-15): Increase the number of tribal, state, and local dental public health programs	Increase the number of health agencies that have a dental public health program directed by a dental professional with public health training. a. State (including the District of Columbia) and local health agencies that serve jurisdictions of 250,000 or more persons. b. Indian Health Service Area and Tribal health programs that serve jurisdictions of 30,000 or more persons.	Number of state, tribal, territorial, and local health agencies with an effective public dental health program (directed by a dental professional with public health education) ASTDD Synopses, ASTDD; IHS, Division of Oral Health
(OH HP2020-17) Increase patients that receive oral health services at community health centers annually	Increase the proportion of patients that receive oral health services at FQHCs each year (newly proposed Healthy People 2020 Oral Health Objective)	% of patients of community health centers receiving dental care Uniformed Data System (UDS), HRSA, BPHC

APPENDIX D-6   HEALTHY PEOPLE: MEASURES TO MONITOR OBJECTIVES AND DATA SOURCES—cont'd

Healthy People 2010 National Health Objective Number* (Healthy People 2020 Proposed National Health Objective Number)†: Objective Topic Summary	Proposed National Oral Health Objective (Healthy People 2020)‡	Measure to Monitor Objective (Healthy People 2010) and Data Source (Healthy People 2020)

Selected National Health Objectives Related to Oral Health

Access to Quality Health Services: HP2010-1-6 (Access to Health Services: AHS HP2020-7): Reduce individuals experiencing difficulties or delays in obtaining necessary medical care, dental care, or prescription medicines	Reduce the proportion of individuals that experience difficulties or delays in obtaining necessary medical care, dental care, or prescription medicines. a. Individuals—medical care, dental care, or prescription medicine b. Individuals—medical care c. Individuals—dental care d. Individuals—prescription medicines	% of individuals that report difficulty or delay in obtaining dental care or did not receive needed dental care MEPS, AHRQ
Access to Quality Health Services: HP2010-1-8 (Public Health Infrastructure: PHI HP2020-11): Increase degrees awarded in the health professions to members of underrepresented racial and ethnic groups, including dentistry	In the health professions, allied and associated health profession fields, and the nursing field, increase the proportion of all degrees awarded to members of underrepresented racial and ethnic groups. a. Health professions, allied and associated health profession fields b. Nursing c. Medicine d. Dentistry e. Pharmacy	% of dental degrees (DDS and DMD) awarded to members of underrepresented racial and ethnic groups Survey of Predoctoral Dental Educational Institutions, American Dental Association (ADA)
Cancer: HP2010-03-6 (Cancer: C HP2020-6): Reduce oropharyngeal cancer deaths	Reduce the oropharyngeal cancer death rate.	Number of oral cancer deaths per 100,000 Population National Vital Statistics System (NVSS), CDC, NCHS

Continued

APPENDIX D-6   HEALTHY PEOPLE: MEASURES TO MONITOR OBJECTIVES AND DATA SOURCES—cont'd

Healthy People 2010 National Health Objective Number* (Healthy People 2020 Proposed National Health Objective Number)†: Objective Topic Summary	Proposed National Oral Health Objective (Healthy People 2020)‡	Measure to Monitor Objective (Healthy People 2010) and Data Source (Healthy People 2020)
Cancer: HP2010-3-10 a, b, c. (Tobacco Use: TU HP2020-17): Increase tobacco cessation counseling in dental care settings	Increase tobacco cessation counseling in health care settings. a. Increase tobacco cessation counseling in office-based ambulatory care settings. b. Increase tobacco cessation counseling in hospital ambulatory care settings. c. Increase tobacco cessation counseling in dental care settings.	Operational definition not specified NCHS—National Ambulatory Medical Care Survey (NAMCS)
Newly proposed Healthy People 2020 Health Objective: Tobacco Use: TU HP2020-19: Increase tobacco screening in health care settings, including dental care settings	Increase tobacco screening in health care settings (newly proposed Healthy People 2020 Health Objective). a. Increase tobacco screening in office-based ambulatory care settings. b. Increase tobacco screening in hospital ambulatory care settings. c. Increase tobacco screening in dental care settings.	Operational definition not specified NCHS—National Hospital Ambulatory Medical Care Survey (NHAMCS)
Diabetes: HP2010-05-15 Diabetes: D HP2020-9: Increase annual dental examination for persons with diabetes	Increase the proportion of persons with diabetes who have at least an annual dental examination.	% of persons (2 years and older) who report ever being diagnosed with diabetes and have had an annual dental visit National Health Interview Survey, CDC, NCHS

APPENDIX D-6   HEALTHY PEOPLE: MEASURES TO MONITOR OBJECTIVES AND DATA SOURCES—cont'd

Healthy People 2010 National Health Objective Number* (Healthy People 2020 Proposed National Health Objective Number)†: Objective Topic Summary	Proposed National Oral Health Objective (Healthy People 2020)‡	Measure to Monitor Objective (Healthy People 2010) and Data Source (Healthy People 2020)
Educational and Community-Based Programs: ECBP HP2020-12: Increase number of preschools and Head Start programs that provide health education to prevent health problems, including dental health	Increase the proportion of preschools and Head Start programs that provide health education to prevent health problems in the following areas: unintentional injury; violence; tobacco use and addiction; alcohol and drug use, unhealthy dietary patterns; and inadequate physical activity, dental health, and safety (developmental). a. Preschool Health Education—All priority areas b. Preschool Health Education—Unintentional injury c. Preschool Health Education—Violence d. Preschool Health Education—Tobacco use and addiction e. Preschool Health Education—Alcohol and other drug use f. Preschool Health Education—Unhealthy dietary patterns g. Preschool Health Education—Inadequate physical activity h. Preschool Health Education—Dental health i. Preschool Health Education—Safety	Operational definition not specified National Head Start Program Survey; National Household Education Surveys Program (NHES); National Survey of Children's Health (potential data sources)
Older Adults: OA HP2020-6: Increase health care work force with geriatric certification, including dentists	Increase the proportion of the health care work force with geriatric certification. a. Physicians b. Geriatric psychiatrists c. Registered nurses d. Dentists (developmental) Newly proposed Healthy People 2020 Health Objective	Operational definition not specified Annual Survey of Dentists, ADA

*Numbers refer to the chapter and objective as referenced in Healthy People 2010. For example, 21-12 is Chapter 21, Objective 12 or 03-6 is Cancer Chapter 3, Objective 6.

†Numbers refer to objective as referenced in Proposed Oral Health Objectives for Healthy People 2020. For example, OH HP2020-14 is Chapter 1, Proposed Objective 14 in the oral health chapter for Healthy People 2020 or Cancer: C HP2020-6 is Cancer Chapter 6 and Proposed Objective 6 for Healthy People 2020.

‡These Healthy People 2020 health objectives were proposed; see the Healthy People 2020 website for the final objectives to be achieved by 2020.

DT, Decayed permanent teeth; DMFT, decayed, missing, and filled permanent teeth; dft, decayed and filled primary teeth; dt, decayed primary teeth; LOA, loss of attachment.

Adapted from U.S. Department of Health and Human Services: Healthy People 2020: Public meetings 2009 draft objectives, Washington DC, 2009, DHHS; Healthy People 2010: Understanding and improving health, ed 2, Washington, DC, 2009, DHHS; U.S. Department of Health and Human Services: Tracking healthy people 2010, Washington, DC, 2000, U.S. Government Printing Office.

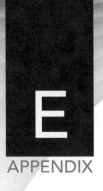

Selected Oral Conditions and Factors Influencing Oral Health that Can Be Assessed in Oral Health Surveys

ORAL CONDITIONS OR FACTORS	VARIABLES THAT CAN BE ASSESSED
Clinical treatment needs	• Dental service needed by type of care (e.g., prevention, restorations, extractions, crowns, etc.) • Treatment urgency
Craniofacial anomalies, including developmental anomalies	• Cleft lip or cleft palate • Craniofacial anomalies • Oral malformations
Dental caries	• Coronal caries • Early childhood caries • DFT, DFS, DMFT, DMFS • Gross loss of tooth structure • Pulpal involvement • Retained roots • Root caries • Untreated tooth (dental) decay • Restoration and Tooth Condition Assessment (RTCA) • Significant Caries Index (SiC Index): World Health Organization
Dental sealants	• Dental sealants on specific teeth (first molars, second molars, primary molars)
Dietary intake	• Healthy Eating Index • Dietary recall and dietary intake questionnaire • Food frequency questionnaire • Food choices and dietary patterns • Bottle feeding practices
Expense and payment source for oral health services	• Dental care expenses • Dental insurance • Medicaid
Fluoride	• Fluoride toothpaste use • Community water fluoridation • Fluoride supplements • Fluoride treatments

Impact of oral health on daily living	• Acute pain • Chronic pain • Eating (e.g., trouble chewing or eating) • Lost work, lost school days, activity change as the result of dental problems • Masticatory function • Mouth pain • Orofacial Pain Assessment: Orofacial pain questionnaire and orofacial pain examination • Salivary function (e.g., dry mouth, Sjögren's syndrome, xerostomia, etc.) • Speech • Swallowing • Temporomandibular dysfunction (TMD) • Temporomandibular Joint (TMJ) Assessment
Malocclusion	• Occlusion and occlusal traits • Orthodontic treatment needs • Dental Aesthetics Index (DAI)
Medications	• Medications prescribed for dental treatment
Oral and pharyngeal cancer	• Receipt of examination to detect oral cancer • Oral cancer diagnosis
Oral health knowledge, beliefs, opinions, attitudes, practices, behaviors, and skills	• Assessments of children, adolescents, and parents • Assessments of younger and older adults • Assessment of oral health care providers • Assessments of health care providers • Assessments of community stakeholders and policymakers
Oral health care providers	• Dental care provider information • Oral health care provider distribution • Oral health care provider training • Staffing of oral health care providers • Types of health care providers seen
Oral health care utilization	• Access to dental care (e.g., cost, travel, time, satisfaction, etc.) • Type of dental provider seen • Dental services by type (e.g., prevention, restorations, extractions, crowns, etc.) • Emergency dental care (e.g., traumatic injuries) • Dental care satisfaction • Frequency of dental visits • Last dental visit (indicating when) • Reason for dental visit • Reason for last dental visit • First dental visit • Frequency of dental visits • Number of dental visits

	• Usual source of dental care
	• Oral health care during pregnancy
	• Centers with oral health services
	• State and local dental programs
Orofacial injury	• Trauma
	• Accident
	• **National Institute for Dental Research** (NIDR) Trauma Index
Perceived oral health status and oral health related quality of life	• Assessment of general oral health status
	• Global Oral Health Assessment Index (GOHAI)
	• Oral Health Impact Profile (OHIP)
	• Child Oral Health Quality of Life Questionnaire
Perceived treatment needs	• Self-perceived need for dental care
Periodontal diseases	• Alveolar bone loss
	• Community Periodontal Index (CPI)
	• Furcations
	• Gingivitis
	• Calculus (e.g., subgingival calculus or supragingival calculus)
	• Gingival bleeding
	• Gingival inflammation
	• Loss of attachment
	• Periodontal index
	• Pocket depth
	• Recession
	• Tooth mobility
Preventive care	• Preventive care by clinician
	• Preventive self-care (e.g., oral hygiene)
Primary/permanent dentition	• Cleaning
	• Oral debris
	• Oral Health Index
Soft tissue lesions	• Mouth sores
	• Oral herpes
	• Oral lesions
	• Oral ulcers
	• Tongue lesions
Tobacco	• Cigarettes
	• Smokeless tobacco
	• Smoking cigars
	• Smoking pipes
	• Tobacco cessation counseling by dental professionals
Tooth loss/edentulism	• Tooth count
	• Denture ownership and use
	• Missing teeth
	• Self-reported dentition status

Bibliography

National Institute for Dental Research and Centers for Disease Control and Prevention: Dental, Oral, and Craniofacial Data Resource Center (DRC). Catalog of oral health surveys and archive of procedures related to oral health. Rockville, MD: NIDR/CDC; 2010.

National Institute for Dental Research and Centers for Disease Control and Prevention: Dental, Oral, and Craniofacial Data Resource Center (DRC). Oral health survey questions: a compilation of dental and oral health questions included on national health surveys. Rockville, MD: NIDR/CDC; 2010.

Bibliography

Commission on Dental Accreditation. *Accreditation Standards for Dental Hygiene Education Programs.* Chicago: American Dental Association; (approved July 1998; effective January 2000).

American Dental Education Association (ADEA). *Competencies for Entry into the Profession of Dental Hygiene: ADEA Section on Dental Hygiene Education.* (Approved March 2003 House of Delegates).

Glossary

Abstract A summary, confined to approximately 200 words, that concisely defines a study's purpose, methods, materials, and results; a brief description of the research, found at the beginning of a manuscript, designed to provide an overview of the study.

Access Assurance that conditions are in place for people to obtain the care they need and want.

Administrator (manager) A supervisory role in which the dental hygienist directs and oversees oral health programs.

Agent factors Biologic or mechanical means of causing disease, illness, injury, or disability, including microbial, parasitic, viral, and bacterial pathogens or vectors; physical or mechanical irritants; chemicals; drugs; trauma; automobiles; and radiation.

Alternative practice A setting outside the private office in which the dental hygienist provides public health services.

ANOVA (analysis of variance) A commonly used test for parametrics; allows comparison among more than two means from different samples and compares interactions among the variability in multiple sample groups to the variability within groups.

Assessment A core public health function that includes the regular and systematic collection, assemblage, and analysis of data and communication regarding the oral health of the community.

Association of State & Territorial Dental Directors (ASTDD) Basic Screening Survey (BSS) A survey used to assess need and referral for dental care; categories include (1) no dental care needed other than routine care, (2) early dental care recommended, and (3) urgent or emergency care recommended.

Assurance A core public health function in which agencies educate, support, and evaluate programs to ensure that the community's oral health needs are addressed.

Basic Screening Survey (BSS) A model for collecting oral health data developed by ASTDD.

BRFSS (Behavioral Risk Factor Surveillance Survey) A state-specific survey developed by the Centers for Disease Control and Prevention (CDC); structured questions are asked over the telephone to assess behaviors that influence health status; an oral health module assesses use of dental services.

Calibration Agreement of examiners who are involved in data collection with a set standard of performance.

Change agent/consumer advocate A role in which the dental hygienist must have the knowledge and skills to work to promote change and advance people's health through legislation, public policy, research, and science.

Chi-square test The most commonly used nonparametric test; is used to analyze questionnaire data and to determine whether a relationship exists between two variables.

Clinical rotation This curriculum-based activity is not necessarily associated with a service outcome and is designed primarily to benefit the student's learning. Students are assigned rotation through clinical experiences to enhance knowledge, skills, and expertise.

Collaboration The process of working together to accomplish a goal.

Community The public or group of people with common interests who live in a specific locality.

Community oral health assessment A multifaceted process of identifying factors that affect the oral health of a selected population to determine resources and interventions for oral health improvement.

Community Organization Theory The idea of involving and activating members of a community or subgroup to identify a common problem or goal, to mobilize resources, to implement strategies, and to evaluate their efforts.

Community Periodontal Index (CPI) An assessment of periodontal status of a population by grades of periodontal disease; measures gingival bleeding, calculus, and periodontal pockets.

Community profile A comprehensive description of the community, including items such as population size, geographic boundaries, community type, and physical conditions.

Community water fluoridation The addition of a controlled amount of fluoride to the public water supply with the intent of preventing dental caries in the population.

Continuous data A type of collected information described as measurements made from a particular value, such as from temperature, scores on tests, or time; can be any value along a continuum.

Control group The group of subjects in a study who do not receive the experimental treatment or intervention.

Convenience sample A group of individuals who are most readily available to be subjects in a study

Correlation A statistical method of determining whether a variation in one variable may be related to a variation in another variable.

Cross-cultural communication Effectively exchanging information with persons of diverse populations.

Cross-cultural encounter Interaction with persons or communities of diverse populations.

Cultural competence Considerations that have an impact on the profession's responsibility to reduce the burden of disease for people of various cultures and backgrounds.

Cultural destructiveness Attitudes, policies, and practices that are detrimental to culture, communities, and individuals.

Cultural diversity The degree to which a population consists of people from varied national, ethnic, racial, and religious backgrounds.

Current status State of affairs or position at the present time.

Data Pieces of information collected from measurements and counts obtained during the course of a research study.

Data collection The process of gathering the information that can be used by the community to make decisions and set priorities.

Decayed, missing, and filled teeth/surfaces (DMFT, DMFS) Index A survey used to count caries in the permanent dentition; dft and dfs are used to count caries in the primary dentition.

Demand Health care services desired by the individual or community.

Dental public health The science and art of preventing and controlling dental disease and promoting dental health through organized community efforts.

Department of Health and Human Services (DHHS) A department of the federal government presiding over agencies that conduct oral health activities.

Dental Health Professional Shortage Areas (Dental HPSA) Geographic areas where the dentist/dental health professional to population ratio is low.

Dental home A continuous accessible source of receiving comprehensive dental care.

Dependent variable The variable thought to depend on or to be caused by the independent variable; the outcome variable of interest.

Descriptive statistics Used to describe and summarize data; determine information only about the sample being studied.

Determinants of health Factors that interact to create circumstances and produce specific health conditions; can be classified as physical (environmental), biologic, behavioral, social, cultural, and spiritual.

Diffusion of Innovations Theory A concept that assesses how new ideas, products, or services spread within a society or to other groups or how innovations are adopted.

Discrete data Collected information that is counted only in whole numbers.

Disparities Uneven distribution of the burden of disease (such as oral disease) throughout the population, especially in the poor, the elderly, and the disabled.

Environmental factors Physical, sociocultural, sociopolitical, and economic components that interact with host and agent.

Epidemiology The study of the distribution and determinants of health-related states and events in specified populations and the application of this study to the control of health problems.

Essential Public Health Services for Oral Health Guidelines describing the roles of state oral health programs; used in the development and evaluation of public health activities at the state level.

Ethics/professional ethics The general science of right and wrong conduct; the code by which the profession regulates actions and sets standards for its members.

Ethnocentrism Judging others by one's own cultural standards.

Evaluation The method of measuring results of a program against objectives developed during the early planning stages.

Evidenced-based dentistry Oral healthcare based on clinically relevant scientific evidence.

Experiential learning An umbrella term that references various models of learning in which experience governs the learning process.

Experimental group The sample group of subjects in a study who receive the experimental treatment or intervention.

Focus group Five to 10 members of the intended target audience who undergo group interviews lasting about 30 to 60 minutes; a moderator with structured questions guides the discussion.

Follow-up/referral An essential component of assessment and screening; without further observation and referral for care, screening is ineffective.

Framing health messages A concept that relates to the cues (e.g., sounds, symbols, words, pictures) that signal how and what to think about an issue.

General supervision Supervision of the dental hygienist in which the dentist does not have to be on the premises, but the patient must be one of record or seen by the dentist previously.

Goal A broad-based statement of changes to take place from which specific objectives are developed.

Health Complete physical and social well-being, not merely the absence of disease.

Health Belief Model An assessment of perceptions of how susceptible one is to a health problem and whether one believes that recommended preventive behaviors will result in less susceptibility

Health education The process in which the client is encouraged to become responsible for personal oral health and is informed of scientifically based methods for preventing dental disease.

Health educator/wellness promoter A role in which the dental hygienist works to prevent disease and to promote oral health through the presentation of scientific information.

Health Insurance Portability and Accountability Act (HIPAA) Regulations governing and protecting the rights and privacy of patients in health care.

Health promotion A broad concept referring to the process of enabling people and communities to increase their control over the determinants of health and, therefore, to improve their own health.

Health security The rights and conditions that enable individuals to attain and enjoy their full potential for a healthy life.

Healthy People 2020 A document that contains national health objectives for prevention of disease and promotion of health.

Host factors Factors that affect a host's (a person's, an animal's, or a plant's) susceptibility and resistance to disease.

Hypothesis A statement that reflects the research question, stated in positive terms, and represents the researcher's prediction or opinion.

Implementation The process of putting a plan into action; monitoring a plan's activities, personnel, equipment, resources, and supplies.

Independent variable The experimental treatment or intervention that is imposed on the experimental group.

Index A graduated numeric scale with upper and lower limits; scores correspond to a specific criterion for individuals or populations.

Inferential statistics Used to draw a generalization between the sample studied and the actual population.

Interrater reliability Agreement of findings by two or more examiners.

Interval scale A scale of measurement that determines quantities; characterized by having order and equal distance between points on the scale.

Intrarater reliability Consistency of findings by one examiner with those previously recorded by the same examiner.

Judgmental sample A sample, provided through personal judgment, of subjects who are most representative of the population.

Learning styles The ways in which people collect and retain knowledge.

Legislative/policy changes New or revised laws on health care that the dental hygienist as Consumer Advocate/ Change Agent helps to create and implement.

Mandala of health Hancock's model of health of the human ecosystem.

Mean Average of the group; a sum of all the values divided by the number of items.

Median The exact middle score or value in a distribution of scores; when the total number of scores is even, the sum of the two middle scores, divided by 2, provides the median.

Medical Expenditure Panel Survey (MEPS) Survey that reports on the number of annual dental visits for various population groups.

Mid-level provider Healthcare provider delivering routine direct care; may or may not be under the supervision of a physician or a dentist.

Mode The score or value that occurs most frequently in a distribution of scores.

National Health and Nutrition Examination Survey (NHANES) A national survey conducted in 1996 in which many aspects of oral health were measured.

National Health Interview Survey (NHIS) A survey that asks questions about a person's health, including edentulous status.

Need Those services deemed by the health professional to be necessary after use of a variety of assessment and diagnostic tools and perhaps, past experience.

Network A system in which information about a common population is shared with other health professionals.

Nominal scale A scale of measurement in which characteristics or numbers are assigned into categories by name only.

Nonparametric test A statistical test used when assumptions about a normal distribution in the population cannot be met or when the level of measurement is nominal or ordinal.

Normal distribution An assumption that approximately 68% of the population falls within 1 standard deviation (SD) of the mean, approximately 95% falls within 2 SDs of the mean, and 99% lies within 3 SDs of the mean.

Null hypothesis An assumption that there is no statistically significant difference between the groups being studied.

Objective The desired end result of program activities, described in a measurable way; more specific than a goal.

Oral Health Coalition A cooperative effort on the part of many individuals and organizations to build systems and to develop programs that improve community oral health.

Oral health education A learning experience directed at assisting people in preventing oral disease.

Oral paper A method of presentation of a topic.

Ordinal scale A scale of measurement that orders data into categories in rank order; the space between these categories is undefined.

Organizational Change: Stage Theory A statement of how organizations pass through a series of stages as they initiate change; organizational structures and processes influence workers' behavior and motivation for change.

Parameter A term relating to numeric characteristics of the population.

Parametrics A technique used when data include interval or ratio scales of measurement; best used when the sample is large and randomized and the population from which the sample is taken is normally distributed.

Pilot study (trial run) A preliminary study performed in preparation for a major study.

Planning An organized response to reduce or eliminate one or more problems.

Planning cycle A model commonly used in public health practice that provides a basic flowchart of steps in the process to assess, plan, implement, and evaluate.

Pluralistic systems Numerous, distinct health care delivery systems that coexist simultaneously.

Policy development A core public health function in which laws are planned and developed to support community oral health issues.

Population The entire group, or whole unit of individuals, having similar characteristics to which the results of an investigation can be generalized.

Population health The health outcomes of a group of individuals, including the distribution of such outcomes within the group.

Poster A method of presentation of a topic.

Power analysis A determination of how many subjects are needed to provide significance; calculated using a specific statistical formula based on what an examiner hopes to observe in a specific number of subjects.

Practicum/internship Activity that is typically longer than a clinical rotation and is designed to benefit the student. The student may be assigned to work in a particular specialty area for an entire academic quarter or semester.

Primary prevention Services that are used to prevent a disease before it occurs; this level includes health education, avoidance of disease, and health protection.

Professional ethics The code by which the profession regulates actions and sets standards for its members.

Public health The science and art of preventing disease, prolonging life, and promoting physical health and efficiency through organized community effort.

***P* value** A declaration of how likely it is that a study could have come to a false conclusion; the probability that the obtained results are due to chance alone.

Qualitative data Information that reflects the quality or nature of things that cannot be numerically measured or analyzed.

Qualitative evaluation A determination of why and how (e.g., why did people participate in the activity, and how do they intend to change their parenting behaviors?)

Quality of life Characteristics of living that are affected by a person's health status; oral disease restricts activities at school, work, and home and often diminishes one's quality of life.

Quantitative data Information that is objective and measurable; can be expressed in a quantity or amount (such as the number of children with dental sealants or the rate of dental caries in young children).

Quantitative evaluation A determination of how many (e.g., how many people increased their knowledge of the causes of early childhood caries?)

Random sample A sample in which each member of a population has an equal chance of being included, thus preventing the possibility of selection bias by the researcher.

Range A measurement of the difference between the highest and lowest values in a distribution of scores.

Ratio scale A scale of measurement that not only has all the qualities of nominal, ordinal, and interval but also has an absolute zero such as age, height, and weight.

Refereed journal A journal in which articles have been reviewed by an editorial board of peers.

Reflection Critical thinking and critical expressions about the Service-Learning experience and the specific encounters. The aim of reflection is to draw meaning from the experience.

Reliability Consistency and stability of the data collected in a study.

Researcher A role in which the dental hygienist uses scientific methods to acquire knowledge on topics relevant to serving the needs of the public's oral health.

Risk management A phrase that suggests that risks can be managed with organizational influence. An affiliation agreement between the service providers and the organization being serviced would be an example.

Roundtable discussion Method of presentation of a topic in which the participants sit in a circular pattern and discuss issues relevant to the topic.

Sample A portion or subset of the entire population.

Sealant A plastic resin material applied to the occlusal surfaces of molars and premolars; an effective primary preventive strategy.

Service-Learning Service-Learning (SL) is an example of an experiential learning method. SL is a jointly structured learning experience in which the course learning objectives (LO) and the community partner's service objectives (SO) are deliberately combined for mutual benefit.

Service provider/clinician A role in which the dental hygienist assesses oral health needs and provides treatment.

Shortage areas Localities where the dentist-to-population ratio shows an unmet need for oral health.

Social Learning Theory The idea that people learn through their own experiences by observing the actions of others and the results of those actions.

Social marketing Use of effective advertising tools from commercial marketing to influence a valued health behavioral change.

Social responsibility A broad term encompassing professionalism, personal and professional ethics, and the role of a profession in the context of the greater society.

Stages of Change Theory The idea that change is a process or cycle that occurs over time rather than as a single event.

Standard deviation The positive square root of the variance.

Statistics Numeric characteristics of samples.

Status State or condition.

Stratified sample Random selection of subjects from two or more subdivisions of the population.

Systematic Approach to Health Improvement Framework describing the interrelated determinants of health, including the goals and objectives necessary to improve health.

Systematic sample Selection of subjects by including every nth person in a list.

Tailoring messages A concept in which specific cues are used to make messages meaningful for a specific individual.

Target population The people from whom information is being collected and to whom the researcher would like to generalize the findings of a study.

Technical assistance The use of the professional skills and knowledge base to provide guidance to nondental community members interested in developing preventive programs.

Theory A set of interrelated concepts, definitions, and propositions that presents a systematic view of events or situations by specifying relations among variables to explain and predict the events or situations.

Trend Inclination or direction on a particular course over a period of time.

t-Test A test used to analyze the difference between two means.

Type I alpha (α) error Based on statistical results, the researcher rejects the null hypothesis when it is true.

Type II beta (β) error Based on statistical results, the researcher accepts the null hypothesis when it is actually false.

Validity The degree to which an instrument measures what it is intended to measure.

Variable A characteristic or concept that varies, or differs, within the population under study.

Variance A method of measuring the way in which individual variables are located around the mean; a common technique of measuring interval and ratio variables.

Volunteerism Activity in which students provide a service to the community that is a major benefit for the community. This activity is not necessarily associated with an academic course.

Xylitol A noncariogenic sugar alcohol used as a sugar substitute in foods.

Index

Page numbers followed by "f" indicate figures, "t" indicate tables, and "b" indicate boxes.